Isabelle Bichindaritz, Sachin Vaidya, Ashlesha Jain, and Lakhmi C. Jain (Eds.)

Computational Intelligence in Healthcare 4

Studies in Computational Intelligence, Volume 309

Editor-in-Chief

Prof. Janusz Kacprzyk
Systems Research Institute
Polish Academy of Sciences
ul. Newelska 6
01-447 Warsaw
Poland
E-mail: kacprzyk@ibspan.waw.pl

Further volumes of this series can be found on our homepage:
springer.com

Vol. 286. Zeev Volkovich, Alexander Bolshoy, Valery Kirzhner,
and Zeev Barzily
Genome Clustering, 2010
ISBN 978-3-642-12951-3

Vol. 287. Dan Schonfeld, Caifeng Shan, Dacheng Tao, and
Liang Wang (Eds.)
Video Search and Mining, 2010
ISBN 978-3-642-12899-8

Vol. 288. I-Hsien Ting, Hui-Ju Wu, Tien-Hwa Ho (Eds.)
Mining and Analyzing Social Networks, 2010
ISBN 978-3-642-13421-0

Vol. 289. Anne Håkansson, Ronald Hartung, and
Ngoc Thanh Nguyen (Eds.)
*Agent and Multi-agent Technology for Internet and Enterprise
Systems*, 2010
ISBN 978-3-642-13525-5

Vol. 290. Weiliang Xu and John Bronlund
Mastication Robots, 2010
ISBN 978-3-540-93902-3

Vol. 291. Shimon Whiteson
Adaptive Representations for Reinforcement Learning, 2010
ISBN 978-3-642-13931-4

Vol. 292. Fabrice Guillet, Gilbert Ritschard,
Henri Briand, Djamel A. Zighed (Eds.)
Advances in Knowledge Discovery and Management, 2010
ISBN 978-3-642-00579-4

Vol. 293. Anthony Brabazon, Michael O'Neill, and
Dietmar Maringer (Eds.)
Natural Computing in Computational Finance, 2010
ISBN 978-3-642-13949-9

Vol. 294. Manuel F.M. Barros, Jorge M.C. Guilherme, and
Nuno C.G. Horta
*Analog Circuits and Systems Optimization based on
Evolutionary Computation Techniques*, 2010
ISBN 978-3-642-12345-0

Vol. 295. Roger Lee (Ed.)
*Software Engineering, Artificial Intelligence, Networking and
Parallel/Distributed Computing*, 2010
ISBN 978-3-642-13264-3

Vol. 296. Roger Lee (Ed.)
*Software Engineering Research, Management
and Applications*, 2010
ISBN 978-3-642-13272-8

Vol. 297. Tania Tronco (Ed.)
New Network Architectures, 2010
ISBN 978-3-642-13246-9

Vol. 298. Adam Wierzbicki
Trust and Fairness in Open, Distributed Systems, 2010
ISBN 978-3-642-13450-0

Vol. 299. Vassil Sgurev, Mincho Hadjiski, and
Janusz Kacprzyk (Eds.)
Intelligent Systems: From Theory to Practice, 2010
ISBN 978-3-642-13427-2

Vol. 300. Baoding Liu (Ed.)
Uncertainty Theory, 2010
ISBN 978-3-642-13958-1

Vol. 301. Giuliano Armano, Marco de Gemmis,
Giovanni Semeraro, and Eloisa Vargiu (Eds.)
Intelligent Information Access, 2010
ISBN 978-3-642-13999-4

Vol. 302. Bijaya Ketan Panigrahi, Ajith Abraham,
and Swagatam Das (Eds.)
Computational Intelligence in Power Engineering, 2010
ISBN 978-3-642-14012-9

Vol. 303. Joachim Diederich, Cengiz Gunay, and
James M. Hogan
Recruitment Learning, 2010
ISBN 978-3-642-14027-3

Vol. 304. Anthony Finn and Lakhmi C. Jain (Eds.)
Innovations in Defence Support Systems, 2010
ISBN 978-3-642-14083-9

Vol. 305. Stefania Montani and Lakhmi C. Jain (Eds.)
Successful Case-based Reasoning Applications, 2010
ISBN 978-3-642-14077-8

Vol. 306. Tru Hoang Cao
Conceptual Graphs and Fuzzy Logic, 2010
ISBN 978-3-642-14086-0

Vol. 307. Anupam Shukla, Ritu Tiwari, and Rahul Kala
Towards Hybrid and Adaptive Computing, 2010
ISBN 978-3-642-14343-4

Vol. 308. Roger Nkambou, Jacqueline Bourdeau, and
Riichiro Mizoguchi (Eds.)
Advances in Intelligent Tutoring Systems, 2010
ISBN 978-3-642-14362-5

Vol. 309. Isabelle Bichindaritz, Sachin Vaidya,
Ashlesha Jain, and Lakhmi C. Jain (Eds.)
Computational Intelligence in Healthcare 4, 2010
ISBN 978-3-642-14463-9

Isabelle Bichindaritz, Sachin Vaidya, Ashlesha Jain, and Lakhmi C. Jain (Eds.)

Computational Intelligence in Healthcare 4

Advanced Methodologies

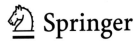 Springer

Prof. Isabelle Bichindaritz
Institute of Technology/Computing and
Software Systems
University of Washington, Tacoma
1900 Commerce Street
Campus Box 358426
Tacoma, WA 98402
USA

Dr. Sachin Vaidya
Flinders Medical Centre
Adelaide, South Australia
Australia

Dr. Ashlesha Jain
Royal Adelaide Hospital
Adelaide, South Australia
Australia

Prof. Lakhmi C. Jain
School of Electrical and Information
Engineering
University of South Australia
South Australia SA 5095
Australia
E-mail: Lakhmi.jain@unisa.edu.au

ISBN 978-3-642-14463-9   e-ISBN 978-3-642-14464-6

DOI 10.1007/978-3-642-14464-6

Studies in Computational Intelligence   ISSN 1860-949X

Library of Congress Control Number: 2010930916

Typeset & Cover Design: Scientific Publishing Services Pvt. Ltd., Chennai, India.

Printed on acid-free paper

9 8 7 6 5 4 3 2 1

springer.com

Preface

Computational Intelligence is comparatively a new field but it has made a tremendous progress in virtually every discipline right from engineering, science, business, management, aviation to healthcare.

Computational intelligence already has a solid track-record of applications to healthcare, of which this book is a continuation. We would like to refer the reader to the excellent previous volumes in this series on computational intelligence in healthcare [1-3].

This book is aimed at providing the most recent advances and state of the art in the practical applications of computational intelligence paradigms in healthcare. It includes nineteen chapters on using various computational intelligence methods in healthcare such as intelligent agents and case-based reasoning. A number of fielded applications and case studies are presented. Highlighted are in particular novel computational approaches to the semantic management of health information such as in the Web 2.0, mobile agents such as in portable devices, learning agents capable of adapting to diverse clinical settings through case-based reasoning, and statistical approaches in computational intelligence.

This book is targeted towards scientists, application engineers, professors, health professionals, professors, and students. Background information on computational intelligence has been provided whenever necessary to facilitate the comprehension of a broad audience including healthcare practitioners.

We are grateful to the authors and reviewers for their contributions. Obviously, this book would not have existed without the excellent contributions of the authors or without the careful comments of the reviewers. Finally, the excellent editorial assistance by the Springer-Verlag is acknowledged.

Isabelle Bichindaritz
USA

Sachin Vaidya
Australia

Ashlesha Jain
Australia

Lakhmi C. Jain
Australia

Preface

References

[1] H. Yoshida, A. Jain, A. Ichalkaranje, L.C. Jain and N. Ichalkaranje (Editors) Advanced Computational Intelligence Paradigms in Healthcare 1, Springer-Verlag, 2007.
[2] S. Vaidya, L.C. Jain and H. Yoshida (Editors) Advanced Computational Intelligence Paradigms in Healthcare 2, Springer-Verlag, 2008
[3] M. Sardo, S. Vaidya and L.C. Jain (Editors) Advanced Computational Intelligence Paradigms in Healthcare 3, Springer-Verlag, 2008.

Table of Contents

Part IV: Sample Applications and Case Studies

Part I
Introduction

Chapter 1
Advances in Computational Intelligence in Healthcare

Isabelle Bichindaritz[1] and Lakhmi C. Jain[2]

[1] University of Washington, Tacoma
WA 98402
USA
[2] University of South Australia
Adelaide
South Australia SA 5095
Australia

Abstract. This chapter presents an introduction to the computational intelligence in medicine as well as a sample of recent advances in the field. A very brief introduction of chapters included in the book is included.

1 Introduction

The tremendous advances in computational intelligence in recent years can be attributed to a variety of reasons such as the cheap and easy availability of computing power and so on. First were developed decision-support systems such as INTERNIST in 1970 and MYCIN in 1976. INTERNIST is classified as a rule-based expert system focused on the diagnosis of complex diseases. It has been commercialized later on as Quick Medical Reference (QMR) to support internists' diagnosis. MYCIN was also a rule-based expert system, but applied to the diagnosis and treatment of blood infections. Created by Ted Shortliffe, this knowledge-based system mapped symptoms to diseases, led to clinical evaluation of its effectiveness, and to the development of an expert system shell EMYCIN. The evolution of artificial intelligence engendered new generations of artificial intelligence systems in medicine, expanding the range of AI methodologies in biomedical informatics, such as implementation of clinical practice guidelines in expert systems, data mining to establish trends and associations between symptoms, genetic information, and diagnoses, and medical image interpretation, to name a few. Researchers stressed the value of early systems for testing artificial intelligence methodologies.

These early systems attempted to model how clinicians reasoned. One major step was to include intelligent systems in clinical practice. Computational intelligence systems in use today are numerous. One of the first one was NéoGanesh, developed to regulate the automatic ventilation system in the Intensive Care Unit (ICU), in use since 1995. Another example is Dxplain, a general expert system for the medical field, associating 4,500 clinical findings, including laboratory test results, with more than 2,000 diseases. Some of these systems are available for routine purchase in medical supplies catalogues. Clinical outcomes have been demonstrated, through

I. Bichindaritz et al. (Eds.): Computational Intelligence in Healthcare 4, SCI 309, pp. 3–7.
springerlink.com

several studies showing the effectiveness of these systems in clinical practice in terms of improving the quality of care, the safety, and the efficiency. One such example is a 1998 computer-based clinical reminder system showing evidence that a particular clinical act – discussing advance directives with a patient – was significantly better performed with the clinical reminders under evaluation than without them. More generally prescription decision-support systems (PDSS) and clinical reminder systems, often based on clinical guidelines implementation, have consistently shown clinical outcomes in several studies. However clinical outcomes are rarely measured, while process variables and user satisfaction are often measured. Obviously computer system intrinsic measures are always reported.

The successful development and deployment of expert systems also called knowledge-based systems in medicine gave tremendous incentive to the researchers to explore this field further. The brittleness of expert systems and the enormous effort involved in the development and maintenance of knowledge bases prompted researchers to look for other approaches. Computational intelligence approaches based on neural networks, fuzzy, logic, case based reasoning, evolutionary computation and the like, filled this perceived need by adding a new dimension to our quest for the application of these techniques in healthcare.

The success of computational intelligence in the healthcare is explained by the shift of focus from centering the system success on the computational performance versus the application domain performance. Indeed successful systems provide a practical solution to a specific healthcare or health research problem. The systems presenting the largest impact, such as the clinical reminders, do not have to represent a challenging conceptual or technical difficulty, but they have to fit perfectly well the clinical domain in which they are embedded – they are application domain driven – versus artificial intelligence driven.

The main purpose of this book is to bring together, under one cover, some of the important developments in the use of computational intelligence to address the challenging problems in the field of healthcare.

2   Chapters Included in the Book

This book is divided into four parts. The first part includes one chapter. This chapter introduces the book and sets a scene related to the advances in computational intelligence in healthcare.

The second part of the book includes five chapters on Artificial Agents in healthcare. Chapter 2 in the book is on Clinical Semantics. It presents the discussion on a flexible and evolving clinical practice supported by open clinical agents for both clinical professionals and patients capable of learning at a human abstraction level. Chapter 3 presents the practical applications of agents in healthcare. The challenges and the future research directions are discussed. Chapter 4 presents three cases regarding the applications of agents in healthcare. The first one is related to the gathering of patient record. The second application involves the retrievial of partial information from an emergency scene. The final application is related to the analysis of the Mobile Agent Electronic Triage Tag System. Chapter 5 is on a joint Bayesian framework for MR Brain scan tissue and structure segmentation based on distributed Markovian agents. Chapter 6 reports the development of an intelligent pedestrian aid for elders. The use of intelligent agents to support mobility and communication in senior citizens is demonstrated.

The third part presents a sample of of Case-Based Reasoning (CBR) paradigms in healthcare. Chapter 7 presents a broad overview of CBR in health sciences. Chapter 8 is on intelligent signal analysis using CBR for decision support in stress management. Chapter 9 is on CBR in a travel medicine application. Chapter 10 presents the application of CBR to implement case-based retrieval as a decision support strategy in healthcare. Chapter 11 presents a framework for model building in image processing by meta-learning based on CBR. Chapter 12 presents a scheme using CBR to explain cases that do not fit a statistical model in healthcare applications. Chapter 13 presents the use of computational intelligence techniques for classification in microarray analysis.

The final part presents a sample of practical applications of the computational intelligence paradigms in healthcare. Chapter 14 presents an overview of Web 2.0 novelties and describes how medical information can be exploited in favour of the community. Chapter 15 presents an approach for the intelligent monitoring in the cardiac domain. Chapter 16 presents a computational intelligence-based approach to analyse the lesions of human organs as well as supporting the management of medical units. Chapter 17 presents a Bayesian network-based approach for multi-view analysis of mammograms. Chapter 18 presents the pattern classification techniques for lung cancer diagnosis by an electronic nose. The final chapter reports a portable wireless solution for back pain telemonitoring.

3 Conclusions

The chapter has provided a brief introduction to the book. The main purpose of the book is to bring together a sample of some of the important developments in the use of computational intelligence in healthcare.

References

[1] Cerrito, P.B.: Choice of Antibiotic in Open Heart surgery. Intelligent Decision Technolo-gies-An International Journal 1(1-2), 63–69 (2007)
[2] De Paz, J.F., et al.: Case-based Reasoning as a Decision Support System for Cancer Di-agnosis: A Case Study. International Journal of Hybrid Intelligent Systems 6(2), 97–110 (2009)
[3] Goel, P., et al.: On the Use of Spiking Neural Networks for EEG Classification. Interna-tional Journal of Knowledge-Based and Intelligent Engineering Systems 12(4), 295–304 (2008)
[4] Hüllermeier, E.: Case Based Approximate Reasoning. Springer, Heidelberg (2007)
[5] Husmeier, D., Dybowski, R., Roberts, S. (eds.): Probabilistic Modelling in Bioinformat-ics and Medical Informatics. In: Wu, X., Jain, L.C. (eds.) Advanced Information and Knowledge Processing Series. Springer, Heidelberg (2005)
[6] Ichalkaranje, N., Ichalkaranje, A., Jain, L.C. (eds.): Intelligent Paradigms for Assistive and Preventive Healthcare. Springer, Heidelberg (2006)

[7] Jain, A., Jain, A., Jain, S., Jain, L.C. (eds.): Artificial Intelligence Techniques in Breast Cancer Diagnosis and Prognosis. World Scientific, Singapore (2000)

[8] Kabassi, K., et al.: Specifying the personalization reasoning mechanism for an intelligent medical e-learning system on Atheromatosis: An Empirical Study. Intelligent Decision Technologies-An International Journal 2(3), 179–190 (2008)

[9] Kang, E., et al.: Remote Control Multiagent System for u-Healthcare Service. In: Nguyen, N.T., Grzech, A., Howlett, R.J., Jain, L.C. (eds.) KES-AMSTA 2007. LNCS (LNAI), vol. 4496, pp. 636–644. Springer, Heidelberg (2007)

[10] Kodogiannis, V.S., et al.: An Intelligent Decision Support Systems for Bacterial Clinical Isolates in Vitro Utisising an Electronic Nose. Intelligent Decision Technologies-An International Journal 3(4), 219–231 (2009)

[11] Kodogiannis, V.S.: Decision Support Systems in Wireless Capsule Endoscopy. Intelligent Decision Technologies-An International Journal 1(1-2), 17–32 (2007)

[12] Koleszynska, J.: GIGISim-The Intelligent Telehealth System: Computer Aided Diabetes Management – A New Review. In: Apoloni, B., Howlett, R.J., Jain, L.C. (eds.) KES 2007, Part I. LNCS (LNAI), vol. 4692, pp. 789–796. Springer, Heidelberg (2007)

[13] Kostakis, H., et al.: A Computational Algorithm for the Risk Assessment of Developing Acute Coronary Syndromes using Online Analytical Process Methodology. International Journal of Knowledge Engineering and Soft Data Paradigms 1(1), 85–99 (2009)

[14] Koutsojannis, C., Hatzillygeroudis, I.: Fuzzy-Evolutionary Synergism in an Intelligent Medical Diagnosis System. In: Gabrys, B., Howlett, R.J., Jain, L.C. (eds.) KES 2006. LNCS (LNAI), vol. 4252, pp. 1313–1322. Springer, Heidelberg (2006)

[15] Mateo, R.M.A., et al.: Mobile Agent Using Data Mining for Diagnostic Support in Ubiquitous Healthcare. In: Nguyen, N.T., Grzech, A., Howlett, R.J., Jain, L.C. (eds.) KES-AMSTA 2007. LNCS (LNAI), vol. 4496, pp. 795–804. Springer, Heidelberg (2007)

[16] Menolascina, F., et al.: Fuzzy rule Induction and Artificial Immune Systems in Female Breast cancer Familiarity Profiling. International Journal of Hybrid Intelligent Systems 5(3), 161–165 (2008)

[17] Nebot, A.: Rule-Based Assistance to Brain Tumor Diagnosis Using LR-FIR. In: Loverek, I., Howlett, R.J., Jain, L.C. (eds.) KES 2008, Part II. LNCS (LNAI), vol. 5178, pp. 173–180. Springer, Heidelberg (2008)

[18] Nejad, S.G., et al.: An Agent-based Diabetic Patient Simulation. In: Nguyen, N.T., Jo, G.S., Howlett, R.J., Jain, L.C. (eds.) KES-AMSTA 2008. LNCS (LNAI), vol. 4953, pp. 832–841. Springer, Heidelberg (2008)

[19] Jeong, C.-W., Kim, D.-H., Joo, S.-C.: Mobile Collaboration Framework for u-Healthcare Agent Services and its Application Using PDAs. In: Nguyen, N.T., Grzech, A., Howlett, R.J., Jain, L.C. (eds.) KES-AMSTA 2007. LNCS (LNAI), vol. 4496, pp. 747–756. Springer, Heidelberg (2007)

[20] Okamoto, T., Ishida, Y.: Towards an Immunity-based System for Detecting Masqueraders. International Journal of Knowledge-based and Intelligent Engineering Systems 13(3,4), 103–110 (2009)

[21] Papageorgiou, E., et al.: Combining Fuzzy Cognitive Maps with Support Vector Machines for Bladder Tumor Grading. In: Gabrys, B., Howlett, R.J., Jain, L.C. (eds.) KES 2006. LNCS (LNAI), vol. 4251, pp. 515–523. Springer, Heidelberg (2006)

[22] Pous, C., et al.: Diagnosing Papients with a Combination of Principal Component Analysis and Cased Based Reasoning. International Journal of Hybrid Intelligent Systems 6(2), 111–122 (2009)

[23] Qian, Y.-W., et al.: An On-line Decision Support System for Diagnosing Hematologic Malignancies by Flow Cytometry Immunophenotyping. International Journal of Medical Engineering and Informatics 1(1), 109–124

[24] Rakus-Andersson, E.: Fuzzy and Rough Techniques in Medical Diagnosis and Medication. Springer, Heidelberg (2007)

[25] Sardo, M., Vaidya, S., Jain, L.C. (eds.): Advanced Computational Intelligence Paradigms in Healthcare, vol. 3. Springer, Heidelberg (2008)

[26] Seta, K., et al.: Learning Environment for Improving Critical Thinking Skills in Nursing Domain. International Journal of Advanced Intelligence Paradigms 1(2) (2008)

[27] Silverman, B., Jain, A., Ichalkaranje, A., Jain, L.C. (eds.): Intelligent Paradigms in Healthcare Enterprises. Springer, Heidelberg (2005)

[28] Tentori, M., et al.: Privacy-Aware Autonomous agents for Pervasive Healthcare. IEEE Intelligent Systems 21(6), 55–62 (2006)

[29] Teodorescu, H.-N., Jain, L.C. (eds.): Intelligent Systems and Technologies in Rehabilitation Engineering. CRC Press, USA (2001)

[30] Teodorescu, H.-N., Kandel, A., Jain, L.C. (eds.): Fuzzy and Neuro-fuzzy Systems in Medicine. CRC Press, USA (1999)

[31] Teodorescu, H.-N., Kandel, A., Jain, L.C. (eds.): Soft Computing in Human Related Sciences. CRC Press, USA (1999)

[32] Tonfoni, G., Jain, L.C. (eds.): Innovations in Decision support Systems, Advanced Knowledge International, ch. 8, 9 (2003)

[33] Vaidya, S., Jain, L.C., Yoshida, H. (eds.): Advanced Computational Intelligence Paradigms in Healthcare, vol. 2. Springer, Heidelberg (2008)

[34] Velikova, M.: A Decision support system for Breast Cancer Detection in Screening Programs. In: Proceedings of the 18th European Conference on Artificial Intelligence, pp. 658–662. IOS Press, Amsterdam (2008)

[35] Wagholikar, K.V., Deshpande, A.W.: Fuzzy Relation Based Modeling for Medical Diagnostic Decision Support: Case Studies. International Journal of Knowledge-Based and Intelligent Engineering Systems 12(5-6), 319–326 (2008)

[36] Yoshida, H., Jain, A., Ichalkaranje, A., Jain, L.C., Ichalkaranje, N. (eds.): Advanced Computational Intelligence Paradigms in Healthcare, vol. 1. Springer, Heidelberg (2007)

Part II
Artificial Agents in Healthcare

Chapter 2
Clinical Semantics

Jari Yli-Hietanen and Samuli Niiranen

Department of Signal Processing, Tampere University of Technology,
POB 553, 33101, Tampere, Finland
{jari.yli-hietanen,samuli.niiranen}@tut.fi

Abstract. We discuss the challenge of efficient and flexible clinical informatics and provide initial results on how to tackle the computerized management of the complex and diverse information space of clinical medicine through an approach coined as open information management. The approach builds on natural language as the core information management tool in place of formal, structured representation. The chapter discusses a flexible, evolving clinical practice supported by open clinical agents for both clinical professionals and patients capable of learning at the human abstraction level. Clinical semantics is not an add-on but rather natively integrated to, and an operational principle behind, the functionality of these agents.

1 Introduction

1.1 Background

Figure 1 presents a framework for health care and life sciences with three key areas of contemporary research activity: personalized medicine, translational medicine and biosurveillance. Biomedical informatics is a well-recognized venue of research within the health care, life sciences and information technology communities and is rightly argued to be a key component in supporting advances in the three major areas of research activity. It is also commonly accepted that the domain is a challenging one from an informatics point-of-view with many open research problems.

Concerning the current status of informatics research in the domain, the application of Semantic Web and related formal, structured approaches has been suggested to be a key component in solving some of the challenges related to the complexity, diversity and fluidity of information inherent to the domain. The thesis is that the use of these technologies for information modeling, sharing and analysis will bring along a way to approach the question of semantics in the domain in a unified and encompassing way.

However, a major practical argument can be made against the Semantic Web approach in bringing computable semantics to health care and life sciences domain information. The argument emerges from the fact that, as an example of weak artificial intelligence, the approach primarily relies on the use of hand-crafted, metadata-based annotations to provide for the semantics of information. In clinical informatics, the approach relies on a massive knowledge and systems engineering effort to manually build integrating ontologies bridging the gaps between biological and clinical

I. Bichindaritz et al. (Eds.): Computational Intelligence in Healthcare 4, SCI 309, pp. 11–24.
springerlink.com © Springer-Verlag Berlin Heidelberg 2010

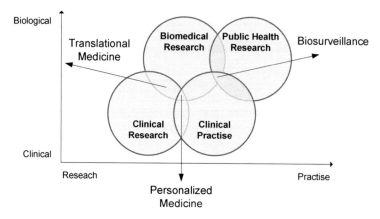

Fig. 1. A framework for health care and life sciences (adapted from [1])

information, to migrate existing domain ontologies and coding systems (e.g., from HL7, UMLS) and diverse, vendor-specific electronic health record systems to support the fully structured approach. Furthermore, apart from the initial construction effort, the approach would necessitate the establishment of a centrally-planned co-ordination effort on a massive scale to account for the inevitable (and hopefully welcomed!) evolution of both information and semantics in the domain. This issue has been practically highlighted by the authors in a system migration evaluation study carried out in co-operation with an industrial partner [2] as discussed later.

The question arising from this discussion is that might there be a way to avoid the complexity of construction and maintenance inherent to the Semantic Web and related approaches? A discussion on some possible answers to this question is the topic of this chapter.

1.2 Open Information Management

Earlier work by the authors has probed into the question of human abstraction level information management and has developed an approach coined as 'open information management'. For a general review of the approach see [3] and for discussion in the scope of health care see [4], [5] and [6]. A textbook edited by the authors on the topic is also available [7].

The fundamentals of this approach can be summarized under three observations:

- The expressive power of natural language
- The associative power of unrestricted linkage
- The descriptive power of direct observation

The basic claim of the approach is that these observations lay the foundation for the development of information management tools capable of learning on the human abstraction level with a principally unbounded case space. In practice, the learning process results from user interactions with expressivity similar to natural language supported by the associative and descriptive powers of the latter two constructs. The implication is that semantics is automatically and natively constructed through a learn-while-use paradigm. In relation to this, further research has been carried out by authors in the domain of language models for clinical medicine. Practical work in this direction has been reported in [8] and is further elucidated in [9], [10] and [11].

The chapter builds on this foundation and discusses a flexible, evolving clinical practice supported by open clinical agents for both clinical professionals and patients capable of learning at the human abstraction level. Clinical semantics is not an add-on but rather natively integrated to, and an operational principle behind, the functionality of these agents. A key technical topic is natural language models specifically in the context of clinical applications.

2   The Challenge of Clinical Informatics

The application of information technology to the computerization of medical records dates back to 1960s when the first attempts were made at developing comprehensive, structured hospital information systems. A prominent example of such technology is MUMPS (Massachusetts General Hospital Utility Multi-Programming System) originally developed by Dr. G. Octo Barnett's lab at the Massachusetts General Hospital. The authors of a research paper [12] reporting early experiences on the use of MUMPS technology at a hypertension clinic state that:

"It is estimated that the data structure developed for hypertension and its complications represents between 1 and 5 per cent of the content of clinical medicine".

This estimate turned out to be a wildly positive one considering all the effort put into developing structured electronic medical records (EMRs) during the last 30+ years. It often seems that the evolution of clinical information outpaces the efforts of system developers. The authors furthermore state that:

"In any system that is developed, mechanisms must be provided for adapting the structure to changing needs, so that is remains relevant and appropriate at all times. It is anticipated that this task of maintaining a structure representation of current knowledge will be a much simpler task than its de novo development. "

In fact, the maintenance problem of a conventionally structured medical record has turned out to be an exceedingly complex one. In the typical clinical setting, different information systems are tightly interconnected so that changes in one system can result in a cascade changes in the entire health information system infrastructure of an institution.

Still, the use of highly structured data remains a key technological goal as the prevalence of free-text, natural language composition is seen as one of the major hindrances in the work towards increased utility of an electronic medical record [9]. System designers often seek to limit the use of free-text compositions as the ambiguity and unbounded nature of natural language results in difficulty in [9]

- validating the correctness and completeness of human-submitted information to be recorded;
- generating descriptive and aggregative reporting and visualizations out of recorded information; and
- developing decision support tools utilizing the recorded information.

As stated earlier, there have been considerable energies expended in an attempt to standardize and formalize clinical information by developing encoding standards and ontologies also for use in structured data entry and management (e.g., within the Health Level 7 (HL7) and Unified Medical Language System (UMLS) initiatives). However, some recent discussion in medical informatics has brought attention to the fact that the overall attempt towards an efficient EMR, wherein this approach is an integral component, has not proven to be a panacea. [9]

Information systems efficiently integrating with clinical work remain an elusive goal. As Wears and Berg state in [13],

"Behind the cheers and high hopes that dominate conference proceedings, vendor information, and large parts of the scientific literature, the reality is that systems that are in use in multiple locations, that have satisfied users, and that effectively and efficiently contribute to the quality and safety of care are few and far between"

In relation to this, EMR's must intertwine information from a multitude of domains and levels of abstraction into a complex and evolving operational context. Clinical operations and decision making requires the application of data that do not always easily fit into a predetermined, rigid and linear set of selections. Restricted expression of clinical information via formulaic constructs often results in a loss of expressivity and limits the capture of important, subtle clinical details. A small fragment of natural language can convey a complex message and is natively understandable, by definition, to humans. In addition, an ever-increasing number of complex user interface components, as typically necessary for structured data entry in clinical systems, have a negative effect on both end-user usability and data entry efficiency. Still, these shortcomings do not take away from the fact structured data entry does suite a number of EMR scenarios, just that it is not applicable universally. [9]

To further illustrate the challenge of clinical informatics, we will next look into two clinical process transitions involving the use of structured electronic medical records. The first one describes a case where a manual data gathering and management process is replaced with a computerized one. The second one involves the architectural migration of an existing computerized clinical process.

2.1 Transition from a Manual to a Computerized Clinical Process

An evaluation study on changes in the quality of care and cost of care resulting from the reorganization (supported by computerization) of a Finnish primary care anticoagulation treatment workflow is described in [14]. In Finland, the anticoagulant effect of warfarin is usually followed up with laboratory testing of venous blood samples guaranteeing that the correct anticoagulation level, measured in P-INR units, is maintained. Follow-up is organized by public primary care health clinics covering the anticoagulated population of a municipality or a number of municipalities [15]. Considering the follow-up media, data have typically been recorded on paper-based anticoagulation notebooks. However, primary health care EMR's increasingly offer basic functionality for the maintenance of anticoagulation follow-up data. The study in question involved the development of a separate, structured system for managing anticoagulation data in an electronic format. Figure 2 shows the architecture of the system.

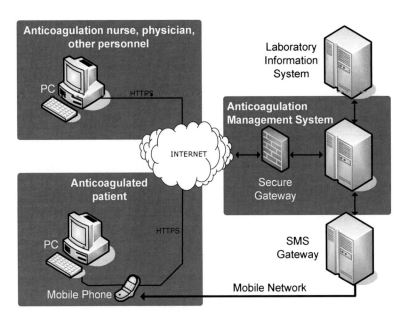

Fig. 2. Architecture of the electronic anticoagulation management system [15]

The primary reorganization methodology was the introduction of an anticoagulation nurse model where routine tasks were transferred to nursing personnel from physicians supported by computerization. The results showed that the quality of care was maintained while the physicians' time allocation was reduced [15]. The latter result represents a potential for cost savings.

However, the paper concludes with the observation that investments into case-specific, highly structured information management tools are potentially difficult to justify. Why is this so? Considering the studied case, the clinic in question already utilized a basic electronic medical record. A separate system was developed for anticoagulation treatment as the basic system didn't include support for the structured entry of these data and the related task management functionality required for the anticoagulation nurse model in a realistic timeframe. This situation is an example of one standard dilemma in clinical informatics. Novel care management models (such as the anticoagulation nurse model) benefitting from the use of integrated information management tools (replacing manual entry) are developed regularly but the system development processes of comprehensive, structured electronic medical records are prohibitively long and cumbersome to support the agile testing and introduction of such models. On the other hand, there is understandable resistance to the introduction of new case-specific systems by health care providers.

Apart from the few academic institutions having the necessary in-house personnel to develop such functionality it can be argued that many innovations requiring information technology tools never take off due to the inflexibility of the information management infrastructure of health care providers.

Ideally, the personnel developing new care management processes would be themselves able to augment supportive functionality to the basic electronic record.

2.2 Transition from a Legacy to a New Computerized Clinical Process

A study presenting the experiences gathered from the migration of an existing and deployed joint replacement surgery information system from a legacy, 2-tier architecture to a new, 4-tier architecture is presented in [2]. The key functionalities of the system are [2]

- structured data entry and aggregate reporting of prosthetic components installed in hip, knee, ankle, shoulder, elbow and wrist joint replacement surgeries. This includes the trade names, types, serial numbers and physical dimensions of the installed components. In addition, details on the operation, such as immediate complications, are also recorded. The data entry is carried by the operating orthopedic hospitals. Aggregate information on the installed components is transferred annually to the National Agency for Medicines for quality assurance and reporting purposes. This functionality replaces manual, paper-based reporting on installed prosthetic components.
- an automated call-up system for alerting post-operative follow-up sites on forthcoming new follow-ups. This functionality removes the reliance on a manual call-up list and enhances information transfer between operative and post-operative follow-up sites.

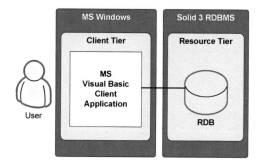

Fig. 3. Legacy architecture of the joint replacement surgery management system [2]

Figures 3 and 4 present the legacy and new architectures of the system. The legacy system based is on a standard 2-tier, fat client architecture while the new system uses a 4-tier, thin client architecture. The benefits of modern multi-tier architectures in health care information system design are well-established. These include reusability, flexibility, reductions in initial system development cost and effort, and, more controversially, provision of an easy, open migration pathway for future change of technology and system redevelopment [16].

The study includes discussion on the motivation for the migration and on the technical benefits of the chosen technical migration path and an evaluation of user experiences. The results from the analysis of clinical end-user and administrator experiences show an increase in the perceived performance and maintainability of the system and a high level of acceptance for the new system version. [2].

Still - the study concludes [2] - despite the success of this architectural migration project, such endeavors often represent one of the major challenges in clinical informatics. The migration process of highly structured information systems does need

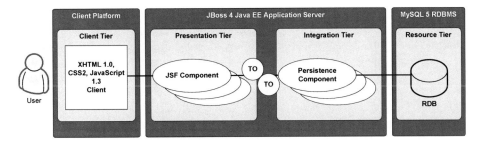

Fig. 4. New architecture of the joint replacement surgery management system [2]

careful planning and execution for successful completion. Without this costly process, there is a high risk for disruptions in system use during and immediately after the migration. Considering the overall need for architectural migrations, there is potential for the emergence of a vicious circle due to an ever increasing number of interconnected, structured clinical systems providing increasingly complex functionality. The migration of a single system to a new architecture often creates a cascade of changes in other interconnected systems.

Ideally, such architectural overhauls would be avoided through technologies allowing for the gradual evolution of system functionality and experience.

3 Open Clinical Agents

Considering the challenges of clinical informatics outlined in the previous section and the fundamentals of open information management presented in the introduction, we will next look at how these help to provide possible answers to the outlined challenges. This will be done in the context of an abstract architecture for open clinical agents building on the three fundamental observations of open information management. We will also look a practical case study involving the management of emergency department chief complaints.

3.1 Abstract Architecture

Looking at information in clinical medicine from the expressivity angle, we note that a level of expressivity similar to natural language is required to represent the diversity of information inherent to the domain. One reflection of this fact are the numerous failures at fully replacing free-text, natural language compositions in electronic medical records with conventionally structured information entry and the maintenance problem inherent to the structured approach. With this in mind, natural language expressions are set down as the fundamental form of representation. The implicated goal is a workable approach for natural language understanding (NLU) within the constraints of clinical medicine.

It can be argued that understanding of natural language derives from the seamless interplay of many components including the lexical semantics (i.e., the possible meanings of words), structural semantics (i.e., the ways of structuring and compositing words, phrases and clauses to convey different meanings) and, most importantly, from the constraints of the clinical domain at hand (i.e., the constraints for meanings defined by the static and dynamic descriptions of the clinical environment and the clinical goal of operation) [9]. The key observation is that, in general, the understanding of natural language cannot be separated from the clinical domain, (i.e., clinical medicine in general and in specific operational environments). Thus, a proposed solution is domain-specific symbolic language modeling as initially developed and studied in [8-11] for emergency department chief complaints.

In the context of open clinical agents, a workable mechanism for natural language understanding has to be capable of learning on the human abstraction level with the implication that semantics can in principle be automatically and natively constructed through a design-while-use paradigm to support gradual evolution of system functionality and experience. In practice, this means the ability to learn, in a principally unbounded case space, through user interactions having the expressivity of natural language. Supporting the understanding and integrated learning process is a constantly augmented and unrestricted linkage of explanations expressed as computable explanations (here natural language labeled ontological relations). Initial work on how this augmentation (i.e., learning) should be done is presented in the chief complaint case study [8-11].

As part of an abstract architecture for reflective clinical agents (Figure 5), the linkage ('*Explanations*') provides the associative power to provide for the semantic disambiguation of both natural language user interactions complementing and working towards the goal of operation (though the physical '*Action interfacer*' component) and natural language labeled ontological relations of the linkage itself.

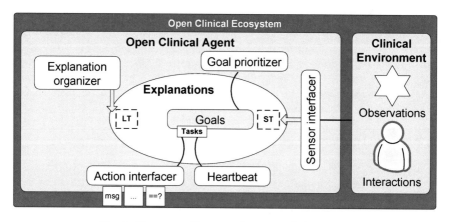

Fig. 5. Abstract architecture of an open clinical agent

Apart from general descriptions of the clinical domain, the linkage embeds a diverse, comprehensive set of direct observations characterizing the clinical domain as well as the clinical goal(s) of operation itself. The descriptive annotations LT and ST denote '*long-term memory*' and '*short-term memory*', concepts widely used in cognitive computing and expert systems research. The observations include anything from ordered laboratory result data to equipment and personnel location data and from genetic information to medical imaging data. A key topic in this context is (semi)automatic feedback from these observations to agent goals (i.e., functionality) supported by high-abstraction level information fusion. The physical sensor interfacer component handles syntactic language constraints in natural language user interactions through the generation of all possible structural phenomena from the interactions on hand. The physical goal prioritizer and explanation organizer components provide high-abstraction level prioritization, ordering and information fusion functionality. The physical action interfacer component serves as a semantic interface to various physical information processing actions, including the physical user interface for an interacting user. The physical, scheduled heartbeat component initiates actions based on the state of the explanations. As a starting point, work towards a prototype of an open clinical agent for emergency medicine has been presented in [8-11] as discussed next.

3.2 The Chief Complaint Agent

Emergency medicine represents a particularly challenging care setting for clinical information management. Rapid and effortless information submission and retrieval are essential to match the pace of a busy emergency department (ED). It is the point-of-entry for a diverse population of patients into the health care system. ED's see patients from newborns through old age, and treat the full range of illnesses and concerns. Patients with acute trauma, chronic disease, potential exposures and social problems can all be encountered on any given night. This wide range of patients and ailments makes it more challenging to develop an efficient mechanism for the entry of discrete medical data for ED encounters. [9]

The chief complaint (CC) is one of the most important components of ED triage decision making. It is a key determinant of the direction and history taking, physical examination, and diagnostic testing in the ED [17]. Still, the chief complaint has a number of flaws. For example, the patient may not always be able to accurately describe their concern (e.g., "I don't feel well"), the same chief complaint can map to a wide range of severity (e.g., 'chest pain' can be either indigestion or a heart attack). Despite its flaws, the chief complaint is the first available description of what's wrong with the patient, and is often electronically accessible in many hospitals. [9]

A number of studies (e.g., [18] and [19]) report activities towards a standard, limited set of encodings for the structured entry of chief complaint information in clinical ED information systems. However, no consensus exists on this matter and it remains a challenging and elusive goal. The purpose of the CC is to record the patient's primary problem, and it is often recorded in his or her own words. Obviously, the implied diversity of expression is difficult to compress into a set of strictly problem-oriented, structured encodings without losing the nuances of original message. This is especially true if one wants to accommodate the rich and informative use of almost an unbounded set of anatomic (e.g., problem related to which body part?) and functional (e.g., problem related to which bodily function?) descriptions and positional and other qualifiers (e.g., "left-sided", "possible", "sports-related", etc.) all of which can be expressed in a number of ways and on varying levels of abstraction with sometimes subtly different semantics. [9]

There are many reasons for gaining understanding of the ED chief complaints in an automated, computable context. Recently, the use of chief complaint information in syndromic surveillance has gathered attention in medical informatics research. This research is carried out in the context of ultimately developing practical applications for monitoring the incidence of certain syndromes associated with bioterrorism and other emerging infections with the goal of timely outbreak detection. In addition, we want the computer to understand the chief complaint (CC) so that we can [9]:

- Quickly group similar cases for research purposes
- Expedite care by suggesting predefined care protocols to be initiated at triage
- Improve patient safety by alerting providers to conditions they might not have considered
- Improve efficiency by pre-selecting documentation templates for physicians

However, if we choose not to abandon collection of free-text chief complaint information, how do we optimize the capture and understanding process? We will next briefly discuss and illustrate the ways to accomplish this with open information management. This is done with the specific goal of distilling categorical information from chief complaints, for example, for automated syndromic surveillance, with a chief complaint agent.

Figure 6 describe the architecture of a system for this purpose.

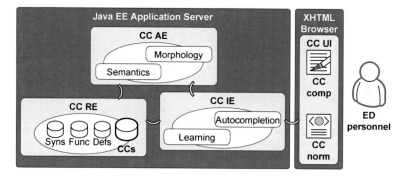

Fig. 6. Overview of the chief complaint agent architecture

The system provides for the capture and storage of chief complaints as natural language compositions maintaining their full expressivity while a computable understanding of them is collaboratively built enabling distillation of categorical information from the CC's. The core of the system is an unrestricted, associative linkage of synonym and category definitions mapping features in free-text chief complaints into higher abstraction level categories[1] as constrained by the operational domain. [9]

In practice, the associative linkage defines the production rules of a rewriting system for a chief complaint language. Figure 7 illustrates the normalization of the

---

[1] P: Problem
   A: Anatomic location/function/property
   Q: Qualifier
   D: Diagnosis
   I: Ignorable
   U: Unknown

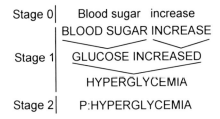

Stage 0| Blood sugar   increase

| BLOOD SUGAR INCREASE

Stage 1| GLUCOSE INCREASED

| HYPERGLYCEMIA

Stage 2| P:HYPERGLYCEMIA

Fig. 7. The rewriting system in practice [11]

original CC 'Blood sugar   increase' into the concept P:HYPERGLYCEMIA via the recursive application of production rules in Stage 1. Extra white space is removed and capitalization is carried out in stage 0. Stage 2 is category assignment. Further details of the three-stage algorithm are presented in [9] and [11].

The current system version can increase its semantic analysis capability through an on-line learning process supported by morphological analysis. This enables through-use evolution of the system's ability to categorize chief complaints, i.e. to increase its power of understanding. The server side architecture of the systems consists of a CC interaction engine (IE), a CC analysis engine (AE), and a CC repository engine (RE). [9] Functional details of these components and the entire system are described in [9].

Figure 8 shows the entry of a new CC with the interaction engine.

Figure 9 illustrates the collaborative learning process of the chief complaint agent.

The performance of the chief complaint agent in distilling categorical information from free-text CC's was evaluated in [8-11]. Table 1 shows the results of the evaluation in [9] where the system was trained with the CC's from one ED and then tested with the CC's of this and four other ED's. Complete normalization means that all free-text terms in the CC were matched with a category and correct normalization refers to whether these normalizations were correct. Not surprisingly, emergency department A, the same from which the training data originated, showed best normalization performance. Overall, the results show that the approach worked reasonably well after extensive initial training. Further evaluations of the system are described in [8], [10] and [11].

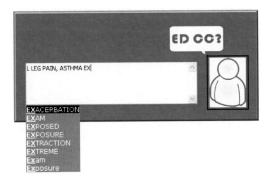

Fig. 8. Assisted entry of chief complaints [9]

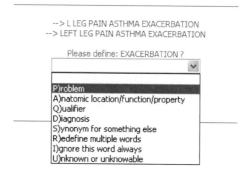

Fig. 9. The collaborative learning facility [9]

Table 1. Automatic normalization performance after initial training (95% CI). (1): without approximate matching, (2): with approximate matching. [9].

	% Completely Normalized (1), N=5000	% Correctly Normalized (1), N=100	% Completely Normalized (2), N=5000	% Correctly Normalized (2), N=100
A	95.7 [95.1-96.3]	100 [96.3-100]	96.9 [96.4-97.4]	100 [96.3-100]
B	88.6 [87.7-89.5]	95.0 [88.8-97.9]	89.9 [89.1-90.7]	95.0 [88.8-97.9]
C	83.1 [82.1-84.1]	99.0 [94.6-99.8]	92.5 [91.8-93.2]	99.0 [94.6-99.8]
D	66.0 [64.7-67.3]	93.0 [86.2-96.6]	69.6 [68.3-70.9]	93.0 [86.2-96.6]
E	73.6 [72.4-74.8]	98.0 [93.0-99.5]	76.8 [75.6-78.0]	98.0 [93.0-99.5]

4 Discussion

The efficient and flexible computerized management of the complex and diverse information space of clinical medicine remains fundamentally an open research question. The mixed record of clinical information system implementations so far tells us that much work remains to be done. Much effort has been poured into the fully formalized, structured approach of information representation. As discussed, this results in a serious maintenance problem as processes, information and semantics of the domain evolve and new systems are introduced and interconnected.

The approach suggested here, open information management, builds around natural language as an expressive, evolving and native clinical information management tool. Human organizations have successfully utilized natural language for a very long time to exchange information. The level of expressivity of natural languages is high and even persons that have never met can understand each other provided they speak the same language. Natural languages have also mechanisms to introduce new words and concepts, i.e. to evolve.

This chapter discussed a flexible, evolving clinical practice supported by open clinical agents for both clinical professionals and patients capable of learning at the human abstraction level. Clinical semantics is not an add-on but rather natively integrated to, and an operational principle behind, the functionality of these agents. Still, the presented work represents a mere beginning with many open questions remaining. For example, the presented case study on emergency department chief complaints involves the use of relatively simple natural language in a very constrained setting. Thus, the developed tool is by no means applicable to most areas of clinical information management. A key future research goal is the development of more advanced and universally applicable natural language tools.

References

1. Semantics for Healthcare and the Life Sciences. In: Tutorial Presentation at the International World Wide Web Conference WWW 2006 (2006)
2. Niiranen, S., Välimäki, A., Yli-Hietanen, J.: Experiences from the architectural migration of a joint replacement surgery information system. Medical Informatics Insights 1, 1–5 (2008)
3. Yli-Hietanen, J., Niiranen, S.: Towards reflective information management. In: Proceedings of the 12th Finnish Artificial Intelligence Conference STeP 2006 (2006)
4. Niiranen, S., Yli-Hietanen, J.: Reflective Information Management for Assisted Home Living. In: Proceedings of the TICSP Workshop on Ambient Multimedia and Home Entertainment at the EuroITV 2006 (2006)
5. Niiranen, S., Yli-Hietanen, J.: Reflective information management in the dissemination of health care practices. In: Proceedings of International Conference on Integration of Knowledge Intensive Multi-Agent Systems, KIMAS 2007 (2007)
6. Yli-Hietanen, J., Niiranen, S.: Towards Open information management in health care. Open Med. Inform J. 2, 42–48 (2008)
7. Niiranen, S., Yli-Hietanen, J. (eds.): Open Information Management Book. IGI Publishing, Hershey (2009)
8. Aswell, M., Niiranen, S., Nathanson, L.: Enhanced normalization of emergency department chief complaints. In: Proceedings of the American Medical Informatics Association 2007 Annual Symposium (2007)
9. Niiranen, S., Yli-Hietanen, J., Nathanson, L.: Towards reflective management of emergency department chief complaint information. IEEE Trans Inf. Technol. Biomed. 12, 763–767 (2008)
10. Niiranen, S., Aswell, M., Yli-Hietanen, J., Nathanson, L.: Domain-specific analytical language modeling – the chief complaint as a case study. In: Proceedings of the First Louhi Conference on Text and Data Mining of Clinical Documents, Louhi 2008 (2008)
11. Yli-Hietanen, J., Niiranen, S., Aswell, M., Nathanson, L.: Domain-specific analytical language modeling-The chief complaint as a case study. Int. J. Med. Inform (2009)
12. Greenes, R., Barnett, O., Klein, S., Robbins, A., Prior, R.: Recording, retrieval and review of medical data by physician-computer interaction. New Engl. J. Med. 282, 307–315 (1970)
13. Wears, R., Berg, M.: Computer technology and clinical work: still waiting for Godot. JAMA 293, 1261–1263 (2005)
14. Niiranen, S., Wartiovaara-Kautto, U., Syrjälä, M., Puustinen, R., Yli-Hietanen, J., Mattila, H., Kalli, S.: Reorganization of oral anticoagulant (warfarin) treatment follow-up. Scand. J. Prim. Health Care 24, 33–37 (2006)

15. Niiranen, S., Yli-Hietanen, J.: Analysis of computer-supported oral anticoagulant treatment follow-up workflow. In: Conf. Proc. IEEE Eng. Med. Biol. Soc., pp. 4330–4332 (2008)
16. Chu, S., Cesnik, B.: A three-tier clinical information systems design model. Int. J. Med. Inform. 57, 91–107 (2009)
17. National Center for Injury Prevention and Control. Data elements for emergency department systems, release 1.0. Centers for Disease Control and Prevention, Atlanta (1997)
18. Aronsky, D., Kendall, D., Merkley, K., James, B., Haug, P.: A comprehensive set of coded chief complaints for the emergency department. Acad. Emerg. Med. 8, 980–989 (2001)
19. Thompson, D., Eitel, D., Fernandes, C., Pines, J., Amsterdam, J., Davidson, S.: Coded Chief Complaints–automated analysis of free-text complaints. Acad. Emerg. Med. 13, 774–782 (2006)

Chapter 3
Agent Technology and Healthcare: Possibilities, Challenges and Examples of Application

David Sánchez, David Isern, and Antonio Moreno

Universitat Rovira i Virgili (URV)
Department of Computer Science and Mathematics
Intelligent Technologies for Advanced Knowledge Acquisition (ITAKA) Research Group
Avinguda Països Catalans, 26. 43007 Tarragona, Catalonia (Spain)
david.sanchez@urv.cat, david.isern@urv.cat,
antonio.moreno@urv.cat

Abstract. Agent technology has emerged as a promising technology to develop complex and distributed systems. They have been extensively applied in a wide range of healthcare areas in the last 10 years. This chapter introduces the basic aspects and properties of agents and multi-agent systems and argues their adequacy to solve different kinds of problems in healthcare. It also describes several healthcare areas in which this technology has been successfully applied, introducing, in each case, some of the most relevant works. The explanation is illustrated with a more detailed description of two agent-based healthcare applications in which the authors have been involved. One of them automates the enactment of clinical guidelines by coordinating several healthcare entities of a medical organization. The other is a Web-based knowledge-driven platform that supports the execution of personalized Home Care services. The benefits that agent technology brings to those approaches are commented and several lines of future research are enounced.

1 Introduction

Healthcare is an area that affects very directly the life quality of all human beings. It is a complex domain which usually involves lengthy procedures, in which a large quantity of professionals with a wide range of expertise, knowledge, skills and abilities (from family doctors to medical specialists, nurses, laboratory technicians or social workers) have to co-ordinate efficiently their activities to provide the best possible care to patients. In this sense, the computerization of administrative and medical assistance processes can help to improve the provision of care services, both from the temporal, medical and economic points of view. However, healthcare is one of the most difficult domains to automate due to its inherent complexity. The lack of standardization between healthcare organizations, the heterogeneous profiles of their users, the reluctance of practitioners to use computerised systems, the enormous amount of data to be handled and their variety of formats, the decentralisation of data

I. Bichindaritz et al. (Eds.): Computational Intelligence in Healthcare 4, SCI 309, pp. 25–48.
springerlink.com

sources, the security issues related to the management of sensitive data and the robustness in front of possible errors are just some of the difficulties which a computerized healthcare system has to face.

Agent technology has emerged in the last 20 years as a promising paradigm for the modelling, design and development of complex systems. *Agents* and, more generally, *multi-agent systems* [47] allow to model in a realistic way complex, heterogeneous and distributed systems and environments. Agents offer a natural solution in which each of the human actors or physical entities are modelled by means of an agent. In the first case, for example, agents may be responsible of storing the human's knowledge, the actions he/she is allowed to perform, the interactions with other actors, and the access and processing of data. In the second case, agents may control the access to the resources, control timetables or implement planning tasks.

Internally, each agent implements the behaviours, the main communicative processes and the methods needed to mimic real-world processes. Moreover, agents can take their own decisions, based on their internal state and the information that they receive from the environment.

When several agents cooperate in the same environment, a multi-agent system may use *distributed problem solving* techniques, allowing to decompose a complex problem in several pieces, which can be concurrently solved in a distributed and decentralised fashion. As a result of the distributed cooperation of several heterogeneous agents, global complex behaviours emerge, allowing realistically modelling and simulating real-world environments, which may be difficult to simulate using other computational paradigms.

As will be argued in section 3, all those possibilities make intelligent agents and multi-agent systems an ideal paradigm to model or simulate healthcare processes. Healthcare entities can be modelled as agents, implementing appropriate behaviours and developing high-level negotiation and communication processes, which represent faithfully real-world medical interactions. The use of intelligent agents in Medicine may be considered a complementary technique to improve the performance of typically ad-hoc and closed medical systems, in terms of interoperability, scalability and flexibility [36].

The contents of this chapter are based in the authors' experience on applying agent technology to healthcare processes. It offers a comprehensive introduction to agent technology from the point of view of a newcomer, illustrating the explanation with several practical examples of agent-based healthcare systems in which authors have been closely involved. As a result of this analysis, several challenges in which research efforts should be put in the following years in order to facilitate the transition of agent technology from the prototypical and research scope to a real-word setting are presented.

The rest of the chapter is organised as follows. Section 2 makes an introduction to the main properties and characteristics of agents and multi-agent systems from a theoretical point of view. Section 3 argues why agent technology is a good option to be applied in the healthcare environment, and presents the main medical areas in which agents have been applied in the last 10 years. Several relevant works applying agents in those areas are also introduced. The benefits that agents can bring to the healthcare domain are also illustrated with two practical examples. Section 4 describes HeCaSe2, a multi-agent system which is able to enact clinical practical guidelines by the coordination of several healthcare entities and to provide personalised healthcare services. Section 5 is devoted to K4Care, a knowledge-driven agent-based platform which provides personalized home-care services for elderly patients following a specially designed European Home Care model. The chapter finishes with some general conclusions on the use of agents in health care, focusing on some lines of future work that could help to move agents from the academic labs to their routine use in clinical settings.

2   Agents and Multi-agent Systems

In the last twenty years, agents have emerged as a promising computer engineering paradigm. In one of the most relevant works in the area, Wooldridge [52] defined an agent as follows:

> *"An agent is an entity that must be able to perceive the physical or virtual world around it using sensors. A fundamental part of perception is the ability to recognize and filter out the expected events and attend to the unexpected ones. Intelligent agents use effectors to take actions either by sending messages to other agents or by calling application programming interfaces or system services directly"*

Agents represent a core idea in modern computing, where cooperation and communication are heavily stressed. The agent paradigm advances the modelling of technological systems, as agents embody a stronger and more natural notion of autonomy and control than objects.

As software entities, agents implement their functionalities in the form of *behaviours* which are initiated by means of an external stimulus (*e.g.,* the reception of a signal from a physical entity or a message from another agent) and execute a series of actions according to the agent's objectives. Those objectives are designed to mimic the behaviour of a real world entity (*e.g.,* a user, a physical resource) that the agent represent, framed in the context of a complex and distributed system. In order to offer a realistic implementation of a real behaviour and an added value to the final user, agents typically incorporate Artificial Intelligence techniques (*e.g.,* data mining, planning techniques, fuzzy logic, etc.) in order to decide the actions to execute in function of the input data or to pre-process or to filter information according to the user profile to which interact.

In order to extend the theoretical definition of agents, Wooldridge and Jennings [53] distinguished the main characteristics and features that intelligent agents may exhibit:

- *Autonomy.* Agents can operate without the direct intervention of humans or others entities, and may have some kind of control over their actions and internal state.
- *Reactivity.* Agents may perceive their environment (physical world, a user, a collection of agents, the Internet, or a combination of all of them) and respond in a timely fashion to changes that occur in it. Those changes may be transmitted to the agent in the form of stimulus, signals or messages.

- *Pro-activeness*. Agents do not simply act in response to their environment, they are able to exhibit goal-directed opportunistic behaviour and take the initiative when appropriate.
- *Social ability*. Agents interact with other agents (and humans) via some kind of agent-communication language when they recognise the necessity of such communication (usually with the aim to complete their own problem solving and to help others with their activities in a coordinated fashion).

Later, the same authors presented a further list of features ([54]) that emphasizes cognitive functions that an agent should implement. Those include the following functionalities:

- Maintaining an explicit model of the state of its environment, and perhaps its own mental state as well.
- Raising and pursuing goals about the state of its environment, or its knowledge of the state of the environment.
- Perceiving events that occur in its environment, recognizing when its goals are not currently satisfied.
- Establishing plans to acquire information about the environment and to create changes, which will be consistent with its goals.
- Implementing these plans by acting upon the environment in order to bring about the desired change.

The advantages that agent technology brings are understood in the context of cooperation between a set of heterogeneous agents. A collection of agents which are able to interact compose a *Multi-agent system* (MAS). MAS are collections of autonomous agents that communicate between them to coordinate their activities in order to be able to solve collectively a problem that could not been tackled by an agent individually.

Being inherently distributed, a MAS has the following interesting properties which offer an added value over classical software engineering paradigms:

- *Modularity*: the different services or functionalities which are involved in a complex problem may be divided, distributed and modelled among diverse agents, depending on their complexity. In addition, a MAS allows for the interconnection and interoperation of multiple existing legacy systems. By building an agent wrapper around such systems, they can be incorporated into an agent society.
- *Efficiency*: due to the parallel and concurrent nature of MAS execution, in which each agent can be deployed in a separate computer node, it enhances overall system performance, specifically along the dimensions of computational efficiency, reliability, extensibility, robustness, maintainability, responsiveness, flexibility, and reuse.
- *General performance*: a MAS can distribute computational resources and capabilities across a network of computers in which a set of interconnected agents are deployed. Whereas a centralized system may be plagued by resource limitations, performance bottlenecks or critical failures, a MAS is decentralized and thus, does not suffer from the single point of failure problem and the hardware bottlenecks associated with centralised systems. Agent technology does not introduce special hardware or software requirements and thus, they can take profit from already existing, obsolete and underused hardware resources of a computer network.

- *Flexibility*: agents may be dynamically created or eliminated according to the needs of the application without affecting to the execution of their environment. Negotiation and knowledge exchange allow the optimization of shared resources.
- *Existence of a standard*: the Foundation for Intelligent Physical Agents (FIPA, [18]) is an IEEE Computer Society standards committee that promotes the agent-based technology and impulses the interoperability with other technologies by definition communication standards. They establish the rules that have to govern the design and implementation of a MAS in order to achieve interoperability among heterogeneous agent-based systems.
- *Existence of agent methodologies*: due to the potential complexity of a MAS, it is important to use a software engineering methodology in order to be able to design an agent architecture with the appropriate agent behaviours which fit with the real-world requirements. Nowadays there exist several agent-oriented engineering methodologies such as INGENIAS [42], Gaia [55] and Prometheus [41].
- *Existence of software development tools*: there are many tools to implement, execute and manage MAS that provide some facilities (graphical tools, APIs, examples, documentation, execution environment, debugging possibilities, etc.) [36, 45]. From all the available tools, the most well-known and widely-used are JADE (Java Agent Development Environment, [5]), Zeus [40], and agentTool III [20].

Thanks to those advantages, MAS may be used in domains in which classical software approaches may be hardly applied or may introduce serious limitations.

On the one hand, problems in which the knowledge required to solve is spatially distributed in different locations may take profit from the inherently distributed nature of agent technology, physically deploying some knowledge oriented agents in the data source location and performing remote request for data or operations with these data.

On the other hand, problems in which several entities, while keeping their autonomous behaviour, have to join their problem solving abilities to solve a complex problem by exploit MAS' modularity in order to divide the problem or replicate it.

As a results of the several advantages which agent technology brings in this kind of systems and their inherent capability of modelling and simulating complex real-world environments in a natural way, multi-agents systems have been considered as the latest software engineering paradigm [4, 5, 39].

Klein *et al.* [33] classified multi-agent systems according to their reliability into closed and open systems. A closed MAS contain well-described agents designed to work together. An open context deals with unreliable infrastructures, non-compliant agents and emergent dysfunctions. Being the healthcare domain a critical environment which typically deals with sensitive and private data, MAS studied in this chapter are closed in terms of reliability and include coordination and cooperation techniques such as auctions, negotiations, and planning methods among the different involved entities.

3   Agents Applied in Healthcare

As introduced above, agents and multi-agent systems provide interesting features that have been used in complex domains such as healthcare. In this section, we analyse the main characteristics of distributed healthcare problems, and then, we discuss the adequacy of agent technology in order to tackle them. Then, we present a brief review of the main fields of healthcare where the agent technology has been applied, summarizing some of the most relevant works.

3.1 Adequacy of Agents Applied in Healthcare Problems

Reviewing the literature [1, 7, 10, 15, 16, 19, 21, 43, 50], some of the most common problems which should be faced in a medical environment are:

- It is very usual that the knowledge and data required to solve a medical problem are spatially distributed in different locations. Also, remote expertise can be required when dealing with complicate cases. This fact adds several constraints in the planning of coordinated actions.
- Treatments and cares are usually given by different providers (physicians, nurses, carers, social workers, etc.) in different stages of the illness. This requires up-to-date information for all health professionals involved. In addition, these professionals have different skills, roles and needs, and are located in different places, usually without the supervision of a single coordinator. Those actors should be able to access to the medical system and interact between them in a remote fashion.
- Many health care problems are quite complex in relation to the amount of entities and variables which should be taken into consideration when implementing a solution. In consequence, finding standard software engineering solutions for them is not straightforward. This complexity can be a bottleneck if it is managed with a centralised system.
- Data managed in medical informatics has a legal framework that protects them when exchanging and storing. Data protection and data security mechanisms should be included in these kinds of systems in order to provide *confidentiality*, *integrity*, *authentication*, *accountability*, and *availability*. In many situations, these data cannot be electronically transmitted and should be managed in a particular place.
- Nowadays, there is a great amount of medical documents, usually called evidences, which are published from many different medical organizations (*e.g.*, Agency for Healthcare Research and Quality (U.S.), Cancer Research UK), becoming a de facto standard. All these documents should be retrieved and processed in order to obtain a knowledge that can be shared and reused in new clinical guidelines.
- Due to the reluctance and preconceptions of individuals involved in healthcare, the penetration of computerized systems (which may automate or aid some processes or decision making) is a hard and slow process. In any case, the interaction between the software and the professionals is crucial in order to supervise critical healthcare process and decisions which should be performed and taken at any time.

Considering the described issues and the added values provided by agent technology, as stated in [39], agent paradigm can be a good option to be used in complex healthcare applications. The main reasons to support this assessment are the following:

- The components of a MAS may be running in different machines, and can be physically located in many different geographical locations. Each of the agents may keep a part of the knowledge required to solve the problem in a distributed manner, such as patient records held in different departments within a hospital. These kind of systems improve the reliability and robustness in comparison with centralised ones [48].
- MAS offer a natural way to include legacy systems such as clinical information systems. For instance, Choe and Yoo [9], propose a secure multi-agent architecture for accessing healthcare information through the Internet from multiple heterogeneous repositories. Agents also enable to process the data locally and only exchange a set of obtained results. For instance, HealthAgents [23] is a network of different medical centres (named contributors) with their local existing databases of cases and classifiers, which are used to diagnose new cases of brain tumours.
- One of the main properties of an intelligent agent is sociability. Agents are able to communicate between themselves, using some kind of standard agent communication language, in order to exchange any kind of information. In that way they can engage in complex dialogues, in which they can negotiate, coordinate their actions and collaborate in the solution of a problem (for example, different care units of a hospital may collaborate in the process of patient scheduling [38]).
- When a problem is too complex to be solved by a single system, it is usual to decompose it in sub-problems (which will probably not be totally independent of each other). MAS inherently support techniques of cooperative problem solving, in which a group of agents may dynamically discuss how to partition a problem, how to distribute the different subtasks to be solved among them, how to exchange information to solve possible dependences between partial solutions, and how to combine the partial results into the solution of the original problem [31, 52]. Thus, MAS can handle the complexity of solutions through decomposition, modelling and organising the interrelationships between components.
- Agents can also be used to provide information to health professionals and patients. There exist information agents, which are specialised in retrieving information from different sources, analysing and processing the obtained data, selecting the information in which the user is especially interested, filtering redundant or irrelevant information, and presenting it to the user with an interface adapted to the user's preferences. Those agents implement in a natural way, AI techniques for data and knowledge processing such as data mining, intelligent data integration, natural language text processing or formal knowledge structures such as ontologies [37, 47]. In addition, as Vieira-Marques *et al.* [51] show, a common relational database for all the agents is often unpractical because of cost and technical requirements, and medical institutions usually prefer to maintain control of their own medical data.
- Another important property of agents is their pro-activity, their ability to perform tasks and execute processes that may be beneficial for the user, even if he/she has not explicitly requested those tasks to be executed. Using this property and taking into consideration information about the user's personal profile, they may find relevant information and show it to the user before he has to request it.

- The basic characteristic of an intelligent agent is its autonomy. Each agent takes its own decisions, based on its internal state and the information that it receives from the environment. Therefore, agents offer an ideal paradigm to implement real-world systems in which each component models the behaviour of a separate entity, which wants to keep its autonomy and independence from the rest of the system (*e.g.,* each unit of the hospital may keep its private data, or each hospital may use a different policy to rank the patients that are waiting for an organ transplant).

Moreover, Fox *et al.* [19] identified other benefits of applying agents to healthcare problems. On the one hand, agent technology offers advanced platforms for building expert systems to assist individual clinicians in their work. On the other hand, distributed agent systems have the potential to improve the operation of healthcare organisations, where failures of communication and coordination are important sources of error.

3.2   Fields of Application of Agents in Healthcare

The reader can find numerous applications of agents in healthcare. From an analysis of those works, Figure 1 summarises several domains of healthcare in which agent technology has been applied. The figure also presents some of the most relevant works performed in each area, which are briefly introduced in this section.

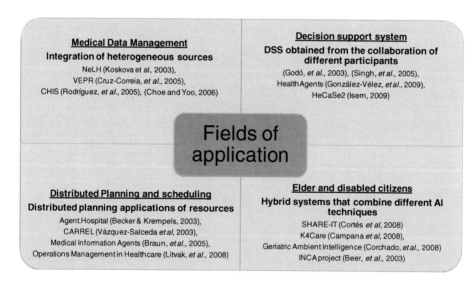

Fig. 1. General overview of main fields where agents have been applied

Medical data management. Systems focused on the retrieval and processing of medical data, such as distributed electronic healthcare records and Web resources. These systems integrate several (heterogeneous) sources that are accessed in a transparent way by a user, or by another decision support system. This approach permits to separate the knowledge source from its use. Examples of this kind of systems are the following projects: the National electronic Library for Health (NeLH) [34], the Virtual Electronic Patient Record (VEPR) [14], the Context-aware Hospital Information System (CHIS) [46], and the proposal made by Choe and Yoo [9]. These systems crawl proactively the sources in order to maintain an up-to-date repository of knowledge, and at the same time, agents coordinate their activities in order to improve the retrieving and processing of data.

Decision support systems. Approaches aimed to assist the professional in the execution of healthcare treatments. In this case, agents are used to retrieve, monitor and decide which information is transmitted to the user. Users are usually represented in the system with his/her particular agent and individual preferences. These systems use a knowledge base to support the inference process. Case-based reasoning and domain ontologies are two of the most used techniques to represent the medical knowledge. Examples of this kind of applications are the following: the proposal made by Godó et al. [22], the Singh's et al. [49] system, the HealthAgents project [23], and the HeCaSe2 system [24]. From the analysis of those systems, the reader can observe the flexibility that agents provide implementing three different topologies. At first, one problem is replicated in parallel among different sources that solve the problem locally and send a (partial) result that is integrated. In a second case, a complex problem is divided into several parts which are solved by individual agents in a grid-like manner, and then, an agent aggregates the received solutions. In last case, the problem is solved co-ordinately by agents exchanging the appropriate medical information.

Planning and resource allocation. Systems centred on the coordination and scheduling of human and material resources. Communication and coordination, which are basic characteristics of agents as stated previously, are extensively exploited in this kind of systems due to the required negotiation among different partners, taking into account different constraints, variables and features (which may introduce potential contractions between them). Good examples of this category are: the Agent.Hospital infrastructure [32], CARREL [13], the Medical Information Agents project [6], and the Operations Management in Healthcare project [35]. The agents of these systems replicate real world behaviours in order to realistically automate processes. Mainly, they decompose a problem in smaller units which are easier to deal with and which are assigned to individual agents [31].

Composite systems. Systems which offer complete and integrated solutions for healthcare management for a concrete organization. These kinds of systems combine different AI techniques with a particular purpose under the umbrella of e-Health. Assistance to elder or disabled citizens (such as the projects SHARE-IT [12], K4Care platform [8], and the Geriatric Ambient Intelligence [10]), and community care (such as the INCA project [3]), are two examples of this area of application. These systems can be considered as final applications meant to substitute traditional and ad hoc solutions currently running in medical organizations. The maturity of some of these systems also shows the feasibility that agent technology can offer to the healthcare domain.

In order to illustrate the benefits that agent technology brings in the healthcare environment, in the following sections we describe in more detail two of the introduced systems in which the authors have been closely participated at the design and implementation stages: HeCaSe2 and K4Care.

4 HeCaSe2

Healthcare Services release 2 (HeCaSe2) is a research prototype designed as a distributed multi-agent system that allows to simulate complex processes in a healthcare organization [24]. HeCaSe2 proposes the inclusion of Clinical Guidelines (CG) with Multi-Agent Systems in order to obtain a prototype that can be used in a real medical environment to improve the current resource management.

The proposal defines an architecture of agents that emulates the behaviours of medical partners in a medical centre. This infrastructure is used by practitioners to execute CGs that describe sequences of steps to be performed over a patient in order to treat a particular pathology. These CGs are generally promoted by governmental institutions, but the practical implementation in real scenarios is difficult due to the lack of interoperability of existing guideline-based execution engines [27]. The use of agents aids to address this issue, allowing to build a flexible and modular application that can be easily customised attending to the particular circumstances of the final medical centre (*e.g.,* the use of a particular electronic health record), and that can facilitate the coordination of activities between different medical centres.

4.1 HeCaSe2 Architecture

The proposed agent-based architecture includes different kinds of agents following the organisational rules of a real healthcare institution (see Figure 2). Each agent acts autonomously with its own knowledge and data. It is decentralised, as there is not any central control node and the number of agents may be configured depending on the specific structure of a healthcare organisation (*e.g.,* doctors, departments, and devices in a medical centre).

At the top of the architecture it is located the patient, who interacts with the system through his *User Agent* (UA). This agent stores static data related to the user (*e.g.,* national health care number, name, address, and access information -login, password, and keys-) and dynamic data (the timetable and the preferences of the user).

The *Broker Agent* (BA) is an agent that knows all the medical centres located in a certain area. It maintains the information of all connected medical centres, and permits the user to search a medical centre according to a criterion (*e.g.,* the centre of a village, or a centre that has a particular department).

A *Medical Centre Agent* (MCA) controls and monitors the outsider accesses to the agents that manage the information of a medical centre. A MCA monitors all of its departments, represented by *Department Agents* (DAs), and a set of general services linked to human or physical resources, represented by *Service Agents* (SAs) (*e.g.,* a blood test service). Each department has a staff of several doctors, modelled through *Doctor Agents* (DRAs), and offers more specific services, also modelled as SAs (*e.g.,* a nurse that can take different observations *in situ*). Both MCAs and DAs are aware of the services they can provide (*i.e.* when a SA enters the system, it sends a message detailing its services to the associated MCA or DA).

In addition, each department contains a *Guideline Agent* (GA) that performs all actions related to guidelines (*e.g.*, it can retrieve the CG associated to a specific disease). This GA contains only CGs associated to the department where it is located, allowing versioning of CGs authored by the practitioners.

The *Ontology Agent* (OA) provides information about the concepts that appear in a guideline - medical and/or organisational terms - (know-what) and their relations (know-how). The OA uses the medical ontology designed to represent all relationships between all kind of actors, their roles, and allowed activities. There is one OA per department in order to locate the information close to the clients, but at the same time, different OAs can use different ontologies, for instance, to represent different roles or responsibilities of the medical staff, or different available resources in a department.

At the bottom of the architecture, a *Medical Record Agent* (MRA) controls the accesses to a database that stores all medical records of the patients of the medical centre. Appropriate security measures have been taken to ensure that only properly authenticated and authorised agents may access and update the medical records.

Agent interactions are implemented over communication protocols and sharing a common knowledge representation. Mainly, agents use well-known protocols such as FIPA-Query, FIPA-Request and FIPA-Contract Net [17]. The MAS has been implemented using JADE, which is compliant with the FIPA specification for agent development [5]. Moreover, HeCaSe2 has been designed following an agent-oriented software engineering methodology (INGENIAS [42]) in order to provide a more general and reusable framework, documenting all the services, and improving further updates [25].

4.2 Task Coordination during the Treatment

One of the main advantages of using agents in healthcare is the possibility of coordinating the activities or tasks that cannot be achieved by one entity due to their inherent complexity [30]. In the case of healthcare, a practitioner may use the facilities provided by the HeCaSe2 system during the treatment of a patient, which consists on the enactment of a CG. A CG incorporates the declarative knowledge related to the treatment of the patient, including the steps to be followed: actions, enquiries and decisions. Depending on the case, the practitioner may require the support of another colleague or an external service.

In addition, HeCaSe2 guides this search taking into account preferences of the user (patient) about a set of criteria such as the medical centres, the days and the period of the day in which a medical test should be performed. This negotiation-based procedure balances the load among centres (agents send different proposals of free slots) and, at the same time, permits the user selecting the most appropriate alternative according to his preferences. This is a flexible approach that allows the managers of the medical centres the analysis and supervision of the waiting lists of patients in particular services.

As said previously, one of the possibilities that a practitioner can find during the execution of a treatment is that the patient requires an *action*. This specifies a medical procedure that should be performed over a patient. At this point the MAS searches

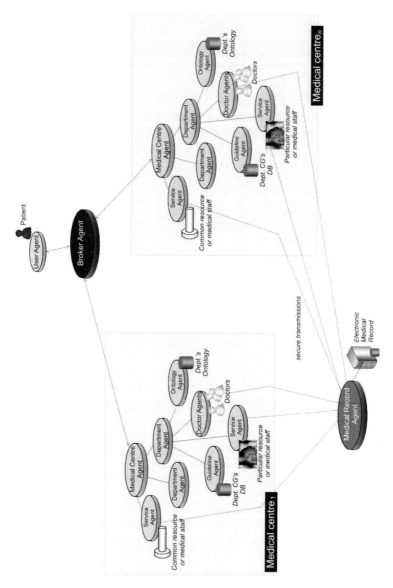

Fig. 2. HeCaSe2 Architecture

who is the responsible of performing this action (by the way of the *ontology agent*). An action can be done by the same practitioner that executes the CG (*e.g.*, prescribe a particular diet, a drug, or perform some basic activities), but it may require a specialist (*e.g.*, to perform a biopsy). On the last case, agents look for specialists that perform the required medical procedure and select the most appropriate one. As Figure 3 shows, this search is performed through the same medical centre (locally) and also through others centres that have the required service (this remote search is performed

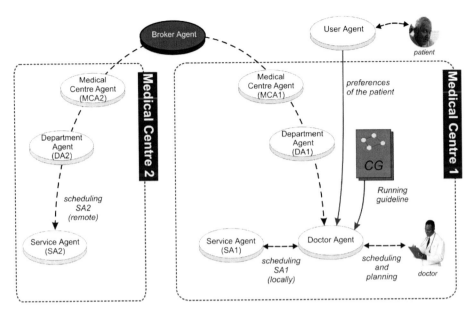

Fig. 3. Communication-based scheduling of resources

using the facilities provided by the *broker* agent). The final ranking and filtering of the set of alternatives received, takes into account the preferences of the user, which selects one of them. The final approval of this alternative and rejection of the rest is also made during this process.

In the case of *enquiries*, the treatment may require some missing values about the patient. Usually, these values are findings, symptoms and syndromes that are used in further steps of the treatment (*e.g.,* if a patient smokes, evaluation of a risk factor for some disease). Also, like in the case of actions, several entries should be referred to specialists. For instance, if an enquiry requires the result of a biopsy (positive or negative), this value should be filled by a surgeon who is able to perform it.

The last item that a practitioner can find in a CG is a *decision* that embeds logical conditions and different paths that can be followed in the future. Decisions are made by practitioners. HeCaSe2 only presents the information to them and waits for their selection (in a supervised fashion). Being a decision support system, HeCaSe2 forwards all the information and data to the expert who decides upon all available possibilities. In this case, it is not necessary to enable inter-communication processes between agents.

4.3 Discussion

HeCaSe2 is a complex agent-based system that simulates the real behaviour of a medical centre. HeCaSe2 guides the execution of daily care activities through the care flow structure defined in CGs. This approach has two main benefits: first, the inclusion of CGs in computerised health information systems, and second, to model a flexible and robust platform with entities running autonomously but cooperating with other partners to manage a more general problem [29].

Taking all these elements into consideration, the practitioner can deal with CGs executed step-by-step. The system permits to retrieve up-to-date patients' data from the medical record and track all the activities done over the patient. At that time, the patient can know exactly where he is (inside of a mid- or long- term treatment) and devise further possible evolutions of his treatment.

This computerised enactment of CGs brings several economical and medical benefits for practitioners and patients, easing, automating and standardising healthcare treatments.

The agent-based platform mimics real relationships and roles of real healthcare organisations, but the management is quite different. The system permits a balance of the load (avoiding or mitigating waiting lists). Also, healthcare managers can identify problems in a particular point and implement different policies in a particular medical resource (*e.g.*, availability 24/7).

An important feature of medical systems is the knowledge representation. HeCaSe2 uses different ontologies that separate the knowledge from its use, and permits to guide the agents' execution with this ontology-based representation.

Another facility promoted with the communication-based execution of CGs is the inclusion of *extra* information in these messages. Concretely, the interaction between practitioners and other services in order to arrange a meeting for this patient uses patient's preferences to guide the search. There is a change for the traditional delivery of services in healthcare where the patient has a passive role. In this case, he can take an active role in the decisions that affect him.

Finally, it is important to note that HeCaSe2 adds security mechanisms to protect all data exchanged in the system. Although there are different agents that can access to the EMR, there is a control over the patient's data accesses and all transmissions are ciphered to assure the privacy and integrity of data.

5   Knowledge Based Home Care eServices for an Ageing Europe (K4Care)

The K4Care European project (*Knowledge based Home Care eServices for an Ageing Europe*, [8]) is a Specific Targeted Research of Innovation Project funded within the Sixth Framework Program of the European Commission that brings together 13 academic and industrial institutions from 7 countries for a period of 3 years starting March 2006. The main goals of the project are, on the one hand, the definition of a HC model which may be incorporated as an European standard, integrating the information, skills and experiences of specialised Home Care centres and professionals of several old and new EU countries and, on the other hand, to incorporate it into a prototype HC platform to provide e-services to health professionals, patients and citizens in general which shows the validity of the model.

While the healthcare information system of a single medical centre is usually rather centralised, medical assistance in Home Care, which is the scope of K4Care, naturally needs a distributed service-oriented architecture, as many kinds of actors from different institutions are involved (*e.g.*, family doctors, physicians, rehabilitation staff, social workers, patients, etc.). Thus, the *K4Care platform*, which implements the proposed generic HC model [8], has been designed in order to meet the needs of decentralization and remote access to distributed sources introduced by the involved actors. Considering these requirements, the execution core of the platform is composed by a multi-agent system which models the real-world entities involved in HC and allow a natural interaction and coordination.

In this section we describe the design and architecture of the K4Care platform, focusing on the multi-agent system aspect and discussing the benefits that the use of this technology brings in front of classical software development paradigms.

5.1 K4Care Architecture and Functionalities

One of the bases of the K4Care model is the medical knowledge representation and exploitation. The idea is to separate the concrete knowledge representation associated to a concrete medical organization from its usage at execution time. Taking this requirement into consideration, the K4Care platform present a knowledge-driven design by means of the definition of a three layered architecture (shown in Figure 4): the *Knowledge Layer*, the *Data Abstraction Layer*, and the *K4Care agent-based platform* [8, 28].

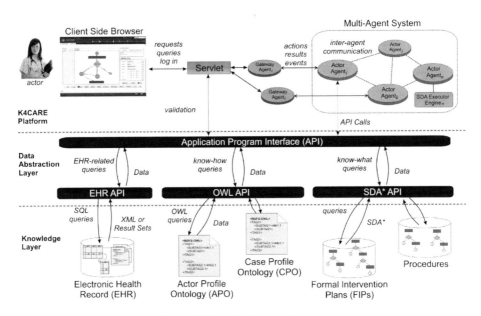

Fig. 4. K4Care platform architecture

The Knowledge Layer [2] includes all the data sources required to specify the HC model and its particular adaptation to a concrete organization. It includes an Electronic Health Record (EHR) which store patient data and clinical histories, the organizational knowledge (*e.g.* actor's skills, permissions and interactions) and medical knowledge (*e.g.* disorders, treatments, symptoms, causes, etc.) required by an organization to execute HC processes represented by means of standard ontologies (*Actor Profile Ontology* –APO- and *Case Profile Ontology* –CPO- respectively) and a repository of careflows (procedures) and formal intervention plans (FIPs), specified in SDA* notation [44] which define the stages to be followed in order to execute administrative and medical processes.

As each knowledge base is expressed in a different format, the intermediate layer (Data Abstraction Layer, [2]) objective is to decouple the generic execution of HC processes by the platform from the way in which the data is stored in the Knowledge Layer. It provides a set of Java-based methods that allow the K4Care entities to retrieve the data and knowledge they need to perform their duties in a transparent manner.

The upper layer of the K4Care platform [26] is implemented by means of a web-based application on the client side (which interacts through a Web browser) and a server side. It is designed to support the interaction with real world actors, allowing a remote access to medical data and services both to HC professionals and patients. The sever side, which implements the execution logic of the platform and relies on the knowledge structures presented above, has been developed extensively using the agent technology.

From the final user point-of-view, the K4Care Platform features the following functionalities:

- Secure access to a patient's EHR: the patient's Electronic Health Record which stores clinical histories and it is stored by means of standard XML documents, is accessed and managed only by the allowed HC actors. Permissions are modelled explicitly within the Actor Profile Ontology and consulted at execution time, making the system automatically adaptable to different health care organisational structures and societies.

- Execution of HC management activities: HC procedures specified in the SDA* formalism indicate the workflow to be followed and the activities to be completed by the different actors in order to execute HC management services. The system is able to interpret those structures and coordinate the execution of the involved entities accordingly.

- Definition and execution of Individual Intervention Plans (see Figure 5): each patient admitted for HC is assigned to an Evaluation Unit, composed by a multidisciplinary team of four people. These actors can use a graphical editor embedded in the platform to define a customised Individual Intervention Plan (IIP) adapted to the patient's personal circumstances (i.e. considering the interaction of several pathologies that the patient may suffer), via the combination and adaptation of several standard Formal Intervention Plans represented in the SDA* notation. The agents in the platform coordinate their activities to efficiently execute these treatments. The platform is responsible of making an intelligent dynamic assignment of the tasks included in the IIP among the available human actors.

- Personalization: actors are also allowed to personalize their interaction with the platform by requesting the modification of some aspects of the HC model (i.e. permissions over clinical data or skills). In this manner, the system can adapt automatically its behaviour to the preferences expressed by an actor for a particular aspect of the HC.

- Web access: actors may have a remote access to the platform using a standard Web browser. The graphical interface permits allowed users to request services, see and attend pending actions, look up the electronic health care record of the patients, fill out documents with results of actions execution, request the updating and personalization of their profile, work as part of a group, define Individual Intervention Plans, etc.

5.2 K4Care Multi-agent System

The agents of the K4Care platform embed all the system logic by personifying the actors involved in HC services (*e.g.*, administrative procedures, careflows, assessments, follow-ups, etc.). The main goal of the MAS is to coordinate the activities enclosed in administrative procedures and individual intervention plans (as presented above) between all involved actors.

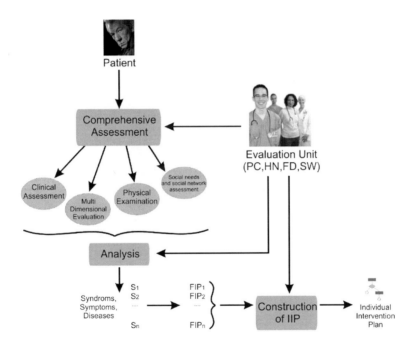

Fig. 5. Definition of an Individual Intervention Plan

Agent's execution is guided by the knowledge and data stored in the knowledge layer at any moment. So a change on that results in immediate changes in the execution logic. Agents act semi-autonomously, in the sense that several actions, such as exchange of information, collection of heterogeneous data concerning a patient (results, current treatment, next recommended step, past history), or the management of actions to execute, are performed by agents without supervision; others, that may have some degree of responsibility (such as decisions taken in the process of healthcare), are supervised by users.

Each user (both patients and healthcare professionals) is represented in the system by a permanent agent (generically represented as *Actor Agents* in Figure 4). Each one owns all the information related to the services in which it is involved and manages all queries and requests coming from the associated user or other Actor Agents. They also incorporate all the details about user's roles and permissions according to the organizational data available in the knowledge bases (specifically, the Actor Profile Ontology). In fact, *Actor Agents'* code is partially created in an automated fashion from the knowledge stored in those structures. Concretely, agent behaviour skeletons are created from the skill definitions stored in the ontologies. In addition to this "static" knowledge, it is also possible to adapt this data in order to personalize the interaction between the user and the system at runtime. This tailoring process is mediated by his/her associated Actor Agent in function of the locally stored profile-related and organizational knowledge.

In order to provide access transparency to end users, the Web interface and the multi-agent system are connected by a bridge constituted by a servlet and a *Gateway Agent* (GA). When an actor logs into the system, the servlet creates a Gateway Agent whose mission is to keep a one-to-one connectivity with the corresponding permanent agent. Considering that the Web and agent environments are not meant to be directly interoperable, GAs act as mediators, translating web request to FIPA-based agent messages. This provides independency between the ubiquitous web accesses from the user's PC or mobile device and the Actor Agent's implementation and execution. Ideally, Actor Agents should be executing in a secure environment and distributed through a computer network in order to provide load balancing in conditions of high concurrency.

Finally, *SDA* Executor Agents* (SDA-Es) allow enacting a care plan by recommending the next step to follow according to the patient's current state. The SDA-E is dynamically created by an Actor Agent in order to enact a SDA* structure corresponding to a healthcare process (like an Individual Intervention Plan) or to a management procedure. The SDA-E agent, after loading a SDA* from the repository, is ready to receive queries about its execution. Those queries are performed by the Actor Agent in order to know the next step to follow. As a result, healthcare actions will be delegated to the appropriate actors considering the organizational knowledge stored in the ontologies and the availability of physical actors represented by means of Actor Agents. Clinical decisions which may arise during the execution of an SDA* will be forwarded to the user in order to implement the healthcare treatment in a supervised manner.

In the same manner as HeCaSe2, the agent-based platform has been implemented with the JADE tool, and using two FIPA-based protocols: FIPA-Request to request actions to be performed to the SDA-E Agent and FIPA-ContractNet to negotiate the execution of a particular action between the available partners.

5.3 Discussion

One of the most interesting aspects of the K4Care platform is the decoupling of the system's implementation from the knowledge structures which represent the HC model and its particular representation on a concrete organization. In this way, the medical and organizational knowledge can be directly modified in order to introduce changes in the HC process, which will immediately be adopted by the actors of the system in execution time. This design provides a high degree of flexibility, reusability and generality, which are fundamental aspects of a system modelling complex and dynamic processes. As an example, in K4Care, the procedures used in potential instantiations of the system in different countries could be adapted to the methods of work in each place, the Formal Intervention Plans used in each medical centre could take into account only the resources they have available or the ontologies can be adapted and extended to model new care units or new procedural or medical knowledge related to the healthcare party without requiring any reprogramming effort. This suppose a great advantage in relation with ad-hoc healthcare systems implemented over legacy systems, which represent a rigid structured hardly adaptable in front of runtime changes.

The use of agent technology, as had been previously argued in [11, 39], certainly seems an interesting option to consider in this kind of distributed systems. K4Care agents model their human counterparts in a realistic and natural way, mimicking their real HC behaviours modelled in the knowledge structures. Agents can be dynamically deployed and managed into the system creating, for example, an Actor Agent associated to a new patient who will immediately allow and manage the interaction of the new user with the system in a personalized manner.

In the K4Care platform, permanent Actor Agents also implement, by relying of the underlying data structures, the persistency necessary to maintain the execution state of user's tasks. In this way, the inherent complexity of HC processes is transparently tackled by decomposing and coordinating individual agent's executions. Actor Agents' behaviour can be also tailored according to user's preferences by locally changing some aspects of the organizational knowledge stored in the common knowledge bases. This adds the high degree of flexibility and adaptability required when managing heterogeneous user profiles from the point of view of different medical organizations.

K4Care agents incorporate behaviours to coordinate their execution and negotiate the delegation of HC actions according to the available data. Planning and data management are the most important issues tackled by the MAS in order to ensure an efficient execution of procedures and intervention plans in a distributed fashion.

The distributed nature of the system also allows to deploy Actor Agents (which may be quite numerous) through a –secured– computer network, allowing an appropriate load balancing, taking profit from underused or obsolete equipment and improving the efficiency and robustness of the platform. The autonomy of the agents executing patient's intervention plans permits to enact and assign tasks avoiding a central monitor or controller which may introduce a serious bottleneck.

Moreover, in order to provide an intuitive and remote interaction with the final user, a web interface is provided. Due to the non-trivial communication between the agent execution environment and the web server which process user's request, an intermediate layer composed by temporal Gateway Agents is introduced, which maintains the logic –session- of the user-agent communication during the logged session and acts as a middleware, translating requests from the web world to the FIPA-compliant agent environment.

6   Future Lines of Work to Promote the Use of Agents in Healthcare

The applications using agent technology in health care (especially the prominent examples mentioned in sections 3.2, 4 and 5), albeit most of them remain at the academic level, show an increasing interest of the research community and prove that multi-agent systems bring a good number of positive properties to the solution of problems in this field.

Particularly, *modularity*, dividing a complex problem in several subtasks which are assigned to specialised agents; *efficiency*, thanks to parallelization of the problem's execution by means of several concurrent agents; *decentralization*, as multi-agent systems are inherently distributed and do not have a centralised control point which may introduce bottlenecks or even fail; *flexibility*, thanks to the dynamic addition/removal of agents at runtime based on the execution requirements; *personalisation*, as each agent may model a particular real-world entity and may have knowledge about its interests and preferences; *distributed planning and management of shared resources*, thanks to the inherently distributed nature which allows to implement distributed problem solving techniques for complex problems; *event management*, as agents may continuously monitor the health status of a patient in a very natural way and react to changes in the environment; *proactiveness*, giving the possibility of providing information or results to the user according to his preferences even before he requests it; *security*, as individual permissions, authorizations and authentication mechanisms (in addition to ciphered inter-agent transmissions) may be incorporated in order to ensure the privacy of private medical data; *adaptive behaviour*, as the agent may adapt its execution dynamically at runtime, depending on the data or knowledge available at each moment or even according to external stimulus such as signals or messages.

However, in opinion of the authors and, considering the experience in developing the agent-based systems shown in sections 4 and 5, we can conclude that there is still a wide gap between the developed systems, which mainly represent academic prototypes or proof-of-concept research initiatives, and the healthcare systems deployed in a real environment and focused in real daily usage.

In order to bridge this gap and make these systems move from University labs to hospitals, some aspects should be taken into account in the next years. First, Agent researchers should be aware of the difficulty of working in a real clinical environment, and should probably aim to start deploying simple systems in a constrained setting (*e.g.*, a single unit of a hospital), rather than trying to make huge projects (*i.e.*, at the hospital-level) from scratch.

In order minimize the reluctance of the users, doctors and patients should be involved from the beginning in the development of the project, from the requirements analysis to the design and the implementation phases. They should be especially involved in the definition of the system's intended functionalities and in the design of a graphical interface with which they feel comfortable.

Many hospitals already incorporate a computerised system to manage data and processes. So, it may be interesting to try to re-use as much as possible all the legacy systems that are currently in use in the hospital (*e.g.*, Electronic Health Records or Hospital Information Systems). Many projects make the mistake of including the design from scratch of these components (*e.g.*, when several hospitals with incompatible EHRs have to be included in the same system), and that makes the project much longer, expensive and technically difficult.

It is also advisable to take into account from the very beginning all the legal aspects concerning the security level that healthcare systems must exhibit. A common mistake is to focus first on the "medical" functionalities of the system and delay "adding" the security aspects until the end of the project. This will hamper the reliability of the prototype system and the introduction of security related mechanisms may require a redesign of already working modules.

The maintenance of the healthcare system once it is deployed is also a very basic issue that is often overlooked. This aspect is critical, since usually the personnel in the computer science unit of the hospital do not know about agent technology, and they can't probably handle the maintenance of the system. Intuitive system management tools should be also developed in order to tackle this aspect.

The use of personalisation techniques and mobile devices should be enhanced, as they clearly help to reduce the usual reluctance that healthcare practitioners (and patients) may have to introduce new technologies in their daily workflow, which on the other hand, bring many advantages in promoting the remote access to healthcare services and in managing Home Care processes.

From the agent community point of view, it would be very interesting to promote the reusability of different parts of these agent-based healthcare systems, so that researchers do not have to start from scratch every time they engage in a project in this field (which is the present situation). FIPA provides standards in order to facilitate this interoperability and re-usability.

In summary, although agent technology is certainly a very promising approach to be used when addressing healthcare problems, in opinion of the authors, there is still much work to be done before agent-based systems are routinely used in medical environments.

Acknowledgements

The work has been supported by a URV grant, and partially supported by the EU funded project K4Care (IST-2004-026968) and the Spanish-funded project Hygia (TIN2006-15453-C04-01).

The authors would also like to acknowledge the work performed by other members of the K4Care project consortium, especially the medical partners, led by Dr. Fabio Campana, and Dr. David Riaño (project co-ordinator and designer of the SDA* formalism).

References

[1] Bakker, A.R.: Healthcare and ICT, partnership is a must. Int. J. Med. Inf. 66(1-3), 51–57 (2002)

[2] Batet, M., Gibert, K., Valls, A.: The Data Abstraction Layer as Knowledge Provider for a Medical Multi-Agent System. In: Riaño, D., Campana, F. (eds.) K4CARE 2007. LNCS (LNAI), vol. 4924, pp. 87–100. Springer, Heidelberg (2007)

[3] Beer, M., Hill, R., Huang, W., Sixsmith, A.: An agent-based architecture for managing the provision of community car - the INCA (Intelligent Community Alarm) experience. AI Commun. 16(3), 179–192 (2003)

[4] Bellazzi, R., Zupan, B.: Predictive data mining in clinical medicine: Current issues and guidelines. Int. J. Med. Inf. 77(2), 81–97 (2008)

[5] Bellifemine, F., Caire, G., Greenwood, D.: Developing multi-agent systems with JADE. John Wiley and Sons, Chichester (2007)
[6] Braun, L., Wiesman, F., van der Herik, J., Hasman, A.: Agent Support in Medical Information Retrieval. In: Cortés, U., Fox, J., Moreno, A., Nealon, J. (eds.) Proc. of 3rd Workshop on Agents Applied in Health Care, IJCAI 2005. AAAI, Edimburgh (2005)
[7] Burgers, J.S., Grol, R., Klazinga, N.S., Makela, M., Zaat, J., Collaboration, A.: Towards evidence-based clinical practice: an international survey of 18 clinical guideline programs. Int. J. Qual. Health Care 15(1), 31–45 (2003)
[8] Campana, F., Moreno, A., Riaño, D., Varga, L.: K4Care: Knowledge-Based Homecare e-Services for an Ageing Europe. In: Annicchiarico, R., Cortés, U., Urdiales, C. (eds.) Agent Technology and e-Health, pp. 95–115. Birkhäuser, Basel (2008)
[9] Choe, J., Yoo, S.K.: Web-based secure access from multiple patient repositories. Int. J. Med. Inf. 77(4), 242–248 (2008)
[10] Corchado, J.M., Bajo, J., Abraham, A.: GerAmi: Improving Healthcare Delivery in Geriatric Residences. IEEE Intell. Syst. 23(2), 19–25 (2008)
[11] Cortés, U., Annicchiarico, R., Urdiales, C.: Agents and Healthcare: Usability and Acceptance. In: Annicchiarico, R., Cortés, U., Urdiales, C. (eds.) Agent Technology and e-Health, pp. 1–4. Birkhäuser Verlag, Basel (2008)
[12] Cortés, U., Annicchiarico, R., Urdiales, C., Barrué, C., Martínez, A., Villar, A., Caltagirone, C.: Supported Human Autonomy for Recovery and Enhancement of Cognitive and Motor Abilities Using Agent Technologies. In: Annicchiarico, R., Cortés, U., Urdiales, C. (eds.) Agent Technology and e-Health, pp. 117–140. Birkhäuser Verlag, Basel (2008)
[13] Cortés, U., Vázquez-Salceda, J., López-Navidad, A., Caballero, F.: UCTx: A Multi-agent Approach to Model a Transplant Coordination Unit. Journal of Applied Intelligence 20(1), 59–70 (2004)
[14] Cruz-Correia, R., Vieira-Marques, P., Costa, P., Ferreira, A., Oliveira-Palhares, E., Araújo, F., Costa-Pereira, A.: Integration of hospital data using agent technologies - A case study. AI Commun. 18(3), 191–200 (2005)
[15] Decker, K., Li, J.: Coordinated Hospital Patient Scheduling. In: Demazeau, Y. (ed.) Proc. of 3rd International Conference on Multi-Agent Systems, ICMAS 1998. IEEE Press, Paris (1998)
[16] EU: Directive 1995/46/EC of the European Parliament and of the Council of 24 October 1995 on the protection of individuals with regard to the processing of personal data and on the free movement of such data (EUR 95/46/EC). Official Journal of the European Communities L281, 31–50 (1995)
[17] FIPA: FIPA Abstract Architecture Specification. Foundation for Intelligent and Physical Agents (FIPA), Geneva, Switzerland (2002),
http://www.fipa.org/specs/fipa00001/
[18] FIPA: The Foundation for Intelligent and Physical Agents (2002),
http://www.fipa.org/
[19] Fox, J., Beveridge, M., Glasspool, D.: Understanding intelligent agents: analysis and synthesis. AI Commun. 16(3), 139–152 (2003)
[20] Garcia-Ojeda, J.C., DeLoach, S.A., Robby: AgentTool Process Editor: Supporting the Design of Tailored Agent-based Processes. In: Proc. of 24th Annual ACM Symposium on Applied Computing, pp. 707–714. ACM Press, Honolulu (2009)
[21] Glasspool, D.W., Oettinger, A., Smith-Spark, J.H., Castillo, F.D., Monaghan, V.E.L., Fox, J.: Supporting Medical Planning by Mitigating Cognitive Load. Methods Inf. Med. 46(6), 636–640 (2007)

[22] Godó, L., Puyol-Gruart, J., Sabater, J., Torra, V., Barrufet, P., Fàbregas, X.: A multi-agent system approach for monitoring the prescription of restricted use antibiotics. Artif. Intell. Med. 27(3), 259–282 (2003)

[23] González-Vélez, H., Mier, M., Julià-Sapé, M., Arvanitis, T.N., García-Gómez, J.M., Robles, M., Lewis, P.H., Dasmahapatra, S., Dupplaw, D., Peet, A., Arús, C., Celda, B., Huffe, S.V., Lluch-Ariet, M.: HealthAgents: distributed multi-agent brain tumor diagnosis and prognosis Appl. Intell. 30(3), 191–202 (2009)

[24] Isern, D.: Agent-Based Management of Clinical Guidelines. An Ontological, Personalised and Practical Approach. VDM Verlag Dr. Müller, Saarbrüken (2009)

[25] Isern, D., Gómez-Alonso, C., Moreno, A.: Methodological Development of a Multi-Agent System in the Healthcare Domain. Communications of SIWN 3, 65–68 (2008)

[26] Isern, D., Millan, M., Moreno, A., Pedone, G., Varga, L.Z.: Agent-based execution of individual intervention plans. In: Moreno, A., Cortés, U., Annicchiarico, R. (eds.) Proc. of Workshop Agents applied in Healthcare collocated in 7th Int. Conference on Autonomous Agents and Multiagent Systems (AAMAS 2008), Estoril, Portugal. IFAAMAS, pp. 31–40 (2008)

[27] Isern, D., Moreno, A.: Computer-Based Execution of Clinical Guidelines: A Review. Int. J. Med. Inf. 77(12), 787–808 (2008)

[28] Isern, D., Moreno, A., Pedone, G., Varga, L.: An Intelligent Platform to Provide Home Care Services. In: Riaño, D., Campana, F. (eds.) K4CARE 2007. LNCS (LNAI), vol. 4924, pp. 149–160. Springer, Heidelberg (2007)

[29] Isern, D., Sánchez, D., Moreno, A.: HeCaSe2: A Multi-agent Ontology-Driven Guideline Enactment Engine. In: Burkhard, H.-D., Lindemann, G., Verbrugge, R., Varga, L.Z. (eds.) CEEMAS 2007. LNCS (LNAI), vol. 4696, pp. 322–324. Springer, Heidelberg (2007)

[30] Isern, D., Sánchez, D., Moreno, A.: An ontology-driven agent-based clinical guideline execution engine. In: Bellazzi, R., Abu-Hanna, A., Hunter, J. (eds.) AIME 2007. LNCS (LNAI), vol. 4594, pp. 49–53. Springer, Heidelberg (2007)

[31] Jennings, N.R.: Coordination techniques for distributed artificial intelligence. In: O'Hare, G., Jennings, N.R. (eds.) Foundations of distributed artificial intelligence, pp. 187–210. John Wiley and Sons, Inc., New York (1996)

[32] Kirn, S., Anhalt, C., Krcmar, H., Schweiger, A.: Agent.Hospital — Health Care Applications of Intelligent Agents. In: Kirn, S., Herzog, O., Lockemann, P., Spaniol, O. (eds.) Multiagent Engineering: Theory and Applications in Enterprises, pp. 199–220. Springer, Heidelberg (2006)

[33] Klein, M., Rodriguez-Aguilar, J.-A., Dellarocas, C.: Using Domain-Independent Exception Handling Services to Enable Robust Open Multi-Agent Systems: The Case of Agent Death Auton. Agents Multi-Agent Syst. 7(1-2), 179–189 (2003)

[34] Kostkova, P., Mani-Saada, J., Madle, G., Weinberg, J.R.: Agent-Based Up-to-date Data Management in National Electronic Library for Communicable Disease. In: Moreno, A., Nealon, J. (eds.) Applications of Software Agent Technology in the Health Care Domain, pp. 105–124. Birkhäuser Verlag, Basel (2003)

[35] Litvak, N., van Rijsbergen, M., Boucherie, R.J., van Houdenhoven, M.: Managing the overflow of intensive care patients. European Journal of Operational Research 185(3), 998–1010 (2008)

[36] Luck, M., McBurney, P., Shehory, O., Willmott, S.: Agent Technology: Computing as Interaction (A Roadmap for Agent Based Computing). AgentLink (2005)

[37] Mohammadian, M. (ed.): Intelligent Agents for Data Mining and Information Retrieval. IGI Global (2004)

[38] Myritz, H., Lindemann, G., Zahlmann, G., Burkhard, H.-D.: Patient Scheduling in Clinical Studies with Multi-Agent Techniques. International Transactions on Systems Science and Applications 1(1), 75–80 (2006)

[39] Nealon, J.L., Moreno, A.: Agent-Based Applications in Health Care. In: Nealon, J.L., Moreno, A. (eds.) Applications of Software Agent Technology in the Health Care Domain, pp. 3–18. Birkhäuser Verlag, Basel (2003)

[40] Nwana, H.S., Ndumu, D.T., Lee, L.C., Collis, J.C.: ZEUS: A Toolkit for Building Distributed Multi-Agent Systems. Appl. Art. Intel. 13(1), 129–185 (1999)

[41] Padgham, L., Winikoff, M.: Developing Intelligent Agent Systems: A Practical Guide. John Wiley and Sons, Chichester (2004)

[42] Pavón, J., Gómez-Sanz, J.J., Fuentes, R.: The INGENIAS Methodology and Tools. In: Henderson-Sellers, B., Giorgini, P. (eds.) Agent-Oriented Methodologies, pp. 236–276. Idea Group, USA (2005)

[43] Quoc Dung, T., Kameyama, W.: Ontology-Based Information Extraction and Information Retrieval in Health Care Domain Tran Quoc. In: Song, I.Y., Eder, J., Nguyen, T.M. (eds.) DaWaK 2007. LNCS, vol. 4654, pp. 323–333. Springer, Heidelberg (2007)

[44] Riaño, D.: The SDA* Model: A Set Theory Approach. In: Kokol, P., Podgorelec, V., Dušanka, M., Zorman, M., Verlic, M. (eds.) Proc. of 20th IEEE International Symposium on Computer-Based Medical Systems, CBMS 2007, pp. 563–568. IEEE Press, Maribor (2007)

[45] Ricordel, P.-M., Demazeau, Y.: From Analysis to Deployment: A Multi-agent Platform Survey. In: Omicini, A., Tolksdorf, R., Zambonelli, F. (eds.) ESAW 2000. LNCS (LNAI), vol. 1972, pp. 93–105. Springer, Heidelberg (2000)

[46] Rodríguez, M.D., Favela, J., Preciado, A., Vizcaíno, A.: Agent-based ambient intelligence for healthcare. AI Commun. 18(3), 201–216 (2005)

[47] Sánchez, D., Isern, D., Moreno, A.: Integrated Agent-Based Approach for Ontology-Driven Web Filtering. In: Gabrys, B., Howlett, R.J., Jain, L.C. (eds.) KES 2006. LNCS (LNAI), vol. 4253, pp. 758–765. Springer, Heidelberg (2006)

[48] Sánchez, D., Isern, D., Rodríguez, Á., Moreno, A.: General purpose agent-based parallel computing. In: Omatu, S., Rocha, M.P., Bravo, J., Fernández, F., Corchado, E., Bustillo, A., Corchado, J.M. (eds.) IWANN 2009. LNCS, vol. 5518, pp. 231–238. Springer, Heidelberg (2009)

[49] Singh, S., Ikhwan, B., Haron, F., Yong, C.H.: Architecture of Agent-Based Healthcare Intelligent Assistant on Grid Environment. In: Liew, K.-M., Shen, H., See, S., Cai, W., Fan, P., Horiguchi, S. (eds.) PDCAT 2004. LNCS, vol. 3320, pp. 58–61. Springer, Heidelberg (2004)

[50] van der Haak, M., Wolff, A.C., Brandner, R., Drings, P., Wannenmacher, M., Wetter, T.: Data security and protection in cross-institutional electronic patient records. Int. J. Med. Inf. 70(2-3), 117–130 (2003)

[51] Vieira-Marques, P.M., Robles, S., Cucurull, J., Cruz-Correia, R.J., Navarro, G., Marti, R.: Secure Integration of Distributed Medical Data Using Mobile Agents. IEEE Intell. Syst. 21(6), 47–54 (2006)

[52] Wooldridge, M.: An Introduction to multiagent systems. John Wiley and Sons, Ltd., West Sussex (2002)

[53] Wooldridge, M., Jennings, N.: Intelligent agents: theory and practice. The Knowledge Engineering Review 10(2), 115–152 (1995)

[54] Wooldridge, M., Jennings, N.R.: Formalizing the cooperative problem solving process. In: Wooldridge, M., Jennings, N.R. (eds.) Readings in agents, pp. 430–440. Morgan Kaufmann, San Francisco (1997)

[55] Zambonelli, F., Jennings, N.R., Wooldridge, M.: Developing Multiagent Systems: The Gaia Methodology. ACM Trans. Soft. Eng. Methodol. 12(3), 317–370 (2003)

Chapter 4

Mobile Agents in Healthcare, a Distributed Intelligence Approach

Abraham Martín-Campillo, Carles Martínez-García, Jordi Cucurull, Ramon Martí, Sergi Robles, and Joan Borrell

Departament of Information and Communications Engineering, Universitat Autònoma de Barcelona, 08193 Cerdanyola del Vallès, Spain
{abraham.martin,carlos.martinez,jordi.cucurull}@uab.cat,
{ramon.marti.escale,sergi.robles,joan.borrell}@uab.cat

1 Introduction

1.1 Introduction

The information in healthcare institutions is generally managed by computer applications deployed in medical centers. Usually, each organization has its own system, which is normally proprietary and makes it difficult the exchange of information with other institutions. This chapter discusses the use of mobile agent technology [51,7] as an enabler of open distributed eHealth applications. More precisely, it describes some successful experiences based on this technology: one regarding integration of medical information, and two concerning emergency scenarios. These three successful cases can be very useful at the time of designing new eHealth systems since they have already solved many of the most common issues in this domain.

The first system that will be presented is MedIGS [49], a mobile agent based application that comprises several important features of current healthcare systems, such as distributed information gathering and interoperation among medical centers. The main goal of the system is achieving a Virtual Electronic Patient Medical Record (VEPMR) [6] out of all the medical data about a patient which are spread over a set of hospitals. The system benefits from the mobile agent technology, which relies on local searches performed by roaming agents avoiding the need of a central repository.

Secondly, an application will be described for retrieving partial information of medical records upon request from an emergency scene [33]. This solution fits well when mobile ad hoc networks are in use, and it is based on the asynchronous communication provided by mobile agents. This system allows, for example, to request remote hospitals for critical information about the victims, such as allergies or infectious diseases, thus facilitating more accurate diagnosis and bringing forward decision making.

Finally, the chapter will analyse the case of the Mobile Agent Electronic Triage Tag system (MAETT) [31][32], which is based on mobile electronic triage tags for emergency situations that makes victim information available at the base of operations as soon as possible, thus allowing an early medical resource allocation and immediate action. The cornerstone of the system is mobile agent technology, which allows information to be transported asynchronously and reliably from terminal to terminal and not

I. Bichindaritz et al. (Eds.): Computational Intelligence in Healthcare 4, SCI 309, pp. 49–80.
springerlink.com

requiring any network infrastructure at all. This approach is ready to be used in the worst case scenario, where only small handheld devices carried by the emergency personnel are available, but also integrates well when synchronous connections are possible, for instance when a mesh network can be created.

The chapter concludes with a discussion of the lessons learnt from the development and deployment of these applications. This discussion includes some best practices for the effective use of mobile agents in the e-health domain.

2   Mobile Agents

2.1   Definition

Mobile agents [51] are a technology which has its origin on two different disciplines. On the one hand, the artificial intelligence community created the concept of intelligent agent [53]. On the other hand, the distributed systems community, with a more pragmatic vision of mobile agents, exploited the code mobility [12].

A valid definition for mobile agents, regarding the two mentioned disciplines, is that they are intelligent software entities that have the ability to stop and resume their execution in different network locations to accomplish a set of tasks. The agents live within environments called agent platforms, which define the boundaries of available locations, and are characterised by a set of properties:

- **Mobility:** Agent ability of suspending its execution in a specific agent platform, and resume it in another agent platform, i.e., in another location. This process is usually called agent migration.
- **Autonomy:** Each agent is driven according to a code specially developed to achieve one or more goals. The agent actions are completely decided according to this code without direct intervention of other parties.
- **Reactivity:** Agents react to the environment changes in order to achieve their goals.
- **Proactivity:** Agents change their environment and take several initiatives to achieve their goals.
- **Sociability:** It is the ability of agents to interact with other agents. This is a key feature, since some agents only can perceive their environment through communication with other agents.

2.2   Agent Architecture

A mobile agent, from an architectural point of view, is an entity with a unique identification that is composed of three main components: code, data, and state. The agents live in an environment called agent platform, which is managed by an agent middleware software layer.

2.2.1   Agent Identification

Each mobile agent has an associated identifier that distinguishes it individually. This identifier is assigned when the agent is created, it should be immutable, and it is unique within the scope of the agent authority. The agent identification is of utmost importance since it is related to the communication among agents.

2.2.2 Agent Components

The *agent code* is the core component of the agent and contains the agent's main functionality. The code is developed and compiled using a programming language and computer architecture supported by the hosting agent middlewares.

The agent code is usually interpreted code, since it must be easily separable from its local agent platform for, later, being incorporated to a remote agent platform. This is the main reason why most of the mobile agent systems run over an interpreter or a virtual machine, e.g., the Java Runtime Environment.

The *agent data* are the movable resources associated to the mobile agent, i.e., all the information used and, maybe, produced by the agent during its life, which is moved along with it. In object oriented systems this is usually associated to the object instance. How this information is encoded is completely dependent on each agent middleware, e.g., in Java mobile agent systems the Java Serialisation mechanism is typically used.

The *agent state* is the information associated to the agent execution from a a operating system point of view. It comprises the program counter, the heap, and so forth. Nonetheless, most of the code interpreters used in mobile agent systems do not support access to this information.

2.2.3 Agent Standards

Since currently several agent middleware implementations exist, a number of organisations have initiated the development of agent standards in an attempt to deal with the problem of incompatibility and interoperability. The most extended agent standards are the ones proposed by *IEEE Foundation for Intelligent Physical Agents (IEEE-FIPA, http://www.fipa.org)*, which is an organisation focused on the management and communication of intelligent agents. The specifications standardised by IEEE-FIPA define the basic components of an agent platform, an agent identification scheme, a complete communication infrastructure, and several agent management services.

2.3 Agent Mobility

Agent mobility is the ability of agents to suspend their execution, move their code, data, and state to another location, and there resume their execution. The set of actions involved in the movement of an agent is called *migration process*. The complexity of this process is variable and depends on the protocols and type of mobility chosen. A mobility mechanism that allows the use of different mobility protocols, and which is based on the IEEE-FIPA standards, is the Inter-Platform Mobility Architecture (IPMA) [7].

2.3.1 Types of Agent Mobility

Not all the agent middlewares can deal with the agent state. Depending on this fact two types of agent mobility [12] can be distinguished: *strong* and *weak* mobility.

Strong mobility allows agents to suspend their execution and resume it exactly at the same point it was suspended. This is an advantage for the agent developer, who do not need to add any special code to continue the execution at the appropriate place of the code, see Algorithm 1 of Figure 1. However, strong mobility is complex to implement because of the need to capture and restore the agent state. Furthemore, this type

Algorithm 1: Strong mobility.	**Algorithm 2**: Weak mobility.

```
begin
    Task A
    doMove();
    Task B
end
```

```
begin
    switch state do
        case 0
            Task A;
            state = 1;
            doMove();
            break;
        case 1
            Task B;
            break;
    end
end
```

Fig. 1. Equivalent algorithms using strong and weak mobility.

of mobility is highly dependent with the underlying computer architectures or virtual machines, which hinders the achievement of interoperable systems.

Weak mobility does not capture the execution state, as a consequence the code is always resumed from the first line of code. This is not a major issue, since part of the agent execution state can be saved as agent data. An example, see Algorithm 2 of Figure 1, is the use of switch control flow statements driven by a simple variable which is updated and saved in each agent execution. Therefore, the execution can be approximately resumed in a specific block of code. This migration type is more difficult to manage by the agent developer, but it is the most flexible and portable alternative.

2.3.2   Agent Itineraries

Agent itineraries are the lists of locations that mobile agents visit during their life. The concept of itinerary was firstly introduced in the Concordia [52] agent middleware. The concept is specially important when security is introduced to mobile agents.

Two basic types of itineraries can be distinguished. On the one hand, there are *static itineraries*, which are decided when the agent is created. They comprise the set of ordered locations that the agent will visit during its life. And, on the other hand, there are *dynamic itineraries*, which are not initially preestablished and are decided during the agent life according to its necessities.

2.4   Advantages

Although there is no application that cannot be conceived without the existence of mobile agents, they ease the implementation of applications which require:

- **Task delegation:** Due to the inherent autonomy of agents and mobile agents, they can be assigned with a set of tasks which the agent performs on behalf of its owner, e.g., in Section 3 is described a medical application where the task of searching for patients information is delegated to an specific agent.
- **Asynchronous processing:** Mobile agent execution is not dependent on a continuous communication with the agent owner or the home agent platform. Therefore,

the agent can freely move through different network locations while it carries out the assigned tasks. An example of this is nomadic computing [30], where agents reside in mobile devices and migrate to other locations to perform tasks without consuming the scarce resources of the mobile device.

- **Dynamic environment adaptation:** Agents perceive environment changes and re-act by adapting their behaviour to them. An example applied to network management can be seen in [43], where a mobile agent is reused without modifications to manage various networks.
- **Flexible interfaces:** Since its ease of adaptability, agents can be used to interact with completely different interfaces, such as it is proposed in [50]. Even, agents can be used as improvised adaptors between two kinds of interfaces.
- **Fault tolerance:** Because of the agents capacity to adapt to changing environments, mobile agents can easily deal with computer and network faults. They are specially suitable for hostile environments, where the agent can decide to visit alternative locations in case of failure. An example of fault tolerance based on mobile agents can be seen in [20].
- **Parallelism:** The autonomous nature of mobile agents, the ability to migrate to different locations, and the capacity of interacting with other agents, make them suitable for parallel applications, where a coordinated group of several agents are used. An example, which uses them as a load balancing mechanism, can be seen in [46].
- **Local data processing:** mobile agents can process data directly where it resides without having to move it from the original location. There are two kinds of ap-plications which benefit from this feature. Firstly, *sea-of-data* applications where there is a large quantity of distributed information to process and the movement of it has an elevated cost [16]. And, secondly, medical applications [49] where moving data from its original location is not legal.

3   MedIGS

In this section it is introduced MedIGS [49], a mobile agent based application that com-prises several important requirements of current healthcare systems, such as distributed information gathering and interoperation among medical centers. The main goal of the system is the generation of Virtual Electronic Patient Records (VEPR) [6] out of all the medical data about a patient spread over a set of hospitals. The system benefits from the mobile agent technology, which relies on local searches performed by roaming agents avoiding the need of a central repository.

3.1   Introduction

Healthcare is information and knowledge driven. Good healthcare depends on taking decisions at the right time and place, according to the right patient data and applica-ble knowledge. Communication is of utmost relevance in today's healthcare settings, as health related activities, such as delivery of care, research and management, depend on information sharing. Indeed, the practice of medicine has been described as being "dominated" by how well information is processed or reprocessed, retrieved, and communicated [2].

As more data on patients are now recorded than ever before [54] the economical impact of their management is high. An estimated 35 to 39 percent of total hospital operating costs has been associated with patient and professional communication activities. In a single healthcare institution, information technologies usually tend to combine different modules or subsystems, resulting in a "best-of-breed" approach [24]. This leads to a great demand on creating efficient integrated electronic patient records that would facilitate the communication process. Nevertheless, centralized solutions are often infeasible and expensive. But, users will not agree on give up the legacy information systems they have been using during years. Thus, integration with these systems is a key issue in order to provide physicians with complete and reliable information. In order to integrate clinical information systems in a way that improves communication process and data use for healthcare delivery, research, and management, many different issues must be handled, e.g., data availability, integrity, and validity. The combination of data from heterogeneous sources takes a great deal of effort because the participating systems usually differ in many respects, such as functionality, presentation, terminology, data representation, and semantics [24]. Interfaces are needed in order to retrieve useful information.

Taking into consideration the intra-institutional level, and departmental systems, Virtual Electronic Patient Medical Records (VEPMR) systems approach can provide for the necessary means for departmental systems integration, enabling, at the point of care, a single integrated view of all patients' clinical information existing on the institution. We could say that at the institution level local information integration could suffice to provide doctors with all the necessary information to deliver care to a given visiting patient. However, patients are mobile entities, they visit multiple institutions during their life time and leave a trail of information scattered around laboratories, primary care units and other hospitals. The patient clinical history available to the doctor should not be resumed only to the information produced locally in the institution but also to the external data. The lack of articulation observed at the institution level, in what information systems integration is concerned, is also present when looking at the inter-institution integration level. Usually data integration relies on patients carrying their paper lab reports, x-rays, and other clinical documents themselves. In order to provide consistent and complete clinical data availability, solutions must be provided for bridging inter-institutional systems integration gap.

MedIGS is a gathering information system for securely integrating distributed medical data using mobile agent technology.

3.1.1   Why Agents in MedIGS?

MedIGS provides new clinical data discovery mechanisms which allow each institution to have access to external complementary patient clinical information. For the development of an inter-institution Virtual Electronic Patients Record system several technologies could be used, such as peer-to-peer, Web services, or mobile agents.

 – Peer-to-Peer is a good technology to efficiently search through a large network in a decentralized way. Unfortunately this technology does not provide the privacy needed in medical environments, because it is based on storing some key data over many computers in the network to ease the searches.

- Web services can be a good solution, but are not flexible enough. They can contact with a set of institutions but it is difficult to dynamically increase it to reach more data. Web services do not have a pro-active nature, and it usually implies working in a synchronous way, so all systems must be available when a request is done.
- Mobile agents can stand as the most well fitted technology for MedIGS. They have pro-active nature, they can be sent to search over a set of data sources in an asynchronous way dealing with resources unavailability or heavy load. And they can choose where and when to go and also dynamically change their itinerary to visit new locations. Although one of the disadvantages of the agents is the complexity of guaranteeing their security, recent agent driven security developments [1] have solved the most important issues related to this fact.

The multi-agent paradigm has been shown to address procedural complexity issues in the health care information systems arena. It can be used with success for modeling complex communication processes, building highly distributed systems and overcoming the cost and technical demand of a central systems approach [42]. Besides all known characteristics of agents such as sociability, pro-activity and adaptive behavior, the mobility of the agents has been used in the healthcare domain in order to ease the development of data integration mechanisms and to provide data availability throughout. Mobility tends also to be used for overcoming issues originating from connectivity instability, load balancing, or complex legacy systems interfacing.

Authors point out several additional reasons as advantages for the use of mobile agents : the ability to optimize computational load distribution, and the ability to handle failure; the need to handle instable or dynamically changing communication channels [45]. Support for a more flexible peer-to-peer model, scalability and decentralization of control and data [27] is also pointed out.

3.1.2 Issues, Challenges, and Requirements

MedIGS arise for networked and distributed medical systems when considering patient mobility. Its architecture is supposed to fulfill the requirements of modern health institutions, where roaming patients contribute to a highly distributed data scenario where useful information is digitally unreachable outside each institutional island. Current situation has important drawbacks:

- Data are distributed and the location where they are actually stored is often unknown.
- A common database is often unfeasible because of its cost and technical requirements.
- Medical institutions usually prefer to keep control of their own medical data.
- Remote on-line data retrieval is not always possible, especially when considering network disruptions, high latencies or specific search procedures.

From this situation, and the need for data integration at the inter-institutional level, several questions arise:

- How to find out which institutions the patient has visited without relying in their volatile memory?
- How to deal with network disruptions, high latencies or complex institutional legacy systems interfacing?
- How to deal with resistance to share data among institutions?
- How to secure the access to stored information in a way that only authorized staff can access it?
- How to secure the data while agents are roaming through the network?

In order to answer these questions we must firstly provide effective and reliable search and interface methods, as well as an adaptive and fault tolerant system behavior. These features, along with strong security enforcement mechanisms, would increase system confidence and solve most of the above questions.

3.2 System

MedIGS is an evolution of current medical information gathering systems, overcoming the main issues described before. This proposal goes far beyond others, such as [42], addressing issues like inter-institution patient health data integration, unavailable on-line remote data retrieval, or secure data access and transportation. Two mainstays support the proposal: mobile agents and agent-driven security. MedIGS is based on the widely used multi-agent platform JADE [3], which is compliant with the IEEE-FIPA agent specifications, together with the JADE Inter-Platform Mobility Service [7] add-on, which allows the agents to move between different platforms. This platform provides the system with the necessary means for inter-institution data discovery, transport, and integration. Information gathering actions will be triggered by consultation appointments, and agents will direct their efforts in order to make patient clinical history available as complete as possible for that event. Integration efforts will be directed to clinical documents and not to the data themselves.

In terms of computer structures there are no major requirements besides the need for an agent platform where the broker agent resides and where mobile agents can move. Regarding existing procedures there is no need for changes on the normal execution of the central system, it is just necessary to have a specific interface behavior that can be executed by the mobile agent to provide for a document retrieval interface from which document references can be retrieved. This interface is in charge of the dynamic report generation with existing data on the fly.

3.2.1 Architecture

The MedIGS proposal defines a common set of agents that exist in all systems. These agents are devoted to event management, data discovery, and data collection. Actions are triggered by scheduled clinical episodes (interventions, outpatient visits) or upon user request. There are five agents present in each system:

- **Mobile Scheduler (MS):** This is the agent in charge of managing scheduled events and launching mobile agent instances that will go in search of patient data references.

- **Collector Agent (CA):** Mobile agent in charge of discovering and collecting document references.
- **Remote Broker (RB):** Agent in charge of attending incoming agents asking for patient references.
- **Local Broker (LB):** Agent that receives mobile agents coming back and takes the medical information provided by them.
- **Document Broker (DB):** Agent that manages the needed documentation about a patient. It will retrieve from other platforms the referenced documents provided by the CA collection actions.

Figure 2 shows an overview of the proposed mobile agent application. The main architectural functional steps are described in more detail below:

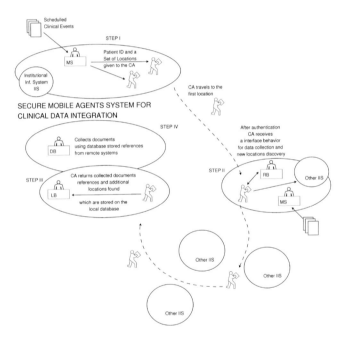

Fig. 2. Overview of the proposed mobile agent application.

Step I - A clinical episode is scheduled creating a new data collection event. This event contains patient information (identification numbers), a date, and a set of known data locations. Based on the scheduled date the MS will start in advance a CA that carries the Patient ID (the National Social Security Number for example) and a set of locations to be visited.

Step II - When the CA reaches the first location it asks for information about the patient it represents. In each institutional system there is a RB which is in charge of attending incoming agents asking for patient data. This RB authenticates the incoming agent, and provides it with the information requested. The CA can request for local patient data and for possible locations with more data. Regarding the patients' data, the agent only retrieves the references to them. Therefore, agents do not need to carry a large amount of data. Regarding the request of other platform locations with more information about the patient, it is returned as a list of new platforms which is included on the agent's itinerary for later visit. After completion, the CA will migrate to the next location and this procedure will be repeated.

Step III - Once CA completes its itinerary it returns to the origin. There all the collected information, e.g., document references and new locations, are managed and stored by the LB.

Step IV - On the home system, a DB is in charge of getting all the referenced documents collected by the CA and making them available locally for the scheduled event.

Since different institutions can communicate inconsistent facts, the system has to include a module to check for contradictory data. For example, if it is known for sure that the patient is male, then he cannot have a pregnancy report; if there is not enough information then the system should keep both facts, let the reader know there is an inconsistence and try to solve the problem by alerting information sources about the inconsistence.

3.2.2   Data Sharing Resistance

Health institutions do not usually have a natural disposition to share data, and this is precisely one issue the proposal overcomes. By using mobile agent technology, data is not directly accessed, but this task is delegated to a mobile agent which performs the actions locally under the security control of the agent platform. This mobile agent searches and collects data references about the scheduled patients, and this makes a difference with a wide and remote access to all the information. On the other hand, in MedIGS the exchange of information is symmetrical between institutions, thus creating a symbiotic relationship in which all profit in the same way. In short, there is not a simple sharing of information here, but a controlled, restricted, and symmetric exchange for which institutions are not believed to object.

As MedIGS deals with clinical information, strong security measures must be put in place in order to ensure protection for both data transportation and collection. For this purpose a set of security mechanisms described in Section 3.3 have been used.

3.3   Security

Security has a paramount importance when designing medical information gathering systems. There are sound and well-known cryptographic mechanisms to guarantee most of the basic security properties (data privacy, integrity, and authenticity). However, having agents that can move along, carrying sensitive data from one execution environment to the next, and acting on behalf of others, raise new security requirements that must be considered.

Three cryptographic techniques face some of the main threats resulting from the utilization of mobile agent technology. These techniques are specific for this type of applications, and are focused in the protection of agent's data and code integrity, and access control:

3.3.1 Self Protected Mobile Agents

In MedIGS scheme, agents protect their code and data by carrying their own protection mechanisms [1]. This approach improves traditional solutions, where protection was managed by the platform. Hence, security is no longer a rigid part of the system, but travels within the agent. Thus, each agent could use its own protection schemes, independently of those supported by the platform. This allows the coexistence of different security mechanisms at the same platform and time.

This solution is based on a public decryption function provided by the platform through a cryptographic service, which is accessed by properly structured agents. It reconciles opposing requirements by introducing a hybrid software architecture that incorporates the advantages of agent driven proposals while limiting the impact of platform driven approaches. Interoperability, code reuse and deployment flexibility concerns are also fully addressed.

3.3.2 Retrieved Medical Information Protection

Another important asset to protect is the information carried by the agent. Although the protection of the agent code is of utmost importance, if the results carried by the agent are not protected against modifications or eavesdroppers the whole security is jeopardized. MedIGS uses a scheme based on hash chains to protect agent's results. Similar mechanisms have been used before to protect agent data, as described in [13]. This type of protection prevents the results from being undisclosed or changed by unauthorized parties. Moreover they allow to check the actual itinerary that the agent has followed.

3.3.3 Access Control

MedIGS purposes a multi-domain scenario where several health institutions come together to share medical data. However, in order to regulate the access to the medical data arises the following problems:

- **Roaming agents act on behalf of unknown users:** When a local user launch a retrieval query, for the rest of the health institutions the user is unknown. However, it can be determined where the query comes from.
- **Credentials are defined locally:** Each independent health institution grants its users with local privileges which are not directly understood in the rest of the health institutions.

In order to solve the above problems, MedIGS purposes a credential conversion mechanism [34] which allows, through conversion policies, the credentials translation from one institution to another. Thus, the Collector Agent privileges are computed in each institution based on the privileges of the local user who launched the query.

4 Mobile Agents for Critical Medical Information Retrieving from the Emergency Scene

Lacking medical information about a victim in the aftermath of an emergency makes the early treatment and the efficient allocation of resources difficult. On the other hand, communication infrastructures are normally disrupted in these situations, thus hindering the gathering of the required information. In this section it is introduced a new application based on mobile agents for retrieving partial information of medical records upon request from the emergency scene. This solution fits well with a mobile ad hoc network environment with asynchronous communications provided by mobile agents. The proposed system allows to request remote hospitals for critical information about the victims, such as allergies or infectious diseases, thus facilitating more accurate diagnosis and bringing forward decision making.

4.1   Introduction

When an emergency occurs, especially in mass casualty incidents, lots of victims need medical attention. Researchers agree that the fast and accurate acquisition and analysis of data, the more effective the answer can be given. That is, the needs will be supplied as soon as possible and the affected population will be reduced. The common point in all cases is the analysis of information. Around it lies the importance of responding to the emergency. Furthermore, information revolves around all stages of disaster: preparation, planning, training, response, recovery and evaluation. [47].

The first responder medical personnel stabilizes the victim before they can be evacuated to a hospital. After it is stabilized, the victim is transferred to a hospital. Normally, while the victim is being stabilized or transferred, the medical personnel search for victim's personal items that could identify them. Discovering who the victim is it is important since with this information, important medical information about the patient can be retrieved from a Virtual Electronic Patient Medical Record (VEPMR) solution, which makes available from any medical institution all the existing medical information about a patient.

The objective of this system is to make VEPMRs available in the emergency scene. This could improve the medical assistance of the victim, since the victim's blood type, chronic and contagious diseases, and so on, can be rapidly obtained. Furthermore, the hospitals can be prepared for the victim's arrival, e.g., special attentions, resources, and so forth.

When incidents like hurricanes, floodings or tsunamis occurs, most communication networks are normally disrupted, being an obvious handicap for quick and coordinated assistance. Some projects propose deploying antennas to have communication networks in all the emergency scene [28]. Others propose using sensor or ad-hoc networks for communication inside the emergency scene [19][41].

We could use any of these systems to make true the VEPMR retrieval from the emergency scene. But, our goal is going a step forward proposing the use of mobile agents on ad-hoc networks to forward requests of VEPMRs to the medical network. This allows the retrieval of the patient's medical record in the place where the emergency has occurred.

4.2   Background

This section describes the state of the art of applications dedicated to emergency management and those that propose solutions to face the lack of infrastructure in the emergency scene.

4.2.1   Emergency Management

Coordination, information sharing, and decision-making are the three fundamental axes for the management of an emergency situation [5] [21]. Optimization of those three axes reduces the response time, one of the objectives of any system for managing the emergency. Several emergency management approaches exist.

AMBULANCE[40] aims to create medical portable devices that allow remote, medium and long distance tele-medicine specialists support. The device allows the transmission of vital signs and patient images from anywhere using the mobile phone network.

ARTEMIS [36] is based on a previous knowledge base to make decisions. It is based on an expert system that follows rules and that, according to the input parameters added, make a decision based on rules applied in other cases available in the knowledge memory.

PHERIS[26] introduces a new protocol to replace the one used in China to deal with the SARS. PHERIS consists of 4 systems: the surveillance, control, action and support. The surveillance system captures emergencies and reports to the control system. The control system decides whether to take measures to raise the alert level and make decisions to meet the emergency. The action system receives the orders from the control system and carries them out in response to the emergency. The support system is responsible for ensuring that all protocol are followed correctly and that the actions are carried out correctly. From the point of view of communication, it creates a virtual network of five layers and three layers. The layers are defined by the magnitude of the organization involved. The levels will depend on the organization.

MASCAL [11] is a system that seeks to integrate a solution based on software and hardware to improve the management of a hospital during a large scale emergency. It integrates TacMedCS (section 5.2.3) and it provides a visual management of hospital resources and their locations supporting different types of views depending on the type of medical center. It also has support for the staff registration and management of individual local areas, such as operating rooms, emergency rooms, radiology, and so on.

CWME [25] is a framework for emergency management that provides a collaborative virtual work space for the organizers of the various fields of emergency. In this way, one can communicate easily and create joint documents defining the plans to deploy.

WIISARD [23] is a project whose main objective is to use wireless networks to assist in the coordination and care of victims in large-scale emergencies. WIISARD proposes providing emergency personnel (medical personnel both in the field and coordinating staff) with medical and tracking data in real-time of all casualties that occur during the emergency. WIISARD proposes to deploy a network of nodes CalMesh as soon as arriving at the emergency scene. This network of nodes can be connected both to the medical devices as well as to classification devices (Section 5.2.3) in the entire area of the emergency. When a victim is found, a tracking and monitoring device is placed on him, and the emergency personnel introduce in it the state of the victim, the treatment and the identification data. These data will travel over the network to the emergency control and management system where they will be sent to all devices in the emergency field through the same network and to the nearest hospital via the Internet. It also shows the list of available resources (hospital beds, medicines, ambulances, and so on) in the area near the emergency. This helps in deciding where each victim must go depending on the resources of the hospital and the condition of the victim. Furthermore, it provides additional information that can help in making decisions in an emergency, such as weather reports, action plans, network status, location of the PDAs, and so forth.

4.2.2 Infrastructure in Emergency Situations

Deploying an infrastructure is something complex in emergencies which require prompt action and when the personnel is engaged in tasks that require greater attention than the deployment of a network. Many of the systems and papers propose the use of wireless networks using mesh nodes installed by first aid teams when arriving at the scene of the accident [28] [8] [17] [41].

Deploying a network is more complicated in places where communication networks are partially operating than in places where no infrastructure exists. This is due to various factors such as interference with existing signals, saturation of these networks, and so on. [29].

The alternative to deploy a network is using mobile ad hoc networks (MANET) (mesh or not) in the devices of the emergency personnel. This way they can communicate each other when they are close enough or if there are devices that behave as routers. A disadvantage is that if the devices are too far they cannot communicate, since their coverage does not reach the coverage of the another device. Several proposals to solve the problem of lack of infrastructure in an emergency scenario exist.

The project IMPROVISA [48] addresses the provision of information services in scenarios which, lacking a fixed communications infrastructure for any reason, require collaboration and performance of human resources and IT. The project provides technological solutions to this problem using MANETs that communicate with each other through wireless links. Furthermore, mobile agents are also used for the management of the deployed network.

The article "A Situation-Aware Mobile System to Support Fire Brigades in Emergency Situations" [28] describes the deployment of network and system support for emergencies, especially fires. For the network deployment, it proposes the use of mesh networks. Fire trucks are provided with wireless network in order to create a mesh network with PDAs carried by firefighters. This mesh network is interconnected to a fixed network (either wired or wireless) through one of its nodes. PDAs are provided with an indicator of the mesh network coverage. When a firefighter sees the coverage level decreases significantly and that it is about to disappear, he is responsible for installing a node to increase the mesh coverage. These nodes are small, portable, battery-operated and can be installed all around the area where necessary.

4.2.3 Decision Support Systems

They also urge the creation and use of a common language among all the teams, understood by all standard signals and of a compatible communication network between groups that help to coordinate the emergency from a decentralized point of view.

To manipulate so much heterogeneous information when designing a system, it must be carefully modeled its structure, the path followed and the decision process of the action. This will produce some tasks that have to be physically carried out by staff. The coordination of these tasks will also be important and will require the involvement of different teams and coordinators of different areas of the emergency (police, social welfare, etc.).

The actions may involve the use of non-personal but material resources. The management of these resources is something that must be taken into account in an emergency as these resources are finite. The number of blood units that are available for victims who needs urgent transfusions, ambulances available to transport the victims to the hospital, the number of beds and operating rooms available at nearby hospitals, etc. are some examples of resources that will necessary have to administer and know its quantity.

The authors of paper [10] aim to integrate the decision-making systems of all the equipment involved in the emergency. The information is automatically shared through the whole devices of the emergency scene and the decisions are based on the scope of the whole emergency.

4.2.4   User Interface

Some systems use specific interfaces on the PDA of the triage staff as a support for the management of information and triage assistance [19,44,36]. At first it seems like a good idea, but a difficult to read or non-intuitive an interface can lead to the opposite.

During an emergency everything is urgent and the staff responsible for the care of the victims cannot spend their time using a tiny keyboard on the PDA or a virtual keyboard on the touchscreen. PDA-personnel interaction should be easy, intuitive, and above all fast. The user of the PDA must comprehend, without reading a long text, what he is doing, what happened, and what the next step is. Therefore it is good to use pictures and intuitive interfaces for data input.

Paper [4] discusses the human-computer interaction related to the systems dedicated to emergency management and how this can influence the response. As a conclusion they define that a human being must be taken into account as part of the system and the hardware as part of the team. Thus, defining a communication between both is an easier task.

4.2.5   Interoperability

Response to an emergency involves different teams: rescue, firefighters, first aid, police. They have to share information and coordinate joint actions to perform. Normally, the action and communication protocols used by them are quite different. Therefore, define standard methods for communication between different emergency teams is of utmost importance if one wants an effective exchange of information and a good coordination [37].

The teams consist of an ad hoc basis by members of different teams with different roles and different priorities. These roles are well defined when these members are within their team. But in emergency situations, in which one must respond quickly and there are involved heterogeneous groups, roles are not predefined and must use improvisation. To deal with improvisation, decision support systems are used.

4.2.6   Agents

Agents can be a good resource to use for emergency management [9], since responding to an emergency requires many complex tasks performed by multiple actors under conditions of time and resource requirements.

During the emergency response agent-based systems can provide a number of important benefits:

- Agents have the ability to operate in highly dynamic environments.
- They can work in decentralized and distributed networks.
- They have the ability to search and collect distributed information, verify, process, analyze, and interpret it for later use and management.
- They are suitable for decision using the data collected by a single agent or exchanged with several agents.

Despite having these advantages, only a few emergency management systems are based on agents [9].

4.3   Communications in the Emergency Scene

The emergency scene is characterized by several zones. The first one is the Zone 0, also called the hot zone, which is the place where the disaster has happened and where the victims are at the beginning. Then there is the Zone 1, with the Advanced Medical Post (AMP) and the Advanced Command Post (ACP), which are improvised medical infrastructures for the emergency. Other zones can be considered outside of the emergency area, such as Zone 2 and Zone 3, for the hospitals which will receive the victims and the medical centers which have treated them before the incident respectively. This last comprises the data which compose the victims' medical records.

Referring to the emergency area, the AMP is the hospital that treat the victims before they can be transferred to a hospital. And the ACP is the place where the coordination team is. From this place, all the decisions about actions to be carried out by rescue and medical teams are taken.

Communications in the emergency scene are getting more and more important. This is due to the greater use of Internet enabled devices and mobile phones by the emergency personnel. Their devices require networks such as mobile phone network (3G) or WiMAX. In most of the emergency cases, hurricanes, terrorist attacks, floodings, and so on, these networks become unstable, unaccessible, overused and even destroyed. As a consequence, emergency personnel cannot use existing network infrastructure. Hence, they should deploy and use their own, or simply use wireless mobile ad-hoc networks (MANETs) or wireless mesh networks. These networks create routes by request of the nodes that are maintained as long as they are needed or the link is available.

If the emergency area is too large, it is possible that the ad-hoc network created by the medical personnel's devices would not be fully connected. As a result, an attempt to communicate between two points of the network could be unsuccessful.

The AMP and ACP always have Internet connection even if the network infrastructures are destroyed or unusable. They use their own deployed network infrastructure, for instance, satellite connections. For the AMP and the ACP, it is very important to have Internet connection for coordination or information communications (f.e. with another coordination point or with hospitals assigned to victims).

4.4   Critical Medical Information Retrieving System

In this section is explained the mechanism to retrieve VEPMRs from the emergency scene. In the context of this system each member of the triage and medical personnel is provided with a mobile device supporting mobile agents. This device allows any member of the triage or medical personnel to create a mobile agent with a VEPMR request when any personal document identification of the victim is found.

4.4.1   Retrieving System

Our proposal takes into account three possible scenarios in the emergency scene. The first one is the existence of a network infrastructure with Internet connection, e.g., cellular phones network infrastructure (GSM, EDGE or 3G). The second and third possible situation lack of a network infrastructure with Internet connection. The second one is a MANET composed of all the neighbor devices of the medical and triage personnel. In this situation, all the mobile devices are close enough each other to create a fully connected MANET and some of the mobile devices are near the AMP or ACP. As a result, all of them are connected Internet through the network infrastructure of the AMP or ACP, taking advantage of the usual usual ad-hoc networks routing protocols. Hence, from any part of the network it is possible to directly send the VEPMR request to the medical network. Finally, the third scenario is similar to the second one but the MANET is not fully connected. Thus clusters of devices without direct Internet access are created.

The application described in this chapter is focused on the third scenario. It is based on creating a mobile agent each time a VEPMR request is done. This mobile agent contains the identification of the victim whose VEPMR is requested. As the MANET is not fully connected, the request cannot be sent directly, thus, the mobile agent have to jump from device to device or cluster to cluster of devices until it reaches the ACP or AMP. Once the mobile agent has arrived, it can communicate the request to the VEPMR system of some hospital of the medical network. Mobile agents have been used to create a mobile agents based MANET. This network uses agent platforms as routers for the mobile agents, which are equivalent to packets in traditional networks. Therefore, the routing process is done in the application layer. Nevertheless, the routing decisions are taken by the mobile agents themselves, accessing and using attributes and values available in the application layer. Hence, it is possible to use specific routing protocols or policies in each agent and depending on the situation.

Using this method it is possible to route a mobile agent between two distinct points of the network despite being isolated in different clusters. In traditional networks this cannot be done because a fully connected network from the origin point to the destiny point is needed. Using mobile agents based MANET, the agents can wait for a connection if there is not, in any part of the network, thus, they can cover a part of the route. Furthermore, they can use different dynamic routing protocols to reach the destination point.

Different dynamic routing protocols can be used in the mobile agents based MANET. In this application, the objective of the mobile agents is to reach the AMP or ACP. So, the routing protocols must the best route spending the minimum time to arrive there. The protocol proposed for this application takes into account the time that the medical personnel expects to stay in the emergency scene to calculate the routing. Then, when a first responder leaves the meeting point they has to state when they will come back. So, each device stores the time when the personnel who carries it expects to return to the AMP. The mobile agent asks for this information for the service's platform of all the neighbor devices and jumps to the one that has the smaller return time value. In this way, the mobile agents arrives to the AMP as soon as possible. This is for security reasons because they will be in a emergency scene where some disaster has occurred and it is not fully safe. Therefore, they foresee a "time to return" (TTR) that they will put into their device.

Some special devices, for instance those installed in an emergency vehicle, can store a special "time to return" value. This is specially useful when an emergency vehicle has to go to the emergency scene and come back to the AMP or ACP, or the first responder has finished their job in the emergency scene and is coming back. In these situations the "time to return" will have a low value. Therefore, all the mobile agents near the platform with low TTR will jump into it because it is the fastest way to reach Internet.

It would wrongly seem that agents are not useful in the first situation, where mobile devices can connect directly to Internet using network infrastructure available in the emergency scene, and in the second situation, where the mobile devices can access to Internet through the fully connected MANET. However, in emergency situations the network infrastructures are usually unstable or over-saturated and mobile agents and the routing protocols implemented can deal with this situation.

When the VEPMR is retrieved, a copy is saved in the AMP and ACP. Then VEPMR will be already available once the victim reaches the AMP or ACP for the medical personnel treating them.

Security has also been taken into account in our system. VEPMRs consist of sensible private medical data. For this reason, this information has to be dealt with carefully using strong security mechanisms, and the communication between ACP, or AMP, and the VEPMR system has to be secure. The problem of security in ad-hoc networks is not fully solved nowadays. Even thought the very agents can protect the data they carry by using mechanisms such as [1]. Thus, the system could be used in insecure networks.

4.4.2 VEPMR for Emergencies

We also propose the creation of a special VEPMR containing only the relevant information for an emergency case. This VEPMR for emergencies (VEPMRE) contains the blood type, hepatitis, AIDS, allergies, and more basic information to treat the patient in an emergency case. Thanks to this, the VEPMRE has a smaller size so it uses less network bandwidth.

An important issue is how a VEPMRE is associated with the victim. An AMP may receive many VEPMRE from requests launched by the mobile agents, so how do the medical personnel know what VEPMRE corresponds to which victim? Our proposal is based on adding the identifier number of the triage tag with each VEPMRE request inside the mobile agent. In this way, once the VEPMRE is received it is possible to identify the victim, since the triage tag is always carried by them.

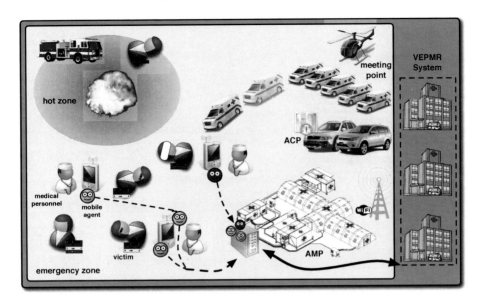

Fig. 3. Emergency scene and VEPMRE retrieval scheme

4.4.3   Implementation

An implementation has been developed as a proof of concept. A Nokia n810 touch screen-based mobile device with a MAEMO Linux distribution has been used as a hardware platform. The programming language used is Java with the JADE Framework [3] as agent platform, together with its FIPA-compliant mobility services [7].

IEEE 802.11g has been used as a network interface. When a device leaves the AMP or ACP, a TTR value is added as can be seen on the left side of Figure 4. When a first responder finds the identity of the victim, it can be introduced in the system and a VEPMRE request is sent (figure 4B). At this moment a mobile agent is created containing the identity of the victim. The mobile agents tries to move from platform to platform following the TTR routing protocol until it reaches the AMP or ACP.

Time To Return

1h : 15m : 55s

Pause return timer

Personal Data

Name:	Dolor Sit Amet
Identification:	879438328
Gender:	○ Female ◉ Male
Age:	32
Address:	

Fig. 4. Implementation screenshots

5 The Mobile Agent Electronic Triage Tag (MAETT)

5.1 Introduction

Once an emergency occurs, the task of the first responder medical personnel arriving to the scene is triageing the victims they find [39] [18]. The triage consists of a protocol to sort victims according to their medical status in order to prioritize their needs for receiving medical attention. When all the victims are triaged, the medical personnel begins to treat them following the color-based prioritization.

The triage of the victims is an important issue to take into account and the implementation through electronic means must meet certain requirements:

- Data from the triage of the victims cannot be lost and its integrity must be guaranteed.
- The time spent to enter the victim information in the mobile device should be as short as possible and must not exceed the time to do it in the traditional triage.
- The triage must be possible under any condition, whether or not there are network or other technical conditions. In addition, the device must be shielded from withstand water, blood, or other fluids which may be in contact with them at the scene of the accident.
- The information should reach the control center, where the emergency is managed, as soon as possible to prepare the required resources for the victims attention on their arrival.

In this section, a system for the electronic triage of the victims using mobile agents [31,32] is explained.

5.2 Background

5.2.1 Introduction
This section describes and analyzes the main protocols for triaging victims in large scale emergency situations. Both, manual and electronic systems are discussed.

5.2.2 Traditional Victims Triage
At present there are different victims triage protocols, the most common protocol used is the START [15]. The protocol consists of the steps depicted in Figure 5. The whole procedure does not take more than 60 seconds for each victim.

As it can be seen in Figure 5 four colors are used to differentiate the possible states of the victim.

- Green color identifies the victim as delayed or low priority.
- Yellow color identifies the victim as urgent priority.
- Red color identifies the victim as immediate priority.
- Black color identifies the victim as deceased.

The triage protocol and the color labels provide an effective visual classification that allows the medical personnel to easily identify the victims which require more urgent attention. The protocol steps are described below:

First it is checked if the victim can walk. If they can, they are labeled with a green triage tag and they are asked to go by their means from the area where the accident or disaster area to where the field hospital is located. Once in the area of the field hospital, they may be treated by the medical staff. If no urgent attention is needed, they recommend the victim to go by themself to a health center where they can be attended.

If the victim has reduced mobility, or there is risk of injury in case of movement, the triage personnel do further checks. First the breathe is checked. If there is no breath, an airway is opened. If they continue without breathing, they are labeled with a black triage tag. If the victim recovers breath thanks to the actions of medical personnel he is labeled with a red triage tag.

In case the patient without mobility breathes, the number of breaths per minute are checked. If they exceed 30 or they are less than 10, the victim is labeled with a red triage tag. Otherwise, the pulse is checked.

The pulse is checked in the wrist. If no pulse is found or if it is over 120 beats per minute, the victim is labeled with a red triage tag. If it is below 120, the response of the victim to some simple commands is checked. If the patient responds correctly to the orders, a yellow triage tag is assigned, otherwise a red one is chosen.

It should be said that wrist pulse may be replaced by a capillary test. The index finger of the victim is pressed for a few seconds and how long filling of blood vessels takes, i.e., the time since the area changes from white color to red again, is measured. If it is under 2 seconds a yellow triage tag is assigned, otherwise it is labeled red.

Triage tags are placed around the neck or wrist of the victim and allow to classify the victims according to their severity, so that when medical help arrives the status of each victim can be easily distinguished.

5.2.3   Electronic Triage Systems

Some systems [35] [22] [14] use as a substitute for the traditional triage tag electronic devices with features that improve the current system. These devices have cardiac

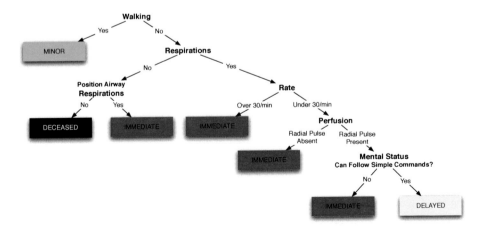

Fig. 5. START Flow

sensors, GPS, wireless network capabilities, the ability to read the data via network, and so on. These characteristics entail clear advantages with respect to paper triage tags. Nonetheless, because of the complexity of the devices and because of the fact that several of them are required, the economic cost of deployment must be carefully considered.

Nevertheless, it must be taken into account that these triage devices are reused. Furthermore, they are exposed to liquid and strokes and may be damaged. The battery of these devices is also an issue to keep in mind, since it must be checked that it is at its maximum capacity before leaving to the emergency. Some of the existing electronic systems for victims triage are described in the next lines.

ARTEMIS [36] is an automated system for the classification and management of casualties that occur in an emergency scene. It uses a network of physiological sensors that are placed on the victim for checking their vital signs and apply the START procedure. It also uses wireless sensor networks to communicate with medical personnel PDAs as well as with the control center located at the base camp.

The CodeBlue project [44] is based on a sensor network for detecting the physiological condition of the patient and transmitting this data to a remote device. With this data one can make an assessment of the patient status and classify them properly.

The Decentralized Electronic Triage System [35] is a system which goal is to create a very low power consumption hardware that emulates the operation of a paper triage tag. This device has buttons to select the patient's condition through some color LEDs for the triage tag. The device can be controlled remotely and provides telemetry to consult data connecting through a wireless network . Each device has a GPS receiver and a radio frequency transmitter to locate victims.

TacMedCS [38] is a military project from the United States to capture and display data in real-time from casualties in the battlefield. It uses radio frequency tags to identify victims and save their data. A mobile device is also used to store data of the victim together with their GPS position and to send them to the database of central server using satellite communications. The information from the victim and their triage travel along them in the RFID tag. In the central server one can check the status of the victim. Besides communications based on mesh networks are used for collaboration through the mobile devices.

The system proposed in [17] is devoted to the triage of casualties using a triage tag with an RFID. The system consists of a traditional triage tag with an attached RFID tag and a mobile device with an RFID reader. Moreover, the PDA has a wireless network interface. Nevertheless, it is required that the PDA has some type of coverage with the wireless network interface device. When the medical staff sorts the victim, he puts the triage tag and reads it with the mobile device. He performs the triage protocol and places the results, comments and processing carried out in the paper triage tag as well as in the mobile device. This information is sent through the wireless network to a central server that stores all information that is collected at the emergency scene. Data from the central server can be consulted by the coordinator of the emergency so that he knows the resources needed to meet the demand. All the equipment are provided with RFID readers and connection to the central server with data associated with the victim's ID from the RFID.

WIISARD [22] also includes an intelligent 802.11 triage tag device. It provides water and handling resistance, wireless networking support, remote operation and a battery of 8 to 12 hours of operation. Victims are triaged by staff with PDAs. After this step, personnel puts this devices on the victim and synchronizes it with the patient data entered in the PDA. The triage tag recognizes and displays the data through its color LEDs for the status of the patient's severity. The wireless network can connect to transmit the position it is. These nodes include GPS to know their position and they use ad hoc network and mesh protocols for the deployment of the network .

5.3   Emergency Zones Definition

The first step towards the definition of a new electronic triage tag mechanism is the modeling of the zones that comprise the place of an emergency and the services they offer.

5.3.1   Zones

The emergency scenario has been split in different zones (Figure 6). The zones range from Zone 0, where the emergency arises, to Zone 3, where the routine medical visits are done.

To better understand the differentiation between these zones, we will put an example. Suppose a tragedy like that of a large earthquake in a major city.

Zone 0

The natural disaster produce some hot spots of different extensions. These hot-spots are what we call Zone 0. There, network infrastructure existence is not guaranteed. Therefore it must be assumed that in practice no available networks exist.

Zone 1

The management of all zones, takes place in Zone 1. Within Zone 1 there are field hospitals, the control center (the place from where the emergency is coordinated and where its information collected), and ambulance and rescue equipment in general. Field hospitals, which are also included in this zone may be associated to one or more Zone 0.

Zone 2

The network of hospitals and medical centers close to the emergency compose Zone 2. This zone is the destination of the victims. It is characterized by having stable communication networks which connect the rest of the hospitals.

Zone 3

This zone comprise the regular medical centers that the victims have visited during their lives. In short, they compose all those actions that have recently featured in the medical record.

The integration of Zone 3 in the proposed scheme may not seem obvious, since it has no apparent direct relationship with the emergency. However, the need to have a minimum medical history for use in emergency situations is the main argument for including the zone in the diagram, as the creation and management of history is intimately linked with the entities that make up the zone. These clinical records contain the minimum basic information from a patient (blood group, chronic or contagious diseases, allergies, and so forth), which may be essential in an emergency situation, e.g., this allows more

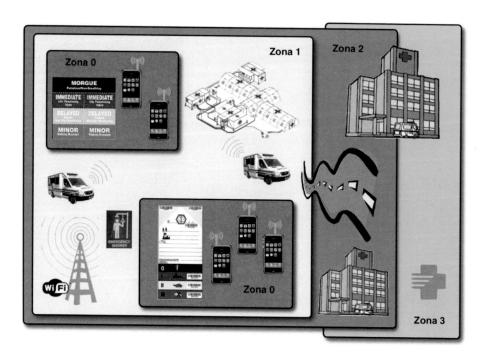

Fig. 6. Emergency zones schema

efficient care to a patient in a state of emergency (to ask for a blood type, medication supplies, and so on) as well as protect the health team of a possible contagion. The system explained in Section 4 provides this functionality.

5.3.2 Services

A key element defining the zones are the services they offer. A list of services are offered by the system in each of them according to their specific needs.

Zone 0 offers localization, triage and basic care of the victims in the emergency.

Zone 1 manages the emergency, such as transport victims, emergency care in field hospitals, management of accidents, calculation of the optimal pathway for transport, and so on.

Zone 2 offers treatment services and basic operations with specialists such as neuro-surgeons, trauma, and so forth.

And finally, Zone 3, provides information about the victims' medical records.

Services are processed and supplied by the emergency system. These services may be required from another part of the emergency system in a manual and automatic way.

5.4   The Mobile Agent Electronic Triage Tag System

5.4.1   System Description

The system aims to manage an emergency from a point of view of the victims. It takes care of managing the resources to search, attend, and transport the victims. The system deals with the tasks comprised from the triage of the victims at the emergency scene to the reservation of the resources needed at the hospital where the victims are transferred.

Let's suppose a scenario with many casualties caused by a large scale emergency, and with the victims spread over a large area. Doctors, caregivers and triage personnel are equipped with identification reflective vests. In addition, triage personnel (staff, from now on) is equipped with bandoliers integrating a PDA, with touch screen tied to an arm, and an additional high capacity battery. This PDA includes a GPS and a RFID reader. The bandoliers contain pockets with first aid equipment to facilitate the task of the emergency personnel, including electronic triage tags, later explained.

When a victim is found, he is labeled with an electronic triage tag, that is composed of a traditional paper triage tag along with a conventional RFID tag that provides the ability to be digitally identified. In this way, reading the RFID tag a unique identifier is obtained to uniquely identify the victim within the emergency. Before labeling the victim, the staff shall approach the electronic triage tag to the PDA that read the incorporated RFID. Then a software wizard to help staff to assess the state of the victim (Figure 7) is activated.

This software provides all the steps required to follow the START protocol (breathing, pulse, responds to simple questions, etc.) and perform the triage (Figure 8).

The software interface of the wizard (Figure 7) is simple, with intuitive icons, short and understandable text, and large buttons that facilitate the use of the touch screen.

Furthermore, its use is optimal for triage because it does not increase the time devoted to follow the START protocol (which must be as short as possible) and benefits from the available data already digitized.

Once the process has been completed, a recommendation of status (color) for the victim is suggested: green for *MINOR)*, yellow for *DELAYED*, red for *IMMEDIATE*, and black for *DECEASED*. This status can be accepted by the staff or may be changed to another one that the staff considers more appropriate.

After selecting the state (color) of the victim, the software will read the GPS device position where the staff, and therefore the victim, is at that time.

5.4.2 Mobile Agent Electronic Triage Tag

The mobile agent crated after the triage will include the status (color of the triage tag) of the victim, the GPS position, the unique identifier of the triage tag, and the patient's vital data (pulse, respiration, and so on).

This mobile agent will stay in the personnel PDAs waiting to arrive to the field hospital for, later, moving to the emergency control center system. During the travel from the Zone 0 to the Zone 1, the mobile agent will try to get to the emergency control center as fast as possible by jumping between the PDAs of the emergency personnel.

The decision of a mobile agent to jump or not to jump to a PDA of another staff or to a computer of an ambulance will depend on the application level routing protocol used by the mobile agent. The use of the TTR routing protocol (see Section 4.4.1) is encouraged.

5.4.3 Additional Services

Apart from the routing service, staff PDAs may offer different specific services. For example, in the event of a medical staff performing triage in Zone 0 is a specialist in any

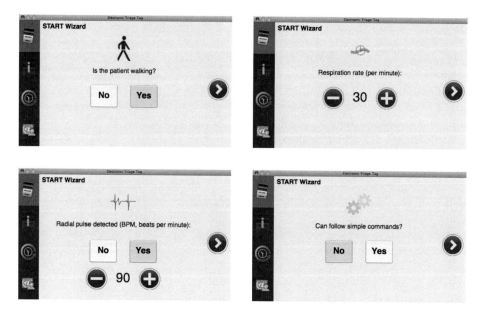

Fig. 7. Software wizard for the triage of victims

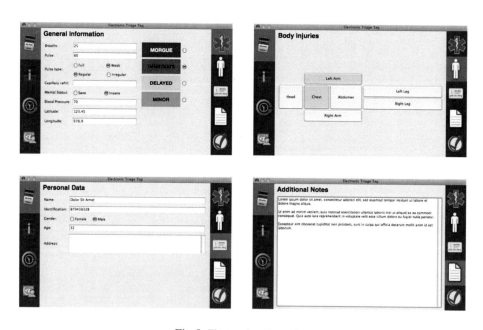

Fig. 8. Electronic Triage Tag

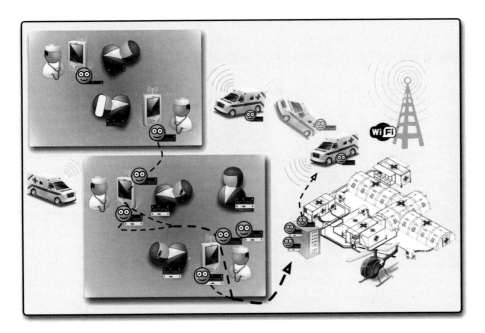

Fig. 9. Electrnic Triage Tag based on Mobile Agents

field of medicine, could provide services associated with his specialty. These may be viewed by the agents and may make requests to be booked by assigning such a victim to a particular specialist. A petition will not always be accepted and may be denied, e.g., because the resource is busy. There is also the option for example of disabling the service, when staff are returning to the control centre or the service has already been reserved by another mobile agent.

Services not only can be unitary, meaning that only pertain to or have a single staff, but there may be services offered by a group. For instance, one can define emergency rescue teams, dedicated to rescuing victims in dangerous floodings or similar. In this case would have the special feature of the service that the entity would be distributed and virtual. This service could be sued by a mobile agent in case that before launching it the staff indicate that a rescue operation to retrieve the victim is required.

5.4.4   Control Center

The control center is responsible of receiving all mobile agents coming from Zone 0. This system may be distributed, i.e., it may comprise more than one server that will be able to exchange data, since they are connected to each other. The control center have a wireless network access point to allow the communication with the arriving PDAs.

Furthermore, the control center keep all the information gathered by the mobile agents. It may know the position of the victims, their status, and whether there are special needs for each one. This eases to plan routes for the collection of the victims by placing higher priority on those that have been selected for such. There may even be a map of the affected area with color dots indicating the status (color) and the position of the victim within the map, which will help the emergency organization and management staff to have a clearer idea of the distribution of victims.

5.4.5   Medical Transportation

After the collection of the victim, personal data from him can be obtained, either because the victim was able to give any of its data or because identification documentation has been found. In this case the new data can be reported inside the agent reading the RFID of the electronic triage tag. Within the rescue vehicles there is a laptop which also allows to update the personal data and/or medicines and treatments provided to the patient.

5.4.6   Shared Medical Record

While the patient is transferred to a hospital or medical center a reservation and preparation of resources can be made. This task may be automatically done by the agent in the area of the emergency. It can contact with the agent in charge of the hospital management and establish an agreement with the institution where the victim is transferred. After the ambulance has picked the victim, the time it takes to get to the hospital may be foreseen so when the victim arrives everything will be ready with the materials and resources needed.

Moreover, if it has been able to collect patient data and added them to the mobile agent, during transit from the collection of the victim to the hospital, he may take advantage of fixed wireless networks, for example, to pass this information to the agent in the hospital.

6   Conclusions

Along this chapter, three eHealth applications using mobile agents have been described. They have shown how mobile agent technology can be successfully applied in this domain, solving some important issues such as interoperability or asynchronous communication.

The first case was based on the integration of medical information. This system provides a global integration of agent-based VEPR systems through secure and standardized mobility and communication mechanism. The system is focused towards a reliable intra-institution integration, allowing a medical doctor from a given institution to have access to all the patient information that can be spread over different medical institutions.

This system makes clear the advantages that agent mobility and agent-driven security add to medical information gathering systems, promoting free patient roaming, up-to-date distributed VEPR access, and other new functionalities such as inter-institution secure information exchange.

The second analysed scenario was a practical application of mobile agents to solve the particular problem of getting critical information about a victim before arriving to a hospital for treatment. It makes it possible to asynchronously retrieve significant information (Virtual Electronic Patients Medical Record for Emergencies, VEPMRE), such as allergies or infectious diseases, from the patient record while the victim is still in transit.

In this case, mobile agents are used to bring critical information forward to the emergency area, thus improving the treatment received by the victim.

Finally, a support system based on the use of mobile agents for the transmission of electronic triage tag information has also been presented. The most important feature of this application is that no end-to-end communication is needed at all, and therefore it can operate without any infrastructure.

All three cases showed common problems in large eHealth systems, and illustrated at the same time how mobile agents can be used to face them. One of the most important conclusions drawn is that agents have been crucial to face the high complexity of these systems. Should traditional technologies had been used to solve these problems, a greater effort in designing would have been required. Besides, the current scalability in all the systems would have been very difficult to achieve, if not impossible.

Basic interoperability problems where solved partially by using the standards defined by IEEE-FIPA (*http://www.fipa.org*). In particular, the Agent Communication Language (ACL) was of great help for designing interactions.

Mobile agents are being used more and more commonly in complex distributed applications, such as complex eHealth systems. However, there is still a long way to run to make the most of mobile agents in this domain. Currently, there are some promising lines of research going on. Integrating different applications to find out interoperability problems is one of them. Also, applying Role Based Access Control (RBAC) to mobile agents in this scenario is being explored. Although the RBAC policies provide for a good access control management, some situations might need additional mechanisms for a more flexible adaptation to sudden changes in the organization or emergency situations. Discretionary delegation of permissions could be of special interest.

The information systems described in this chapter could also be used in different domains other than eHealth, such as public administration or universities. In these scenarios, there exist heterogeneous distributed information sources that could benefit from the results of this work, showing another advantage of using the paradigm of mobile agents: re-usability.

References

1. Ametller, J., Robles, S., Ortega-Ruiz, J.A.: Self-protected mobile agents. In: 3rd International Conference on Autonomous Agents and Multi Agents Systems, July 2004, vol. 1, pp. 362–367. ACM Press, New York (2004)
2. Barnett, O.: Computers in medicine. In: JAMA, vol. 263, pp. 2631–2633 (1990)
3. Bellifemine, F.L., Caire, G., Greenwood, D.: Developing Multi-Agent Systems with JADE, January 2006. Wiley, Chichester (2006)
4. Carver, L., Turoff, M.: Human-computer interaction: the human and computer as a team in emergency management information systems. Commun. ACM 50(3), 33–38 (2007)
5. Chen, R., Sharman, R., Rao, H.R., Upadhyaya, S.J.: Design principles of coordinated multi-incident emergency response systems. In: Kantor, P., Muresan, G., Roberts, F., Zeng, D.D., Wang, F.-Y., Chen, H., Merkle, R.C. (eds.) ISI 2005. LNCS, vol. 3495, pp. 81–98. Springer, Heidelberg (2005) Times Cited: 0

6. Cruz-Correia, R., Vieira-Marques, P., Costa, P., Ferreira, A., Oliveira-Palhares, E., Araújo, F., Costa-Pereira, A.: Integration of hospital data using agent technologies - a case study. AI Commun. 18(3), 191–200 (2005)

7. Cucurull, J., Martí, R., Navarro-Arribas, G., Robles, S., Overeinder, B.J., Borrell, J.: Agent mobility architecture based on IEEE-FIPA standards. Computer Communications 32(4), 712–729 (2009)

8. Demchak, B., Chan, T.C., Griswold, W.G., Lenert, L.A.: Situational awareness during mass-casualty events: command and control. In: AMIA Annu. Symp. Proc., p. 905 (2006) Times Cited: 0

9. Fiedrich, F., Burghardt, P.: Agent-based systems for disaster management. Commun. ACM 50(3), 41–42 (2007)

10. French, S., Turoff, M.: Decision support systems. Commun. ACM 50(3), 39–40 (2007)

11. Fry, E.A., Lenert, L.: Mascal: Rfid tracking of patients, staff and equipment to enhance hospital response to mass casualty events. In: AMIA Annual Symposium Proceedings, pp. 261–265 (2005)

12. Fuggetta, A., Picco, G.P., Vigna, G.: Understanding code mobility. IEEE Trans. Softw. Eng. 24(5), 342–361 (1998)

13. Asokan, N., Karjoth, G., Gülcü, C.A.: Protecting the computation results of free-roaming agents. In: Rothermel, K., Hohl, F. (eds.) MA 1998. LNCS, vol. 1477, p. 195. Springer, Heidelberg (1998)

14. Gao, T., White, D.: A next generation electronic triage to aid mass casualty emergency medical response. In: 28th Annual International Conference of the IEEE Engineering in Medicine and Biology Society, EMBS 2006, 30 2006-September 3, pp. Supplement:6501–6504 (2006)

15. Gebhart, M.E., Pence, R.: Start triage: Does it work? Disaster Management and Response 5(3), 68–73 (2007)

16. Gray, J.: Distributed computing economics. In: Herbert, A., Jones, K.S. (eds.) Computer Systems: Theory, Technology and Applications, December 2003, pp. 93–101. Springer, Heidelberg (2003), Also MSR-TR-2003-24, March 2003

17. Inoue, S., Sonoda, A., Oka, K., Fujisaki, S.: Emergency healthcare support: Rfid based massive injured people management. In: Pervasive Healthcare Workshop in Ubicomp 2006 (Ubi-Health), September 2006, p. 9 (2006)

18. Kennedy, K., Aghababian, R.V., Gans, L., Lewis, C.P.: Triage: Techniques and applications in decisionmaking. Annals of Emergency Medicine 28(2), 136–144 (1996)

19. Killeen, J.P., Chan, T.C., Buono, C., Griswold, W.G., Lenert, L.A.: A wireless first responder handheld device for rapid triage, patient assessment and documentation during mass casualty incidents. In: AMIA Annu. Symp. Proc., pp. 429–433 (2006)

20. Kim, G.S., Eom, Y.I.: Domain-based mobile agent fault-tolerance scheme for home network environments. In: Chen, K., Deng, R., Lai, X., Zhou, J. (eds.) ISPEC 2006. LNCS, vol. 3903, pp. 269–277. Springer, Heidelberg (2006)

21. Kopena, J.B., Sultanik, E.A., Lass, R.N., Nguyen, D.N., Dugan, C.J., Modi, P.J., Regli, W.C.: Distributed coordination of first responders. IEEE Internet Computing 12(1), 45–47 (2008)

22. Lenert, L., Palmer, D., Chan, T., Rao, R.: An intelligent 802.11 triage tag for medical response to disasters. In: AMIA Annual Symposium Proceedings, pp. 440–444 (2005)

23. Lenert, L., Chan, T.C., Griswold, W., Killeen, J., Palmer, D., Kirsh, D., Mishra, R., Rao, R.: Wireless internet information system for medical response in disasters (wiisard). In: AMIA Annual Symposium Proceedings, pp. 429–433 (2006)

24. Lenz, R., Kuhn, K.A.: Integration of heterogeneous and autonomous systems in hospitals. In: Data Management and Storage Technology (2002)

25. Li, Y.D., He, H.G., Xiao, B.H., Wang, C.H., Wang, F.Y.: Cwme: A framework of group support system for emergency responses. In: Mehrotra, S., Zeng, D.D., Chen, H., Thuraisingham, B., Wang, F.-Y. (eds.) ISI 2006. LNCS, vol. 3975, pp. 706–707. Springer, Heidelberg (2006) Times Cited: 0
26. Liang, H.G., Xue, Y.J.: Investigating public health emergency response information system initiatives in china. International Journal of Medical Informatics 73(9-10), 675–685 (2004) Times Cited: 5
27. Oliveira, A.-I., Camarinha-Matos, L.M., Rosas, J.: Tele-care and collaborative virtual communities in elderly care. In: Proceedings of the 1st International Workshop on Tele-Care and Collaborative Virtual Communities in Elderly Care, TELECARE 2004 (2004)
28. Luyten, K., Winters, F., Coninx, K., Naudts, D., Moerman, I.: A situation-aware mobile system to support fire brigades in emergency situations. In: Meersman, R., Tari, Z., Herrero, P. (eds.) OTM 2006 Workshops. LNCS, vol. 4278, pp. 1966–1975. Springer, Heidelberg (2006)
29. Manoj, B.S., Baker, A.H.: Communication challenges in emergency response. Commun. ACM 50(3), 51–53 (2007)
30. Marsa-Maestre, I., Lopez, M.A., Velasco, J.R., Navarro, A.: Mobile personal agents for smart spaces. In: ACS/IEEE International Conference on Pervasive Services, pp. 299–302 (2006)
31. Martí, R., Robles, S., Martín-Campillo, A., Cucurull, J.: Method and system for information management and victims classification, based on its condition, in emergency situations. Spanish Patent Pending P200803741 (2008)
32. Martí, R., Robles, S., Martín-Campillo, A., Cucurull, J.: Providing early resource allocation during emergencies: the mobile triage tag. In: Journal of Network and Computer Applications (2009) (accepted)
33. Martín-Campillo, A., Martí, R., Robles, S., Martínez-García, C.: Mobile agents for critical medical information retrieving from the emergency scene. In: 7th International Conference on Practical Applications of Agents and Multi-Agent Systems, Advances in Intelligent and Soft Computing. Springer, Heidelberg (2009)
34. Martínez-García, C., Navarro-Arribas, G., Borrell, J., Martín-Campillo, A.: An access control scheme for multi-agent systems over multi-domain environments. In: 7th International Conference on Practical Applications of Agents and Multi-Agent Systems. Advances in Intelligent and Soft Computing. Springer, Heidelberg (2009)
35. Massey, T., Gao, T., Welsh, M., Sharp, J.H., Sarrafzadeh, M.: The design of a decentralized electronic triage system. In: AMIA Annual Symposium Proceedings, pp. 544–548 (2006)
36. McGrath, S., Grigg, E., Wendelken, S., Blike, G., De Rosa, M., Fiske, A., Gray, R.: Artemis: A vision for remote triage and emergency management information integration. Dartmouth University (November 2003)
37. Mendonça, D., Jefferson, T., Harrald, J.: Collaborative adhocracies and mix-and-match technologies in emergency management. Commun. ACM 50(3), 44–49 (2007)
38. US Navy. Tactical medical coordination system (tacmedcs),
    http://www.namrl.navy.mil/clinical/projects/tacmedcs.htm
39. National Association of Emergency Medical Technicians U.S. and American College of Surgeons. PHTLS–basic and advanced prehospital trauma life support, 4th edn., Mosby, St. Louis (1999)
40. Pavlopoulos, S., Kyriacou, E., Berler, A., Dembeyiotis, S., Koutsouris, D.: A novel emergency telemedicine system based on wirelesscommunication technology-ambulance. IEEE Transactions on Information Technology in Biomedicine 2(4), 261–267 (1998)
41. Portmann, M., Pirzada, A.A.: Wireless mesh networks for public safety and crisis management applications. IEEE Internet Computing 12(1), 18–25 (2008)
42. Costa, P., Cruz-Correia, R., Vieira-Marques, P.: Integration of hospital data using agent technologies - a case study. AICom 18, 191–200 (2005)

43. Satoh, I.: Building reusable mobile agents for network management. IEEE Transactions on Systems, Man and Cybernetics, Part C: Applications and Reviews 33(3), 350–357 (2003)

44. Shnayder, V., rong Chen, B., Lorincz, K., Fulford Jones, T.R.F., Welsh, M.: Sensor networks for medical care. In: SenSys 2005: Proceedings of the 3rd international conference on Embedded networked sensor systems, pp. 314–314. ACM, New York (2005)

45. Barnett, G.O., Murphy, S.N., Rabbani, U.H.: Using software agents to maintain autonomous patient registries for clinical research. In: Proc. AMIA Annu. Fall Symp., pp. 71–75 (1997)

46. Thant, H.A., San, K.M., Tun, K.M.L., Naing, T.T., Thein, N.: Mobile agents based load balancing method for parallel applications. In: Proceedings of 6th Asia-Pacific Symposium on Information and Telecommunication Technologies, APSITT 2005, November 2005, pp. 77–82 (2005)

47. Van de Walle, B., Turoff, M.: Decision support for emergency situations. Information Systems and E-Business Management 6(3), 295–316 (2008), M3: 10.1007/s10257-008-0087-z

48. Velasco, J.R., López-Carmona, M.A., Sedano, M., Garijo, M., Larrabeiti, D., Calderon, M.: Role of multi-agent system on minimalist infrastructure for service provisioning in ad-hoc networks for emergencies. In: Proceedings of AAMAS 2006, pp. 151–152 (2006)

49. Vieira-Marques, P., Robles, S., Cucurull, J., Cruz-Correia, R., Navarro, G., Martí, R.: Secure integration of distributed medical data using mobile agents. IEEE Intelligent Systems 21(6), 47–54 (2006)

50. De Capitani Di Vimercati, S., Ferrero, A., Lazzaroni, M.: Mobile agent technology for remote measurements. IEEE Transactions on Instrumentation and Measurement 55(5), 1559–1565 (2006)

51. White, J.E.: Telescript technology: Mobile agents. In: Bradshaw, J. (ed.) Software Agents, AAAI Press/MIT Press, Menlo Park (1996)

52. Wong, D., Paciorek, N., Walsh, T., DiCelie, J., Young, M., Peet, B.: Concordia: An infrastructure for collaborating mobile agents. In: Rothermel, K., Popescu-Zeletin, R. (eds.) MA 1997. LNCS, vol. 1219. Springer, Heidelberg (1997)

53. Wooldridge, M., Jennings, N.R.: Intelligent agents: Theory and practice. Knowledge Engineering Review 10(2), 115–152 (1995)

54. Wyatt, J.C.: Clinical data systems, part 1: Data and medical records. Lancet 344, 1543–1547 (1994)

Chapter 5

A Joint Bayesian Framework for MR Brain Scan Tissue and Structure Segmentation Based on Distributed Markovian Agents

Benoit Scherrer[1,3,4], Florence Forbes[2], Catherine Garbay[3], and Michel Dojat[1,4]

[1] INSERM U836, 38706 La Tronche, France
{benoit.scherrer,michel.dojat}@ujf-grenoble.fr
[2] INRIA, Laboratoire Jean Kuntzman, MISTIS Team, 38041 Montbonnot, France
florence.forbes@inrialpes.fr
[3] Laboratoire d'Informatique de Grenoble, 38041 France
catherine.garbay@imag.fr
[4] Université Joseph Fourier, Institut des Neurosciences Grenoble,
38706 La Tronche, France

Abstract. In most approaches, tissue and subcortical structure segmentations of MR brain scans are handled globally over the entire brain volume through two relatively independent sequential steps. We propose a fully Bayesian joint model that integrates within a multi-agent framework local tissue and structure segmentations and local intensity distribution modeling. It is based on the specification of three conditional Markov Random Field (MRF) models. The first two encode cooperations between tissue and structure segmentations and integrate *a priori* anatomical knowledge. The third model specifies a Markovian spatial prior over the model parameters that enables local estimations while ensuring their consistency, handling this way nonuniformity of intensity without any bias field modeling. The complete joint model provides then a sound theoretical framework for carrying out tissue and structure segmentations by distributing a set of local agents that estimate cooperatively local MRF models. The evaluation, using a previously affine-registered atlas of 17 structures, was performed using both phantoms and real 3T brain scans. It shows good results and in particular robustness to nonuniformity and noise with a low computational cost. The innovative coupling of agent-based and Markov-centered designs appears as a robust, fast and promising approach to MR brain scan segmentation.

Keywords: Medical Imaging, Multi-Agents, Medical Image Processing.

1 Introduction

Difficulties in automatic MR brain scan segmentation arise from various sources. The nonuniformity of image intensity results in spatial intensity variations within each tissue, which is a major obstacle to an accurate automatic tissue segmentation. The automatic segmentation of subcortical structures is a challenging task

I. Bichindaritz et al. (Eds.): Computational Intelligence in Healthcare 4, SCI 309, pp. 81–101.
springerlink.com   © Springer-Verlag Berlin Heidelberg 2010

as well. It cannot be performed based only on intensity distributions and requires the introduction of *a priori* knowledge. Most of the proposed approaches share two main characteristics. First, tissue and subcortical structure segmentations are considered as two successive tasks and treated relatively independently although they are clearly linked: a structure is composed of a specific tissue, and knowledge about structure locations provides valuable information about local intensity distributions. Second, tissue models are estimated globally through the entire volume and then suffer from imperfections at a local level. Alternative local procedures exist but are either used as a preprocessing step [1] or use redundant information to ensure consistency of local models [2]. Recently, good results have been reported using an innovative local and cooperative approach [3], [4]. The approach is implemented using a multi-agent framework. It performs tissue and subcortical structure segmentation by distributing through the volume a set of local agents that compute local Markov Random Field (MRF) models which better reflect local intensity distributions. Local MRF models are used alternatively for tissue and structure segmentations and agents cooperate with other agents in their neighborhood for model refinement. Although satisfying in practice, these tissue and structure MRF's do not correspond to a valid joint probabilistic model and are not compatible in that sense. As a consequence, important issues such as convergence or other theoretical properties of the resulting local procedure cannot be addressed. In addition, in [4], cooperation mechanisms between local agents are somewhat arbitrary and independent of the MRF models themselves. In this paper, we aim at filling in the gap between an efficient distributed system of agents and a joint modeling accounting for their cooperative processing in a formal manner. Markov models with the concept of conditional independence, whereby each variable is related locally (conditionally) to only a few other variables, are good candidates to complement the symbolic level of the agent-based cooperations with the numerical level inherent to the targeted applications.

Following these considerations, we propose a fully Bayesian framework in which we define a joint model that links local tissue and structure segmentations but also the model parameters. It follows that both types of cooperations, between tissues and structures and between local models, are deduced from the joint model and optimal in that sense. Our model, originally introduced in [5] and described in details in this chapter, has the following main features: 1) cooperative segmentation of both tissues and structures is encoded via a joint probabilistic model specified through conditional MRF models which capture the relations between tissues and structures. This model specifications also integrate external *a priori* knowledge in a natural way; 2) intensity nonuniformity is handled by using a specific parameterization of tissue intensity distributions which induces local estimations on subvolumes of the entire volume; 3) global consistency between local estimations is automatically ensured by using a MRF spatial prior for the intensity distributions parameters. Estimation within our framework is defined as a maximum *a posteriori* (MAP) estimation problem and is carried out by adopting an instance of the Expectation Maximization (EM) algorithm [6]. We show that such a setting can adapt well to our conditional models formulation and simplifies into alternating and cooperative estimation procedures for standard Hidden MRF models that can be implemented efficiently via a two agent-layer architecture.

The chapter is organized as follows. In Section 2, we explain the motivation in coupling agent-based and Markov-centered designs. In Section 3, we introduce the probabilistic setting and inference framework. The joint tissue and structure model is described in more details in Section 4. An appropriate estimation procedure is proposed in Section 5. Experimental results are reported in Section 6 and a discussion ends the chapter.

2 Distributed Cooperative Markovian Agents

While Markov modeling has largely been used in the domain of MRI segmentation, agent-based approaches have seldom been considered. Agents are autonomous entities sharing a common environment and working in a cooperative way to achieve a common goal. They are usually provided with limited perception abilities and local knowledge. Some advantages of multi-agent systems are among others [7] their ability to handle knowledge from different domains, to

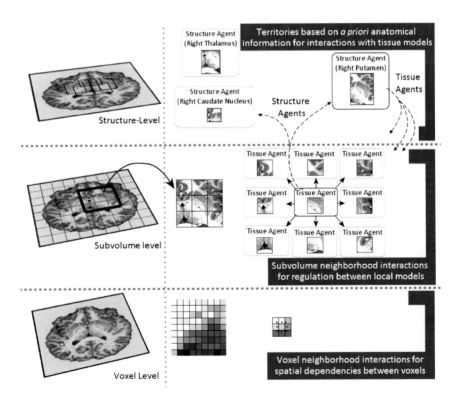

Fig. 1. Symbolic multi-level design of our approach

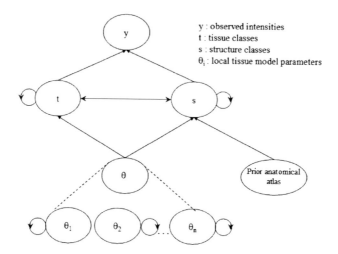

y : observed intensities
t : tissue classes
s : structure classes
θ_i : local tissue model parameters

Fig. 2. Graphical model illustrating the joint dependencies between local intensity models, and tissue and structure segmentations

design reliable systems able to recover from agents with low performance and wrong knowledge, to focus spatially and semantically on relevant knowledge, to cooperate and share tasks between agents in various domains, and to reduce computation time through distributed and asynchronous implementation.

Previous work has shown the potential of multi-agent approaches for MRI segmentation along two main directions: first of all as a way to cope with grey level heterogeneity and bias field effects, by enabling the development of local and situated processing styles [8] and secondly, as a way to support the cooperations between various processing styles and information types, namely tissue and structure information [9], [10]. Stated differently, multi-agent modeling may be seen as a robust approach to identify the main lines along which to distribute complex processing issues, and support the design of situated cooperative systems at the symbolic level as illustrated in Figure 1. A designing approach has been furthermore proposed [10] to benefit from both Markov-centered and agent-based modeling toward robust MRI processing systems. In the course of this work, however, we pointed out the gap existing between the symbolical level of the agent-based cooperations and the numerical level of Markov optimization, this gap resulting in a difficulty to ground formally the proposed design. In particular the mutual dependencies between the Markov variables (tissue and structure segmentations on one hand, local intensity models on the other hand) were handled through rather *ad hoc* cooperation mechanisms.

The point here is then to start from the observation that Markov graphical modeling may be used to visualize the dependencies between local intensity models, and tissue and structure segmentations, as shown in Figure 2. According to this Figure, the observed intensities **y** are seen as reflecting both tissue-dependent and structure dependent information. Tissues and structures are considered as mutually dependent, since structures are composed of tissues.

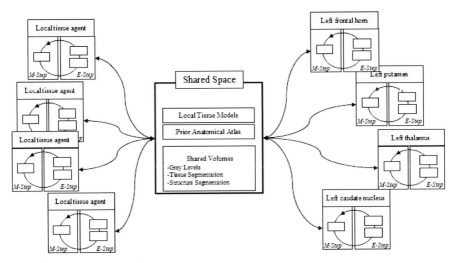

Fig. 3. Implementation using a two agent-layer architecture and a shared space for communication

Also, the observed variations of appearance in tissues and structures reflect the spatial dependency of the tissue model parameters to be computed. Figure 2 then illustrates the hierarchical organization of the variables under consideration and its adequation with the agent hierarchy at a symbolic level. In the following section, we show that this hierarchical decomposition can be expressed in terms of a coherent systems of probability distributions for which inference can be carried out. Regarding implementation, we adopt subsequently the two agent-layer architecture, as illustrated in Figure 3, where tissue and structure agents cooperate through shared information including tissue intensity models, anatomical atlas, tissue and structure segmentations.

3   Hierarchical Analysis Using the EM Algorithm

Hierarchical modeling is, in essence, based on the simple fact from probability that the joint distribution of a collection of random variables can be decomposed into a series of conditional models. That is, if $\mathbf{Y}$, $\mathbf{Z}$, θ are random variables, then we write the joint distribution in terms of a factorization such as $p(\mathbf{y}, \mathbf{z}, \theta) = p(\mathbf{y}|\mathbf{z}, \theta)p(\mathbf{z}|\theta)p(\theta)$. The strength of hierarchical approaches is that they are based on the specification of coherently linked system of conditional models. The key elements of such models can be considered in three stages, the data stage, process stage and parameter stage. In each stage, complicated dependence structure is mitigated by conditioning. For example, the data stage can incorporate measurement errors as well as multiple datasets. The process and parameter stages can allow spatial interactions as well as the direct inclusion of scientific knowledge. These modeling capabilities are especially relevant to tackle the task of MRI brain scan segmentation. In image segmentation problems, the question of interest is to recover an unknown image $\mathbf{z} \in \mathcal{Z}$, interpreted as a classification into a finite number K of labels, from an image $\mathbf{y}$ of observed intensity values. This classification usually requires values for a vector parameter $\theta \in \Theta$ considered in a Bayesian setting as a random variable. The idea is to approach the problem by breaking it into the three primary stages mentioned above. The first data stage is concerned with the observational process or data model $p(\mathbf{y}|\mathbf{z}, \theta)$, which specifies the distribution of the data $\mathbf{y}$ given the process of interest and relevant parameters. The second stage then describes the process model $p(\mathbf{z}|\theta)$, conditional on usually other parameters still denoted by θ for simplicity. Finally, the last stage accounts for the uncertainty in the parameters through a distribution $p(\theta)$. In applications, each of these stages may have multiple sub-stages. For example, if spatial interactions are to be taken into account, it might be modeled as a product of several conditional distributions suggested by neighborhood relationships. Similar decompositions are possible in the parameter stage.

Ultimately, we are interested in the distribution of the process and parameters updated by the data, that is the so-called posterior distribution $p(\mathbf{z}, \theta \mid \mathbf{y})$. Due to generally too complex dependencies, it is difficult to extract parameters θ from the observed data $\mathbf{y}$ without explicit knowledge of the unknown true segmentation $\mathbf{z}$. This problem is greatly simplified when the solution is determined within an EM framework. The EM algorithm [11] is a general technique for finding maximum likelihood solutions in the presence of missing data. It consists in two steps usually described as the E-step in which the expectation of the so-called complete log-likelihood is computed and the M-step in which this expectation is maximized over θ. An equivalent way to define EM is the following. Let $\mathcal{D}$ be the set of all probability distributions on $\mathcal{Z}$. As discussed in [6], EM can be viewed as an alternating maximization procedure of a function F defined, for any probability distribution $q \in \mathcal{D}$, by

$$F(q, \theta) = \sum_{\mathbf{z} \in \mathcal{Z}} \ln p(\mathbf{y}, \mathbf{z} \mid \theta) \, q(\mathbf{z}) + I[q], \tag{1}$$

where $I[q] = -E_q[\log q(\mathbf{Z})]$ is the entropy of q (E_q denotes the expectation with regard to q and we use capital letters to indicate random variables while their realizations are denoted with small letters). When prior knowledge on the parameters is available, the Bayesian setting consists in replacing the maximum likelihood estimation by a maximum a posteriori (MAP) estimation of θ using the prior knowledge encoded in distribution $p(\theta)$. The maximum likelihood estimate of θ ie. $\hat{\theta} = \arg\max_{\theta \in \Theta} p(\mathbf{y}|\theta)$ is replaced by $\hat{\theta} = \arg\max_{\theta \in \Theta} p(\theta|\mathbf{y})$. The EM algorithm can also be used to maximize the posterior distribution. Indeed, the likelihood $p(\mathbf{y}|\theta)$ and $F(q, \theta)$ are linked through $\log p(\mathbf{y}|\theta) = F(q, \theta) + KL(q, p)$ where $KL(q, p)$ is the Kullback-Leibler divergence between q and the conditional distribution $p(\mathbf{z}|\mathbf{y}, \theta)$ and is non-negative,

$$KL(q, p) = \sum_{\mathbf{z} \in \mathcal{Z}} q(\mathbf{z}) \log \left(\frac{q(\mathbf{z})}{p(\mathbf{z}|\mathbf{y}, \theta)} \right).$$

Using the equality $\log p(\theta|\mathbf{y}) = \log p(\mathbf{y}|\theta) + \log p(\theta) - \log p(\mathbf{y})$ it follows $\log p(\theta|\mathbf{y}) = F(q,\theta) + KL(q,p) + \log p(\theta) - \log p(\mathbf{y})$ from which, we get a lower bound $\mathcal{L}(q,\theta)$ on $\log p(\theta|\mathbf{y})$ given by $\mathcal{L}(q,\theta) = F(q,\theta) + \log p(\theta) - \log p(\mathbf{y})$. Maximizing this lower bound alternatively over q and θ leads to a sequence $\{q^{(r)}, \theta^{(r)}\}_{r\in\mathbb{N}}$ satisfying $\mathcal{L}(q^{(r+1)}, \theta^{(r+1)}) \geq \mathcal{L}(q^{(r)}, \theta^{(r)})$. The maximization over q corresponds to the standard E-step and leads to $q^{(r)}(\mathbf{z}) = p(\mathbf{z}|\mathbf{y}, \theta^{(r)})$. It follows that $\mathcal{L}(q^{(r)}, \theta^{(r)}) = \log p(\theta^{(r)}|\mathbf{y})$ which means that the lower bound reaches the objective function in $\theta^{(r)}$ and that the sequence $\{\theta^{(r)}\}_{r\in\mathbb{N}}$ increases $p(\theta|\mathbf{y})$ at each step. It then appears that when considering our MAP problem, we replace (see eg. [12]) the function $F(q,\theta)$ by $F(q,\theta) + \log p(\theta)$. The corresponding alternating procedure is: starting from a current value $\theta^{(r)} \in \Theta$, set alternatively

$$q^{(r)} = \arg\max_{q\in\mathcal{D}} F(q, \theta^{(r)}) = \arg\max_{q\in\mathcal{D}} \sum_{\mathbf{z}\in\mathcal{Z}} \log p(\mathbf{z}|\mathbf{y}, \theta^{(r)}) \, q(\mathbf{z}) + I[q], \qquad (2)$$

and

$$\theta^{(r+1)} = \arg\max_{\theta\in\Theta} F(q^{(r)}, \theta) + \log p(\theta) = \arg\max_{\theta\in\Theta} \sum_{\mathbf{z}\in\mathcal{Z}} \log p(\mathbf{y}, \mathbf{z}, \theta) \, q^{(r)}(\mathbf{z}) + \log p(\theta)$$

$$= \arg\max_{\theta\in\Theta} \sum_{\mathbf{z}\in\mathcal{Z}} \log p(\theta|\mathbf{y}, \mathbf{z}) \, q^{(r)}(\mathbf{z}) \, .$$

The last equality in (2) comes from $p(\mathbf{y}, \mathbf{z}|\theta) = p(\mathbf{z}|\mathbf{y}, \theta)p(\mathbf{y}|\theta)$ and the fact that $p(\mathbf{y}|\theta)$ does not depend on $\mathbf{z}$. The last equality in (3) comes from $p(\mathbf{y}, \mathbf{z}|\theta) = p(\theta|\mathbf{y}, \mathbf{z}) \, p(\mathbf{y}, \mathbf{z})/p(\theta)$ and the fact that $p(\mathbf{y}, \mathbf{z})$ does not depend on θ. The optimization with respect to q gives rise to the same E-step as for the standard EM algorithm, because q only appears in $F(q,\theta)$. It can be shown (eg. [12] p.319) that EM converges to a local mode of the posterior density except in some very special cases. This EM framework appears as a reasonable framework for inference. In addition, it appears in (2) and (3) that inference can be described in terms of the conditional models $p(\mathbf{z}|\mathbf{y}, \theta)$ and $p(\theta|\mathbf{y}, \mathbf{z})$. In the following section, we show how to define our joint model so as to take advantage of these considerations.

4   A Bayesian Model for Robust Joint Tissue and Structure Segmentations

In this section, we describes the Bayesian framework that enables us to model the relationships between the unknown linked tissue and structure labels, the observed MR image data and the tissue intensity distributions parameters.

We consider a finite set V of N voxels on a regular 3D grid. We denote by $\mathbf{y} = \{y_1, \ldots, y_N\}$ the intensity values observed respectively at each voxel and by $\mathbf{t} = \{t_1, \ldots, t_N\}$ the hidden tissue classes. The t_i's take their values in $\{e_1, e_2, e_3\}$ where e_k is a 3-dimensional binary vector whose k^{th} component is 1, all other components being 0. In addition, we consider L subcortical structures and denote by $\mathbf{s} = \{s_1, \ldots, s_N\}$ the hidden structure classes at each voxel. Similarly, the s_i's take their values in $\{e'_1, \ldots, e'_L, e'_{L+1}\}$ where e'_{L+1} corresponds to an additional background class. As parameters θ, we consider the parameters describing the intensity distributions for the $K = 3$ tissue classes. They are denoted by $\theta = \{\theta_i^k, i \in V, k = 1 \ldots K\}$. We write for all $k = 1 \ldots K$, $\theta^k = \{\theta_i^k, i \in V\}$ and for all $i \in V$, $\theta_i = {}^t(\theta_i^k, k = 1 \ldots K)$ (^{t} means transpose). Note that we describe here the most general setting in which the intensity distributions can depend on voxel i and vary with its location. Standard approaches usually consider that intensity distributions are Gaussian distributions for which the parameters depend only on the tissue class. Although the Bayesian approach makes the general case possible, in practice we consider θ_i^k's equal for all voxels i in some prescribed regions. More specifically, our local approach consists in dividing the volume V into a partition of subvolumes and consider the θ_i^k constant over each subvolume (see Section 4.2).

To explicitly take into account the fact that tissue and structure classes are related, a *generative* approach would be to define a complete probabilistic model, namely $p(\mathbf{y}, \mathbf{t}, \mathbf{s}, \theta)$. To define such a joint probability is equivalent to define the two probability distributions $p(\mathbf{y})$ and $p(\mathbf{t}, \mathbf{s}, \theta|\mathbf{y})$. However, in this work, we rather adopt a *discriminative* approach in which a conditional model $p(\mathbf{t}, \mathbf{s}, \theta|\mathbf{y})$ is constructed from the observations and labels but the marginal $p(\mathbf{y})$ is not modeled explicitly. In a segmentation context, the full generative model is not particularly relevant to the task of inferring the class labels. This appears clearly in equations (2) and (3) where the relevant distributions are conditional. In addition, it has been observed that conditional approaches tend to be more robust than generative models [13], [14]. Therefore, we focus on $p(\mathbf{t}, \mathbf{s}, \theta|\mathbf{y})$ as the quantity of interest. It is fully specified when the two conditional distributions $p(\mathbf{t}, \mathbf{s}|\mathbf{y}, \theta)$ and $p(\theta|\mathbf{y}, \mathbf{t}, \mathbf{s})$ are defined. The following subsections 4.1 and 4.2 specify respectively these two distributions.

4.1   A Conditional Model for Tissues and Structures

The distribution $p(\mathbf{t}, \mathbf{s}|\mathbf{y}, \theta)$ can be in turn specified by defining $p(\mathbf{t}|\mathbf{s}, \mathbf{y}, \theta)$ and $p(\mathbf{s}|\mathbf{t}, \mathbf{y}, \theta)$. The advantage of the later conditional models is that they can capture in an explicit way the effect of tissue segmentation on structure segmentation and vice versa. Note that on a computational point of view there is no need at this stage to describe explicitly the joint model that can be quite complex. In what follows, notation $^txx'$ denotes the scalar product between two vectors x and x'. Notation $U_{ij}^T(t_i, t_j; \eta_T)$ and $U_{ij}^S(s_i, s_j; \eta_S)$ denotes pairwise potential functions with interaction parameters η_T and η_S. Simple examples for $U_{ij}^T(t_i, t_j; \eta_T)$ and $U_{ij}^S(s_i, s_j; \eta_S)$ are provided by adopting a Potts model which corresponds to

$$U_{ij}^T(t_i, t_j; \eta_T) = \eta_T \; {}^t t_i t_j \quad \text{and} \quad U_{ij}^S(s_i, s_j; \eta_S) = \eta_S \; {}^t s_i s_j \; .$$

Such a model captures, within each label set $\mathbf{t}$ and $\mathbf{s}$, interactions between neighboring voxels. It implies spatial interaction within each label set.

Structure conditional Tissue model. We define $p(\mathbf{t}|\mathbf{s},\mathbf{y},\theta)$ as a Markov Random Field in $\mathbf{t}$ with the following energy function,

$$H_{T|S,Y,\Theta}(\mathbf{t}|\mathbf{s},\mathbf{y},\theta) = \sum_{i \in V} \left({}^{t}t_i \gamma_i(s_i) + \sum_{j \in \mathcal{N}(i)} U_{ij}^T(t_i, t_j; \eta_T) + \log g_T(y_i; {}^{t}\theta_i t_i) \right), \quad (3)$$

where $\mathcal{N}(i)$ denotes the voxels neighboring i, $g_T(y_i; {}^{t}\theta_i t_i)$ is the Gaussian distribution with parameters θ_i^k if $t_i = e_k$ and the external field γ_i depends on s_i and is defined by $\gamma_i(s_i) = e_{T^{s_i}}$ if $s_i \in \{e'_1, \ldots, e'_L\}$ and $\gamma_i(s_i) = \mathbf{0}$ otherwise, with T^{s_i} denoting the tissue of structure s_i and $\mathbf{0}$ the 3-dimensional null vector. The rationale for choosing such an external field, is that depending on the structure present at voxel i and given by the value of s_i, the tissue corresponding to this structure is more likely at voxel i while the two others tissues are penalized by a smaller contribution to the energy through a smaller external field value. When i is a background voxel, the external field does not favor a particular tissue. The Gaussian parameters $\theta_i^k = \{\mu_i^k, \lambda_i^k\}$ are respectively the mean and precision which is the inverse of the variance. We use similar notation such as $\mu = \{\mu_i^k, i \in V, k = 1 \ldots K\}$ and $\mu^k = \{\mu_i^k, i \in V\}$, etc.

Tissue conditional structure model. *A priori* knowledge on structures is incorporated through a field $f = \{f_i, i \in V\}$ where $f_i = {}^{t}(f_i(e'_l), l = 1 \ldots L + 1)$ and $f_i(e'_l)$ represents some prior probability that voxel i belongs to structure l, as provided by a registered probabilistic atlas. We then define $p(\mathbf{s}|\mathbf{t},\mathbf{y},\theta)$ as a Markov Random Field in $\mathbf{s}$ with the following energy function,

$$H_{S|T,Y,\Theta}(\mathbf{s}|\mathbf{t},\mathbf{y},\theta) = \sum_{i \in V} \left({}^{t}s_i \log f_i + \sum_{j \in \mathcal{N}(i)} U_{ij}^S(s_i, s_j; \eta_S) + \log g_S(y_i|t_i, s_i, \theta_i) \right) (4)$$

where $g_S(y_i|t_i, s_i, \theta_i)$ is defined as follows,

$$g_S(y_i|t_i, s_i, \theta) = [g_T(y_i; {}^{t}\theta_i e_{T^{s_i}}) \, f_i(s_i)]^{w(s_i)} \, [g_T(y_i; {}^{t}\theta_i t_i) \, f_i(e'_{L+1})]^{(1-w(s_i))} (5)$$

where $w(s_i)$ is a weight dealing with the possible conflict between values of t_i and s_i. For simplicity we set $w(s_i) = 0$ if $s_i = e'_{L+1}$ and $w(s_i) = 1$ otherwise but considering more general weights could be an interesting refinement. Other parameters in (3) and (4) include interaction parameters η_T and η_S which are considered here as hyperparameters to be specified (see Section 6).

4.2   A Conditional Model for Intensity Distribution Parameters

To ensure spatial consistency between the parameter values, we define also $p(\theta|\mathbf{y},\mathbf{t},\mathbf{s})$ as a MRF. In practice however, in our general setting which allows different values θ_i at each i, there are too many parameters and estimating them accurately is not possible. As regards estimation then, we adopt a local approach as in [4]. The idea is to consider the parameters as constant over subvolumes of the entire volume. Let $\mathcal{C}$ be a regular cubic partitioning of the volume V in a number of non-overlapping subvolumes $\{V_c, c \in \mathcal{C}\}$. We assume that for all

$c \in \mathcal{C}$ and all $i \in V_c$, $\theta_i = \theta_c$ and consider a pairwise MRF on $\mathcal{C}$ with energy function denoted by $H_\Theta^{\mathcal{C}}(\theta)$ where by extension θ denotes the set of distinct values $\theta = \{\theta_c, c \in \mathcal{C}\}$. Outside the issue of estimating θ in the M-step, having parameters θ_i's depending on i is not a problem. For the E-steps, we go back to this general setting using an interpolation step specified in Section 5.2. It follows that $p(\theta|\mathbf{y}, \mathbf{t}, \mathbf{s})$ is defined as a MRF with the following energy function,

$$H_{\Theta|Y,T,S}(\theta|\mathbf{y}, \mathbf{t}, \mathbf{s}) = H_\Theta^{\mathcal{C}}(\theta) + \sum_{c \in \mathcal{C}} \log \prod_{i \in V_c} g_S(y_i|t_i, s_i, \theta_c),$$

where $g_S(y_i|t_i, s_i, \theta_c)$ is the expression in (5). The specific form of the Markov prior on θ is specified in Section 5.

5   Estimation by Generalized Alternating Minimization

The particularity of our segmentation task is to include two label sets of interest, $\mathbf{t}$ and $\mathbf{s}$ which are linked and that we would like to estimate cooperatively using one to gain information on the other. We denote respectively by $\mathcal{T}$ and $\mathcal{S}$ the spaces in which $\mathbf{t}$ and $\mathbf{s}$ take their values. Denoting $\mathbf{z} = (\mathbf{t}, \mathbf{s})$, we apply the EM framework introduced in Section 3 to find a MAP estimate $\hat{\theta}$ of θ using the procedure given by (2) and (3) and then generate $\mathbf{t}$ and $\mathbf{s}$ that maximize the conditional distribution $p(\mathbf{t}, \mathbf{s}|\mathbf{y}, \hat{\theta})$. Note that this is however not equivalent to maximizing over $\mathbf{t}, \mathbf{s}$ and θ the posterior distribution $p(\mathbf{t}, \mathbf{s}, \theta|\mathbf{y})$. Indeed $p(\mathbf{t}, \mathbf{s}, \theta \mid \mathbf{y}) = p(\mathbf{t}, \mathbf{s}|\mathbf{y}, \theta) \, p(\theta|\mathbf{y})$ and in the EM setting, θ is found by maximizing the second factor only.

However, solving the optimization (2) over the set $\mathcal{D}$ of probability distributions $q_{(T,S)}$ on $\mathcal{T} \times \mathcal{S}$ leads for the optimal $q_{(T,S)}^{(r)}$ to $p(\mathbf{t}, \mathbf{s}|\mathbf{y}, \theta^{(r)})$ which is intractable for the joint model defined in Section 4. We therefore propose an EM variant appropriate to our cooperative context and in which the E-step is not performed exactly. The optimization (2) is solved instead over a restricted class of probability distributions $\tilde{\mathcal{D}}$ which is chosen as the set of distributions that factorize as $q_{(T,S)}(\mathbf{t}, \mathbf{s}) = q_T(\mathbf{t}) \, q_S(\mathbf{s})$ where q_T (resp. q_S) belongs to the set $\mathcal{D}_T$ (resp. $\mathcal{D}_S$) of probability distributions on $\mathcal{T}$ (resp. on $\mathcal{S}$). This variant is usually referred to as Variational EM [15]. It follows that the E-step becomes an approximate E-step,

$$(q_T^{(r)}, q_S^{(r)}) = \arg \max_{(q_T, q_S)} F(q_T q_S, \theta^{(r)}) .$$

This step can be further generalized by decomposing it into two stages. At iteration r, with current estimates denoted by $q_T^{(r-1)}, q_S^{(r-1)}$ and $\theta^{(r)}$, we consider the following updating,

E-T-step: $q_T^{(r)} = \arg \max_{q_T \in \mathcal{D}_T} F(q_T \, q_S^{(r-1)}, \theta^{(r)})$

E-S-step: $q_S^{(r)} = \arg \max_{q_S \in \mathcal{D}_S} F(q_T^{(r)} \, q_S, \theta^{(r)}).$

The effect of these iterations is to generate sequences of paired distributions and parameters $\{q_T^{(r)}, q_S^{(r)}, \theta^{(r)}\}_{r \in \mathbb{N}}$ that satisfy $F(q_T^{(r+1)} q_S^{(r+1)}, \theta^{(r+1)}) \geq F(q_T^{(r)} q_S^{(r)}, \theta^{(r)})$. This variant falls in the modified Generalized Alternating Minimization (GAM) procedures family for which convergence results are available [6].

We then derive two equivalent expressions of F when q factorizes as in $\tilde{\mathcal{D}}$. Expression (1) of F can be rewritten as $F(q, \theta) = E_q[\log p(\mathbf{T}|\mathbf{S}, \mathbf{y}, \theta)] + E_q[\log p(\mathbf{S}, \mathbf{y}|\theta)] + I[q]$. Then,

$$F(q_T\, q_S, \theta) = E_{q_T}[E_{q_S}[\log p(\mathbf{T}|\mathbf{S}, \mathbf{y}, \theta)]] + E_{q_S}[\log p(\mathbf{S}, \mathbf{y}|\theta)] + I[q_T\, q_S]$$
$$= E_{q_T}[E_{q_S}[\log p(\mathbf{T}|\mathbf{S}, \mathbf{y}, \theta)]] + I[q_T] + G[q_S],$$

where $G[q_S] = E_{q_S}[\log p(\mathbf{S}, \mathbf{y}|\theta)] + I[q_S]$ is an expression that does not depend on q_T. Using the symmetry in $\mathbf{T}$ and $\mathbf{S}$, it is easy to show that similarly,

$$F(q_T\, q_S, \theta) = E_{q_S}[E_{q_T}[\log p(\mathbf{S}|\mathbf{T}, \mathbf{y}, \theta)]] + E_{q_T}[\log p(\mathbf{T}, \mathbf{y}|\theta)] + I[q_T\, q_S]$$
$$= E_{q_S}[E_{q_T}[\log p(\mathbf{S}|\mathbf{T}, \mathbf{y}, \theta)]] + I[q_S] + G'[q_T],$$

where $G'[q_T] = E_{q_T}[\log p(\mathbf{T}, \mathbf{y}|\theta)] + I[q_T]$ is an expression that does not depend on q_S. It follows that the E-T and E-S steps reduce to,

E-T-step: $q_T^{(r)} = \arg \max_{q_T \in \mathcal{D}_T} E_{q_T}[E_{q_S^{(r-1)}}[\log p(\mathbf{T}|\mathbf{S}, \mathbf{y}, \theta^{(r)})]] + I[q_T]$ (6)

E-S-step: $q_S^{(r)} = \arg \max_{q_S \in \mathcal{D}_S} E_{q_S}[E_{q_T^{(r)}}[\log p(\mathbf{S}|\mathbf{T}, \mathbf{y}, \theta^{(r)})]] + I[q_S]$ (7)

and the **M-step** $\theta^{(r+1)} = \arg \max_{\theta \in \Theta} E_{q_T^{(r)} q_S^{(r)}}[\log p(\theta|\mathbf{y}, \mathbf{T}, \mathbf{S})]$.

More generally, we adopt in addition, an incremental EM approach [6] which allows re-estimation of the parameters (here θ) to be performed based only on a sub-part of the hidden variables. This means that we incorporate an M-step (5) in between the updating of q_T and q_S. Similarly, hyperparameters could be updated there too.

It appears in equations (6), (7) and (5) that for inference the specification of the three conditional distributions $p(\mathbf{t}|\mathbf{s}, \mathbf{y}, \theta)$, $p(\mathbf{s}|\mathbf{t}, \mathbf{y}, \theta)$ and $p(\theta|\mathbf{t}, \mathbf{s}, \mathbf{y})$ is necessary and sufficient.

5.1   Structure and Tissue Conditional E-Steps

Then, steps E-T and E-S have to be further specified by computing the expectations with regards to $q_S^{(r-1)}$ and $q_T^{(r)}$. Using the structure conditional model definition (3), it comes,

$$E_{q_S^{(r-1)}}[\log p(\mathbf{T}|\mathbf{S}, \mathbf{y}, \theta^{(r)})] = -E_{q_S^{(r-1)}}[\log W_T]$$
$$+ \sum_{i \in V} {}^t T_i E_{q_S^{(r-1)}}[\gamma_i(S_i)] \quad + \sum_{j \in \mathcal{N}(i)} U_{ij}^T(T_i, T_j; \eta_T) + \log g_T(y_i; {}^t\theta_i^{(r)} T_i) , \quad (8)$$

where W_T is a normalizing constant that does not depend on $\mathbf{T}$ and can be omitted in the maximization of step E-T. The external field term leads to

$$E_{q_S^{(r-1)}}[\gamma_i(S_i)] = \sum_{l=1}^{L} e_{T^l} q_{S_i}^{(r-1)}(e_l')$$
$$= {}^t(\sum_{l \, st. T^l = 1} q_{S_i}^{(r-1)}(e_l'), \sum_{l \, st. T^l = 2} q_{S_i}^{(r-1)}(e_l'), \sum_{l \, st. T^l = 3} q_{S_i}^{(r-1)}(e_l')) .$$

The kth ($k = 1 \ldots 3$) component of the above vector represents the probability that voxel i belongs to a structure whose tissue class is k. The stronger this probability the more a *priori* favored is tissue k. Eventually, we notice that step E-T is equivalent to the E-step one would get when applying EM to a standard Hidden MRF over $\mathbf{t}$ with Gaussian class distributions and an external field parameter fixed to values based on the current structure segmentation. To solve this step, then, various inference techniques for Hidden MRF's can be applied. In this paper, we adopt Mean field like algorithms [16] used in [4] for MRI brain scans. This class of algorithms has the advantage to turn the initial intractable model into a model equivalent to a system of independent variables for which the exact EM can be carried out. Following a mean field principle, when spatial interactions are defined via Potts models, these algorithms are based on the approximation of $U_{ij}^T(t_i, t_j; \eta_T)$ by $\tilde{U}_{ij}^T(t_i, t_j; \eta_T) = \eta_T {}^t\tilde{t}_i\tilde{t}_j$ where $\tilde{t}$ is a particular configuration of $\mathbf{T}$ which is updated at each iteration according to a specific scheme. We refer to [16] for details on three possible schemes to update $\tilde{t}$.

Similarly, using definitions (4) and (5),

$$E_{q_T^{(r)}}[\log p(\mathbf{S}|\mathbf{T}, \mathbf{y}, \theta^{(r)})] = -E_{q_T^{(r)}}[\log W_S]$$
$$+ \sum_{i \in V} {}^t S_i f_i + \sum_{j \in \mathcal{N}(i)} U_{ij}^S(S_i, S_j; \eta_S)$$
$$+ E_{q_T^{(r)}}[\log g_S(y_i|T_i, S_i, \theta_i^{(r)}] \quad (9)$$

where the normalizing constant W_S does not depend on S and can be omitted in the maximization in step E-S. The last term can be further computed,

$$E_{q_T^{(r)}}[\log g_S(y_i|T_i, S_i, \theta_i^{(r)})] = \log g_S'(y_i|S_i, \theta_i^{(r)}),$$

where

$$g_S'(y_i|s_i, \theta_i) = [g_T(y_i; {}^t\theta_i e_{T^{s_i}}) \, f_i(s_i)]^{w(s_i)} \, [(\prod_{k=1}^{3} g_T(y_i; \theta_i^k)^{q_{T_i}^{(r)}(e_k)}) f_i(e_{L+1}')]^{(1-w(s_i))} .$$

In this later expression, the product corresponds to a Gaussian distribution with

mean $\sum_{k=1}^{3} \mu_i^k \lambda_i^k q_{T_i}^{(r)}(e_k) / \sum_{k=1}^{3} \lambda_i^k q_{T_i}^{(r)}(e_k)$ and precision $\sum_{k=1}^{3} \lambda_i^k q_{T_i}^{(r)}(e_k)$.

It follows that step E-S can be seen as the E-step for a standard Hidden MRF with class distributions defined by g_S' and an external field incorporating prior structure knowledge through f. As already mentioned, it can be solved using techniques such as those described in [16].

5.2   Updating the Tissue Intensity Distribution Parameters

As mentioned in Section 4.2, we now consider that the θ_i's are constant over subvolumes of a given partition of the entire volume. The MRF prior on $\theta = \{\theta_c, c \in \mathcal{C}\}$ is $p(\theta) \propto \exp(H_\Theta^\mathcal{C}(\theta))$ and (5) can be written as,

$$\theta^{(r+1)} = \arg\max_{\theta \in \underline{\Theta}} p(\theta) \prod_{i \in V} \prod_{k=1}^{K} g_T(y_i; \theta_i^k)^{a_{ik}} =$$

$\arg\max_{\theta \in \underline{\Theta}} p(\theta) \prod_{c \in \mathcal{C}} \prod_{k=1}^{K} \prod_{i \in V_c} g_T(y_i; \theta_c^k)^{a_{ik}}$, where $a_{ik} = q_{T_i}^{(r)}(e_k) q_{S_i}^{(r)}(e_{L+1}') + \sum_{l \, st. T^l = e_k} q_{S_i}^{(r)}(e_l)$. The second term in a_{ik} is the probability that voxel i belongs to one of the structures made of tissue k. The a_{ik}'s sum to one (over k) and a_{ik} can be interpreted as the probability for voxel i to belong to the tissue class k when both tissue and structure segmentations information are combined. Using the additional natural assumption that $p(\theta) = \prod_{k=1}^{K} p(\theta^k)$, it is equivalent to solve for each $k = 1 \dots K$, $\theta^{k\,(r+1)} = \arg\max_{\theta^k \in \underline{\Theta}^k} p(\theta^k) \prod_{c \in \mathcal{C}} \prod_{i \in V_c} g_T(y_i; \theta_c^k)^{a_{ik}}$.

However, when $p(\theta^k)$ is chosen as a Markov field, the exact maximization (5.2) is still intractable. We therefore replace $p(\theta^k)$ by a product form given by its *modal-field* approximation [16]. This is actually equivalent to use the ICM [17] algorithm. Assuming a current estimation $\theta^{k\,(\nu)}$ of θ^k at iteration ν, we consider in turn,

$$\forall c \in \mathcal{C}, \quad \theta_c^{k\,(\nu+1)} = \arg\max_{\theta_c^k \in \underline{\Theta}^k} p(\theta_c^k \mid \theta_{\mathcal{N}(c)}^{k\,(\nu)}) \prod_{i \in V_c} g_T(y_i; \theta_c^k)^{a_{ik}} , \qquad (10)$$

where $\mathcal{N}(c)$ denotes the indices of the subvolumes that are neighbors of subvolume c and $\theta_{\mathcal{N}(c)}^k = \{\theta_{c'}^k, c' \in \mathcal{N}(c)\}$. At convergence, the obtained values give the updated estimation $\theta^{k\,(r+1)}$.

The particular form (10) above guides the specification of the prior for θ. Indeed, Bayesian analysis indicates that a natural choice for $p(\theta_c^k \mid \theta_{\mathcal{N}(c)}^k)$ has to be among conjugate or semi-conjugate priors for the Gaussian distribution $g_T(y_i; \theta_c^k)$. We choose to consider here the latter case. In addition, we assume that the Markovian dependence applies only to the mean parameters and consider that $p(\theta_c^k \mid \theta_{\mathcal{N}(c)}^k) = p(\mu_c^k \mid \mu_{\mathcal{N}(c)}^k) \, p(\lambda_c^k)$, with $p(\mu_c^k \mid \mu_{\mathcal{N}(c)}^k)$ set to a Gaussian distribution with mean $m_c^k + \sum_{c' \in \mathcal{N}(c)} \eta_{cc'}^k (\mu_{c'}^k - m_{c'}^k)$ and precision λ_c^{0k}, and $p(\lambda_c^k)$

set to a Gamma distribution with shape parameter α_c^k and scale parameter b_c^k. The quantities $\{m_c^k, \lambda_c^{0k}, \alpha_c^k, b_c^k, c \in \mathcal{C}\}$ and $\{\eta_{cc'}^k, c' \in \mathcal{N}(c)\}$ are hyperparameters to be specified. For this choice, we get valid joint Markov models for the μ^k's (and therefore for the θ^k's) which are known as auto-normal [18] models. Whereas for the standard Normal-Gamma conjugate prior the resulting conditional densities fail in defining a proper joint model and caution must be exercised.

Standard Bayesian computations lead to a decomposition of (10) into two maximizations: for μ_k^c, the product in (10) has a Gaussian form and the mode is given by its mean. For λ_k^c, the product turns into a Gamma distribution and its mode is given by the ratio of its shape parameter over its scale parameter. After some straightforward algebra, we get the following updating formulas:

$$\mu_c^{(\nu+1)\,k} = \frac{\lambda_c^{(\nu)\,k} \sum_{i \in V_c} a_{ik} y_i + \lambda_c^{0k} (m_c^k + \sum_{c' \in \mathcal{N}(c)} \eta_{cc'}^k (\mu_{c'}^{(\nu)\,k} - m_{c'}^k))}{\lambda_c^{(\nu)\,k} \sum_{i \in V_c} a_{ik} + \lambda_c^{0k}} \quad (11)$$

$$\text{and} \quad \lambda_c^{(\nu+1)\,k} = \frac{\alpha_c^k + \sum_{i \in V_c} a_{ik}/2 - 1}{b_c^k + 1/2[\sum_{i \in V_c} a_{ik}(y_i - \mu_c^{(\nu+1)\,k})^2]} \quad (12)$$

In these equations, quantities similar to the ones computed in standard EM for the mean and variance parameters appear weighted with other terms due to neighbors information. Namely, standard EM on voxels of V_c would estimate μ_c^k as $\sum_{i \in V_c} a_{ik} y_i / \sum_{i \in V_c} a_{ik}$ and λ_c^k as $\sum_{i \in V_c} a_{ik} / \sum_{i \in V_c} a_{ik}(y_i - \mu_c^k)^2$. In that sense formulas (11) and (12) intrinsically encode cooperations between local models.

From these parameters values constant over subvolumes we compute parameter values per voxel by using cubic splines interpolation between θ_c and $\theta_{c'}$ for all $c' \in \mathcal{N}(c)$. We go back this way to our general setting which has the advantage to ensure smooth variation between neighboring subvolumes and to intrinsically handle nonuniformity of intensity inside each subvolume.

The key-point emphasized by these last derivations of our E and M steps is that it is possible to go from a joint cooperative model to an alternating procedure in which each step reduces to an intuitive well identified task. The goal of the above developments was to propose a well based strategy to reach such derivations. When cooperation exists, intuition is that it should be possible to specify stages where each variable of interest is considered in turn but in a way that uses the other variables current information. Interpretation is easier because in each such stage the central part is played by one of the variable at a time. Inference is facilitated because each step can be recast into a well identified (Hidden MRF) setting for which a number of estimation techniques are available.

6   Results

We choose not to estimate the parameters η_T and η_S but fixed them to the inverse of a decreasing temperature as proposed in [17]. In expressions (11) and (12), we considered a general case but it is natural and common to simplify the derivations by setting the m_c^k's to zero and $\eta_{cc'}^k$ to $|\mathcal{N}(c)|^{-1}$ where $|\mathcal{N}(c)|$ is the number of subvolumes in $\mathcal{N}(c)$. This means that the distribution $p(\mu_c^k|\mu_{\mathcal{N}(c)}^k)$ is a Gaussian centered at $\sum_{c'\in\mathcal{N}(c)}\mu_{c'}^k/|\mathcal{N}(c)|$ and therefore that all neighbors c' of c act with the same weight. The precision parameters λ_c^{0k} is set to $N_c\lambda_g^k$ where λ_g^k is a rough precision estimation for class k obtained for instance using some standard EM algorithm run globally on the entire volume and N_c is the number of voxels in c that accounts for the effect of the sample size on precisions. The α_c^k's were set to $|\mathcal{N}(c)|$ and b_c^k to $|\mathcal{N}(c)|/\lambda_g^k$ so that the mean of the corresponding Gamma distribution is λ_g^k and the shape parameter α_c^k somewhat accounts for the contribution of the $|\mathcal{N}(c)|$ neighbors. Then, the size of subvolumes is set to $20 \times 20 \times 20$ voxels. The subvolume size is a mildly sensitive parameter. In practice, subvolume sizes from $20 \times 20 \times 20$ to $30 \times 30 \times 30$ give similar good results on high resolution images ($1\ mm^3$). On low resolution images, a size of $25 \times 25 \times 25$ may be preferred.

Evaluation was then performed following the two main aspects of our model. The first aspect is the partitioning of the global clustering task into a set of local clustering tasks using local MRF models. The advantage of our approach is that, in addition, a way to ensure consistency between all these local models is dictated by the model itself. The second aspect is the cooperative setting which is relevant when two global clustering tasks are considered simultaneously. It follows that we first assessed the performance of our model considering the local aspect only. We compared (Section 6.1) the results obtained with our method, restricted to tissue segmentation only, with other recent or state-of-the-art methods for tissue segmentation. We then illustrate more of the modeling ability of our approach by showing results for the joint tissue and structure segmentation (Section 6.2). As in [19], [20], [21], for a quantitative evaluation, we used the Dice similarity metric [22] measuring the overlap between a segmentation result and the gold standard.

6.1 A Local Method for Segmenting Tissues

We first carried out tissue segmentation only (FBM-T) and compare the results with LOCUS-T [4], FAST [23] from FSL and SPM5 [19] on both BrainWeb [24] phantoms (Table 1) and real 3T brain scans (Figure 4). Our method shows

Table 1. FBM-T. Mean Dice metric and mean computational time (M.C.T) values on BrainWeb over 8 experiments for different values of noise (3%, 5%, 7%, 9%) and nonuniformity (20%, 40%)

	CSF	GM	WM	M.C.T
FBM-T	79.9 %	91.6 %	93.6 %	$\approx$ 4min
LOCUS-T	79.8 %	91.8 %	93.7 %	$\approx$ 4min
SPM5	79.5 %	89.2 %	90.4 %	$\approx$ 12min
FAST	79.6 %	91.3 %	94.1 %	$\approx$ 8min

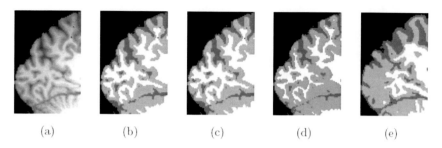

Fig. 4. FBM-T. Segmentations respectively by FBM-T (b), LOCUS-T (c), SPM5 (d) and FAST (e) of a highly nonuniform real 3T image (a)

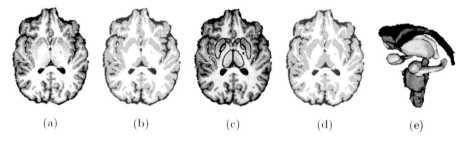

Fig. 5. Evaluation of FBM-TS on a real 3T brain scan (a). For comparison the tissue segmentation obtained with FBM-T is shown in (b). Images (c) and (d): structure segmentation by FBM-TS and corresponding improved tissue segmentation. Image (e): 3-D reconstruction of the 17 segmented structures: the two lateral ventricules, caudates, accumbens, putamens, thalamus, pallidums, hippocampus, amygdalas and the brain stem. The computational time was $< 15min$ after the registration step

very satisfying robustness to noise and intensity nonuniformity. On BrainWeb images, it is better than SPM5 and comparable to LOCUS-T and FAST, for a low computational time. The mean Dice metric over all eight experiments and for all tissues is 86% for SPM5, 88% for FAST and 89% for LOCUS-T and FBM-T. The mean computation times for the full 3-D segmentation were 4min for LOCUS-T and FBM-T, 8min for FAST and more than 10min for SPM5. On real 3T scans, LOCUS-T and SPM5 also give in general satisfying results.

6.2   Joint Tissue and Structure Segmentation

We then evaluated the performance of the joint tissue and structure segmentation (FBM-TS). We introduced *a priori* knowledge based on the Harvard-Oxford subcortical probabilistic atlas[1]. Figures 5 and 6 show an evaluation on real 3T brain scans, using FLIRT [25][2] to affine-register the atlas. In Figures 5 and 6,

---

[1] http://www.fmrib.ox.ac.uk/fsl/

[2] http://www.fmrib.ox.ac.uk/fsl/flirt/

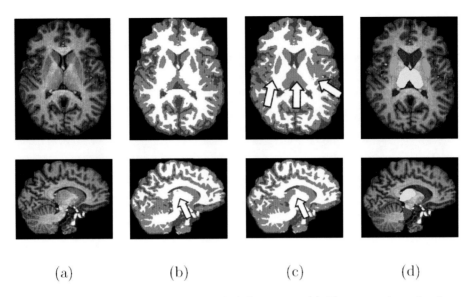

(a)   (b)   (c)   (d)

Fig. 6. Evaluation of FBM-TS on a real 3T brain scan (a). For comparison the tissue segmentation obtained with FBM-T is shown in (b). The tissue segmentation obtained with FBM-TS is given in (c). Major differences between tissue segmentations (images (b) and (c)) are pointed out using arrows. Image (d) shows the structure segmentation with FBM-TS

the gain obtained with tissue and structure cooperation is particularly clear for the putamens and thalamus.

We also computed via STAPLE [26] a structure gold standard using three manual expert segmentations of BrainWeb images. We considered the left caudate, left putamen and left thalamus which are of special interest in various neuroanatomical studies and compared the results with LOCUS-TS [4] and FreeSurfer (see Table 2). FBM-TS lower results for the caudate were due to a bad registration of the atlas in this region. For the putamen and thalamus the improvement is respectively of 14.7% and 20.3%. Due to high computational times, only the 5% noise, 40% nonuniformity image was considered with Freesurfer. For this image, results obtained for FBM-TS were respectively 74%,

Table 2. FBM-T. Mean Dice metric and mean computational time (M.C.T) values on BrainWeb over 8 experiments for different values of noise (3%, 5%, 7%, 9%) and nonuniformity (20%, 40%)

	CSF	GM	WM	M.C.T
FBM-T	79.9 %	91.6 %	93.6 %	≈ 4min
LOCUS-T	79.8 %	91.8 %	93.7 %	≈ 4min
SPM5	79.5 %	89.2 %	90.4 %	≈ 12min
FAST	79.6 %	91.3 %	94.1 %	≈ 8min

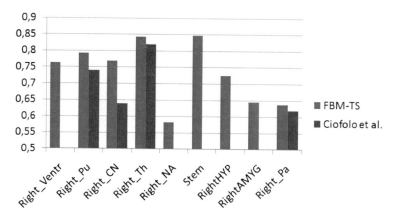

Fig. 7. Evaluation of FBM-TS on IBSR v2 (9 right structures) and comparison with [27]. Y axis = Mean Dice metric

84%, 91% for caudate, putamen and thalamus. We then considered 18 images from the IBSR v2 database. The mean Dice metric for the 9 right structures (17 were segmented) is reported in Figure 7.

7   Discussion

The results obtained with our approach are very satisfying and compare favorably with other existing methods. The strength of our fully Bayesian joint model is to be based on the specification of a coherently linked system of conditional models for which we make full use of modern statistics to ensure tractability. The tissue and structure models are linked conditional MRF's that capture several level of interactions. They incorporate 1) spatial dependencies between voxels for robustness to noise, 2) relationships between tissue and structure labels for cooperative aspects and 3) *a priori* anatomical information via the MRF external field parameters for consistency with expert knowledge.

Besides, the addition of a conditional MRF model on the intensity distribution parameters allows us to handle local estimations for robustness to nonuniformities. In this setting, the whole consistent treatment of MR brain scans is made possible using the framework of Generalized Alternating Minimization (GAM) procedures that generalize the standard EM framework. Another advantage of this approach is that it is made of steps that are easy to interpret and could be enriched with additional information. In particular, results currently highly depend on the atlas registration step which could be introduced in our framework as in [28]. A step in this direction is proposed in [29]. Also a different kind of prior knowledge could be considered such as the fuzzy spatial relations used in [4].

Other on going work relates to the interpolation step we added to increase robustness to nonuniformities at a voxel level. We believe this stage could be generalized and incorporated in the model by considering successively various degrees of locality, mimicking a multi resolution approach and refining from coarse partitions of the entire volume to finer ones.

Also considering more general weights w, to deal with possible conflicts between tissue and structure labels, is possible in our framework and would be an interesting refinement. Eventually, our choice of prior for the intensity distribution parameters was guided by the need to define appropriate conditional specifications $p(\theta_c^k | \theta_{\mathcal{N}(c)}^{k(\nu)})$ in (10) that lead to a valid Markov model for the θ^k's. Nevertheless, incompatible conditional specifications can still be used for inference, $eg.$ in a Gibbs sampler or ICM algorithm with some valid justification (see [30] or the discussion in [31]). In applications, one may found that having a joint distribution is less important than incorporating information from other variables such as typical interactions. In that sense, conditional modeling allows enormous flexibility in dealing with practical problems. However, it is not clear when incompatibility of conditional distributions is an issue in practice and the theoretical properties of the procedures in this case are largely unknown and should be investigated.

In terms of algorithmic efficiency, our agent-based approach enables us to by-pass computationally intensive implementations usually inherent to MRF models. It results in very competitive computational times unusual for such structured models.

References

1. Shattuck, D.W., Sandor-Leahy, S.R., Schaper, K.A., Rottenberg, D.A., Leahy, R.M.: Magnetic resonance image tissue classification using a partial volume model. NeuroImage 13(5), 856–876 (2001)
2. Rajapakse, J.C., Giedd, J.N., Rapoport, J.L.: Statistical approach to segmentation of single-channel cerebral MR images. IEEE Trans. Med. Imag. 16(2), 176–186 (1997)
3. Scherrer, B., Dojat, M., Forbes, F., Garbay, C.: LOCUS: LOcal Cooperative Unified Segmentation of MRI brain scans. In: Ayache, N., Ourselin, S., Maeder, A. (eds.) MICCAI 2007, Part I. LNCS, vol. 4791, pp. 1066–1074. Springer, Heidelberg (2007)
4. Scherrer, B., Forbes, F., Garbay, C., Dojat, M.: Distributed Local MRF Models for Tissue and Structure Brain Segmentation. IEEE Trans. Med. Imag. 28, 1296–1307 (2009)
5. Scherrer, B., Forbes, F., Garbay, C., Dojat, M.: Fully Bayesian Joint Model for MR Brain Scan Tissue and Structure Segmentation. In: Metaxas, D., Axel, L., Fichtinger, G., Székely, G. (eds.) MICCAI 2008, Part II. LNCS, vol. 5242, pp. 1066–1074. Springer, Heidelberg (2008)
6. Byrne, W., Gunawardana, A.: Convergence theorems of Generalized Alternating Minimization Procedures. J. Machine Learning Research 6, 2049–2073 (2005)
7. Shariatpanahi, H.F., Batmanghelich, N., Kermani, A.R.M., Ahmadabadi, M.N., Soltanian-Zadeh, H.: Distributed behavior-based multi-agent system for automatic segmentation of brain MR images. In: International Joint Conference on Neural Networks, IJCNN 2006 (2006)
8. Richard, N., Dojat, M., Garbay, C.: Distributed Markovian segmentation: Application to MR brain scans. Pattern Recognition 40(12), 3467–3480 (2007)

 9. Germond, L., Dojat, M., Taylor, C., Garbay, C.: A cooperative framework for segmentation of MRI brain scans. Artificial Intelligence in Medicine 20, 77–94 (2000)
10. Scherrer, B., Dojat, M., Forbes, F., Garbay, C.: Agentification of Markov model based segmentation: Application to magnetic resonance brain scans. Artificial Intelligence in Medicine 46, 81–95 (2009)
11. McLachlan, G.J., Krishnan, T.: The EM Algorithm and Extensions. Wiley, Chichester (1996)
12. Gelman, A., Carlin, J.B., Stern, H.S., Rubin, D.B.: Bayesian Data Analysis, 2nd edn. Chapman and Hall, Boca Raton (2004)
13. Lafferty, J., McCallum, A., Peirera, F.: Conditional Random Fields: Probabilistic models for segmenting and labelling sequence data. In: 18th Inter. Conf. on Machine Learning (2001)
14. Minka, T.: Discriminative models not discriminative training. Tech. Report MSR-TR-2005-144, Microsoft Research (2005)
15. Jordan, M.I., Ghahramani, Z., Jaakkola, T.S., Saul, L.K.: An introduction to variational methods for graphical models. In: Jordan, M.I. (ed.) Learning in Graphical Models, pp. 105–162. The MIT Press, Cambridge (1999)
16. Celeux, G., Forbes, F., Peyrard, N.: EM procedures using mean field-like approximations for Markov model-based image segmentation. Pat. Rec. 36, 131–144 (2003)
17. Besag, J.: On the statistical analysis of dirty pictures. J. Roy. Statist. Soc. Ser. B 48(3), 259–302 (1986)
18. Besag, J.: Spatial interaction and the statistical analysis of lattice systems. J. Roy. Statist. Soc. Ser. B 36(2), 192–236 (1974)
19. Ashburner, J., Friston, K.J.: Unified Segmentation. NeuroImage 26, 839–851 (2005)
20. Shattuck, D.W., Sandor-Leahy, S.R., Schaper, K.A., Rottenberg, D.A., Leahy, R.M.: Magnetic resonance image tissue classification using a partial volume model. NeuroImage 13, 856–876 (2001)
21. Van Leemput, K., Maes, F., Vandermeulen, D., Suetens, P.: Automated model-based bias field correction in MR images of the brain. IEEE Trans. Med. Imag. 18, 885–896 (1999)
22. Dice, L.R.: Measures of the amount of ecologic association between species. Ecology 26, 297–302 (1945)
23. Zhang, Y., Brady, M., Smith, S.: Segmentation of brain MR images through a hidden Markov random field model and the Expectation-Maximisation algorithm. IEEE Trans. Med. Imag. 20, 45–47 (2001)
24. Collins, D.L., Zijdenbos, A.P., Kollokian, V., Sled, J.G., Kabani, N.J., Holmes, C.J., Evans, A.C.: Design and construction of a realistic digital brain phantom. IEEE Trans. Med. Imag. 17, 463–468 (1998)
25. Jenkinson, M., Smith, S.M.: A global optimisation method for robust affine registration of brain images. Medical Image Analysis 5, 143–156 (2001)
26. Warfield, S.K., Zou, K.H., Wells, W.M.: Simultaneous truth and performance level estimation (STAPLE): An algorithm for the validation of image segmentation. IEEE Trans. Med. Imag. 23, 903–921 (2004)
27. Ciofolo, C., Barillot, C.: Atlas-based segmentation of 3d cerebral structures with competitive level sets and fuzzy control. Medical Image Analysis 13, 456–470 (2009)
28. Pohl, K.M., Fisher, J., Grimson, E., Kikinis, R., Wells, W.: A Bayesian model for joint segmentation and registration. NeuroImage 31, 228–239 (2006)

29. Scherrer, B., Forbes, F., Garbay, C., Dojat, M.: A Conditional Random Field approach for coupling local registration with robust tissue and structure segmentation. In: Yang, G.-Z., Hawkes, D., Rueckert, D., Noble, A., Taylor, C. (eds.) MICCAI 2009. LNCS, vol. 5762, pp. 540–548. Springer, Heidelberg (2009)
30. Heckerman, D., Chickering, D.M., Meek, C., Rounthwaite, R., Kadie, C.: Dependency networks for inference, collaborative filtering and data visualization .J Machine Learning Research 1, 49–75 (2000)
31. Arnold, B.C., Castillo, E., Sarabia, J.M.: Conditionally specified distributions: an introduction. Statistical Science 16(3), 249–274 (2001)

Chapter 6
The i-Walker: An Intelligent Pedestrian Mobility Aid

C. Barrué[1], R. Annicchiarico[2], U. Cortés[1], A. Martínez-Velasco[1],
E.X. Martín[1], F. Campana[3], and C. Caltagirone[2,4]

[1] Universitat Politècnica de Catalunya, Spain
{cbarrue,ia}@lsi.upc.edu
[2] Fondazione Santa Lucia, Italy
r.annicchiarico@hsantalucia.it
[3] Centri Assistenza Domiciliare, Italy
fcampana@tiscali.it
[4] Universita Tor Vergata, Italy

Abstract. In this chapter we focus on the development of an intelligent pedestrian mobility aid for the elders that we call *i-Walker*. The target population includes, but is not limited to, persons with low vision, visual field neglect, spasticity, tremors, and cognitive deficits. The *SHARE-it* architecture will provide an Agent-based Intelligent Decision Support System to aid the elders.

1 Introduction

Already in 1993, Stephanidis *et al* [25] identified two key factors which have had a profound impact on society and have influenced demographic changes: the rapid technological advances and the dramatic improvements in medical treatment and care. Both have led to a reduction of the mortality rate of disease or accident stricken patients, and have contributed to a general increase of life expectancy of the population at large. These effects have, in turn, precipitated a significant increase of the proportion of the population that is characterised by some handicap with respect to the surrounding environment, either as a consequence of some impairment resulting from disability, or as a consequence of some impairment resulting from old age.

It is clear that one of the most important and critical factors in quality of life (QoL) for the elderly is their ability to move about independently and safely. Mobility issues, both inside and outside the home, included challenges to personal mobility in terms of walking in the neighbourhood and use of public transport. Mobility impairments due to age, injury or disease cause a downward trend in their QoL. Lack of independence and exercise can have dramatic results. One of the *SHARE-it*, an EU-funded research project, main objectives is concerned with developing intelligent mobility tools for the elders. Among those tools we have developed an Intelligent Walker, that we called *i-Walker*, to assist the elderly and increase the ease and safety of their daily mobility. The benefits to the user include assistance avoiding dangerous situations (obstacles, drops, *etc.*) and help with navigation through cluttered but well-known environments. Many older adults use walkers to improve their stability and safety while walking. It is hoped

I. Bichindaritz et al. (Eds.): Computational Intelligence in Healthcare 4, SCI 309, pp. 103–123.
springerlink.com

that this assistance will provide the users with a feeling of safety and autonomy that will encourage them to move about more, incurring the benefits of walking and helping them to carry out the activities of daily living (ADLs).

Another related problem is the lack of strength in target population. Doctors make us conscious of the possible uneven loss of strength in the extremities. This of course is the main reason for having troubles in arising from a chair, in walking, being unable to steer a normal walker, being unable to standing still, *etc.*

We have developed a robotically augmented walker to reduce fall risk and confusion, and to increase walker convenience and enjoyment. Among of the *SHARE-it* objectives were to build different *i-Walker* workbench platforms, oriented to demonstrate their feasibility, and gain the confidence to support the specific disabilities [6].

The idea of building robotic walking aids is not new. This robotic aids are equipped with mechanisms for communication, interaction, and behaviors are employed more and more outside the industrial and experimental settings and are arriving to serve elder citizens or people with disabilities to make them less dependable and therefore augmenting their personal autonomy. Most existing robotic devices are active aids – meaning that they are capable to share control over motion with the user – and are aimed at obstacle avoidance and path navigation. Two inspiring works in this line for pedestrian aids are [10][29].

1.1 Plan of the Chapter

The rest of this chapter is organized as follows: In section 2 we make a general description of the target population. In section 3 we introduce our ideas on Shared Autonomy related with the support to the elders. In section 4 we introduce our new intelligent pedestrian mobility aid that we call *i-Walker*. We also introduce in this section the agent-based control elements.

In section 5 we introduce the generic scenarios and in section 6 the *i-Walker* benchmark is described where the *i-Walker* is currently in limited testing, to assure its safeness and soundness, before to go to a full-scale testing with real users from the target population. In section 7 we present our conclusions and future plans for this research in the frame of *SHARE-it*.

2 Aging and Mobility

Transportation and mobility are closely linked to autonomy, well being, and quality of life. A critical factor in an older person's ability to function independently is mobility, the ability to move without assistance [12,9] . Older people who lose mobility are less likely to remain in the community, have higher rates of morbidity and mortality, have more hospitalizations, and experience a poorer QoL [1].

In fact, mobility in addition to represent one of the most important Basic ADL – like defined in the Bartel Index [16] – is directly involved in many basic and instrumental ADL activities like transferring, grooming, toileting, housekeeping, etc. For adults, independent mobility is an important aspect of self-esteem and plays a pivotal role in *aging in place* [24]. For example- as Simpson suggest- if older people find it increasingly difficult to walk or wheel themselves to the commode, they may do so less often or they may drink less fluid to reduce the frequency of urination. If they become unable to walk or wheel themselves to the commode and help is not routinely available in the home when needed, a move to a more enabling environment (*e.g.*, assisted living) may be necessary. Moreover, impaired mobility often results in decreased opportunities to socialize, which leads to social isolation, anxiety, and depression [13]. This is why we focused our attention in mobility and their related activities as crucial issue to guarantee autonomy in elderly and disabled people.

In order to quantify residual autonomy and level of disability of individuals, it is commonly accepted to talk in terms of Functional Disability and Functional Status. In fact, Functional Status is usually conceptualized as the *ability to perform self-care, self-maintenance and physical activities*. Behind that, physical, neurological, and mental functions, and conditions and diseases affecting such functions are to be taken into account as well.

Subjects affected by chronic diseases or outcomes of acute events, (stroke, arthritis, hypertension, cancer, degenerative bone/joint disease, coronary artery disease) represent a heterogeneous category of individuals. Each patient may be affected by at least one of these symptoms: ambulatory impairment, memory loss, staggering gait, ataxia, visuo-spatial dysfunction, aphasia, etc. Moreover, each and every one of these features can be often combined differently and with different severity in individual patients, impairing their self-dependency and worsening their quality of life. Global declines and alterations in motor coordination, spatial perception, visual and auditory acuity, gait, muscle and bone strength, mobility, and sensory perceptions of environmental stimuli (heat, cold) with increasing age are well documented, as are increases in chronic diseases and their disabling sequels [7].

The simultaneous presence of cognitive and mobility impairments has a multiplicative effect, worsening global function more than expected by the sum of the single conditions.

Cognition and mobility heavily affect the capacity of daily planning. For an activity to be effective implies that the person is capable of performing it when he/she wants to or when it is necessary: the possibility of successfully performing daily life connected activities implies the chance of remaining or not in the community.

As a consequence, the capacity of performing ADLs becomes an important indicator of self-dependency or disability, is used as a comprehensive measure in disabled people, and can be chosen as a marker of Functional Status.

It is then mandatory to consider age-related Functional Status impairment among senior citizens when developing devices to improve disability, and to judge their effectiveness in maintaining and improving self-dependency in terms of ADLs.

According to these premises is quite manifest that independent mobility is critical to individuals of any age. While the needs of many individuals with mobility restrictions can be satisfied with standard wheelchairs or power wheelchairs and with standard walkers, some citizens with disabilities find it difficult or impossible to operate a standard aid for mobility. This population includes, but is not limited to, individuals with low vision, visual field neglect, tremors, or cognitive deficits. In these cases, a caregiver is required to grant mobility. In order to minimize caregiver support requirements for providing mobility, aids for mobility can be equipped with an autonomous navigation architecture to assist the user in the control of the aid (like the *i-Walker*, see Figure §1).

- real environments are hard to predict and highly dynamic (people move around, doors open and close, schedules change, emergencies arise, *etc.*);
- platforms should be such that they can be easily reused and adapted to already available resources; and
- it is of key importance to adapt to the users needs and to avoid providing more support than necessary or to disregard his/her wishes to prevent emotional distress; hence, in most cases control is *shared* between the user and the autonomous navigation system and the amount of control exerted by the system depends of the users condition, which may change depending on his/her actual physical/mental condition.

2.1   Acceptability

Finding the right assistive device for each person is not an easy task. Assistive tools have the potential to narrow the gap between an individuals capacity and their environment, and therefore to make it easier for people to remain in his/her preferred environment. The extent to which these tools can narrow the gap depends on elders willingness to use it [18]. The extent to which AT can narrow the gap depends on older peoples willingness to use it, which in turn depends on several complex factors :

- the needs that people perceive,
- safety, may be the most important the perceived usefulness of the AT,
- soundness and,
- degree of autonomy that the assistive tool guarantees to the user

That is why among the *SHARE-it* objectives we pursue the idea of personalization. Personalization implies a large amount of knowledge about the user's abilities and limitations, his/her environment, his/her clinical information, *etc* in order to identify which elements of the aiding tool have to be adapted, when and by whom. Personalization should be a sound, safe and easy and adaptive process. Agents have shown to be a solid option to accomplish this aim.

An open research topic is the acceptability of this technology among elders [19]. Senior citizens facing some disabilities need to find this technology *easy* to learn to use as well as be confident with its usage in their preferred environment. This implies an effort to provide the appropriate infrastructure elsewhere. Also, it should be easy and affordable to adapt these technological solutions to different existing environments.

3   Shared Autonomy: A Vision

Autonomy for the elderly or people with disabilities does not only rely on mobility terms, but on a set of domains influenced by functioning, activity limitations, participation restrictions and environmental factors [28]. Life areas related to activities and participation are such as learning and applying knowledge, general tasks and demands, communication, mobility, self-care, interpersonal interactions and relationships as well as community and social life. All these domains can be affected by aging or disabilities and are the base of personal autonomy and the satisfactory participation on them reflects on the self well-being. Assistive Technologies (AT) are of special interest, as the average age of the population increases fast [4,22]. AT can participate in these activities in order to enhance the user's autonomy, gathering all the environmental information and making use of it properly.

Our idea is based on the notion of a *Shared Autonomy* between the user and its own agent-based mediator with any information system at hand. Existing telematic healthcare systems that provide integrated services to users are not, to our taste, enough flexible to allow a real personalization and maybe now it is too expensive to change them.

The shared autonomy concept is scarcely explored in literature and often it is misunderstood as shared control (*e.g.*, [27,14]). In the personal autonomy and disability context, two different scenarios of the shared autonomy can be elicitaded.

- People presenting mainly physical impairments are able to define their own goals, but due to their restrictions they usually are not able to execute them, suffering a limitation in their autonomy. In this scenario the contribution of AT focus on physical devices, mostly mobility hardware, that allow them to reach their objectives. These devices may be controlled by multi-agent systems or through an agent supervised shared control if the user motor capabilities are not severely damaged. In this scenario, user interfaces are very important to detect the user intention, which is critical to define goals for the wheelchair to be able to assist him/her.
- People presenting mostly cognitive impairments may require a different kind of assistive aids, which may lead even a more relevant role in the sharing of personal autonomy. In this scenario the user probably does not have very clear goals or is not capable of achieving them because he/she cannot remember *how* to do them. In these cases, AT may empower and complement their autonomy using agents that offer them a set of services, like reminding what kind of activities they can or should perform at a certain moment of the day or pointing them out how to achieve these activities. The main idea is to offer the users a set of cognitive aids, either rational or memory based, that can ease their daily living.

Roboticists have developed a number of mobility-enhancing assistive technologies. Most of these are active aids, meaning as said before, that they share control over motion with the user. Most are aimed at obstacle avoidance and path navigation [26][10][15].

4   i-Walker

With this context in mind, we introduced in [6] the design of an integrated architecture aimed at helping citizens with disabilities to improve their autonomy in structured, dynamic environments. The main element of this architecture is an intelligent agent layer that mediates between different technology components (robotic devices –as the *i-Walker*– ubiquitous computing, and interfaces) in order to provide the subject with the necessary degree of independent mobility to benefit from different assistive services and to reach goals determined by either the subject himself/herself or by medical staff.

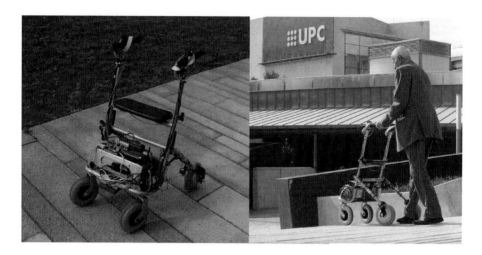

Fig. 1. i-Walker

The agent based control system provides an excellent means to model the different required autonomous elements in the patient's environment (from control elements in the walker to care-giving services). Agents probe to be efficient in coordinating heterogeneous domain-specific elements with different levels of autonomy. Addressing the mobility problem and keeping in mind that different users need different degrees of help, a part of this agent based control layer has been focused on the development of a shared control for the robotic walker that adapts to the user needs.

The *i-Walker* is an assistive device with four conventional wheels and two degrees of freedom (see figure 1). Two of these wheels, the ones placed closest to the user, are fixed wheels driven by independent motors. The other two wheels, the ones placed on the front part, are castor-wheels. They can freely rotate around their axis and are self-oriented. The *i-Walker* has two handles, that the user holds with both hands, to interact with it. The *i-Walker* is a passive robot as it will only move if the user moves it.

The mechanical analysis of the Intelligent Walker is focused on the interaction between a generic user and the vehicle, in addition to how the rear wheel motors -which are the only active control available- can modify the user's behaviour and his/her perception of the followed path. For safety reasons, these motors will never result in pulling the *i-Walker* by themselves.

4.1   i-Walker Control Concept

The walker has been designed to be passive, cooperative and submissive (see figure 2).

- Passive because it can only adjust the facing direction of its front wheel, *i.e.* it can steer. However, it has no forward drive motors and so relies on the user for motive force. This allows the walker to move at the user's pace and provides for the user's feeling of control.
- Cooperative because it attempts to infer the user's path and uses this inference to decide *how* to avoid any obstacles in the user's path.

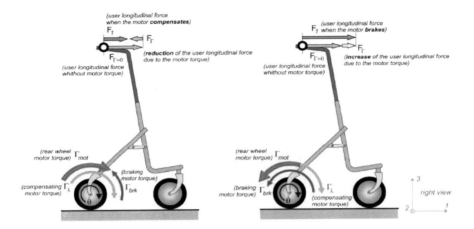

Fig. 2. *i-Walker* Control

- Submissive because it monitors the user to see if s/he is resisting the actions (steering/braking) selected by the walker. If they are, the movements are adjusted. This cycle continues until the user agrees with the motion (*i.e.* does not resist it) or manually over-rides it. This interaction forms the basis of the feedback loop between the user and the agent. Similar approach can be found in [29].

The manual brakes have also been replaced with an automated braking system. The walker can sense the user's steering input via sensors in the handles that detect the difference in force on the two handles.

- Pushing with more force on one handle (left or right), the walker will turn in the opposite direction.
- Applying of equal force on both handles will move the walker straight forward or backward (which direction can be determined by the *i-Walker*'s wheel encoders).

One of the main objectives of *SHARE-it* is helping the users in orienting them when handling the *i-Walker* in a known environment as their home or neighbourhood. The user will receive help from a screen, but the innovative idea will be steering by moderate braking, for helping in navigation. Apart from the multi-modal (in particular speech) interface, we will experiment with moderate brake on the *i-Walker*'s wheels to gain the experience on *how* to better guide the user by allowing s/he sharing with the computer the steering actions.

4.2   Agent Layer

Agents can be defined to be autonomous, problem-solving computational entities capable of effective operation in dynamic and open environments. In Artificial Intelligence research, agent-based systems technology has been hailed as a new paradigm for conceptualizing, designing, and implementing software systems. Agents are often deployed in environments in which they interact, and maybe cooperate with other agents (including both people and software) that have possibly conflicting aims. Such environments are known as multi-agent systems. Agents can be distinguished from objects (in the sense of object-oriented software) in that they are autonomous entities capable of exercising choice over their actions and interactions.

As presented in [17], Multi-agent systems (MAS) are based on the idea that a cooperative distributed working environment comprising synergistic software components can cope with problems which are hard to solve using the traditional centralized approach to computation. Smaller software entities – software agents – with special capabilities are used instead to interact in a flexible and dynamic way to solve problems more efficiently.

Agents are considered to be autonomous (*i.e.*, independent, not-controllable), reactive (*i.e.*, responding to events), pro-active (*i.e.*, initiating actions of their own volition), and social (*i.e.*, communicative). Agents vary in their abilities; *e.g.* they can be static or mobile, or may or may not be intelligent. Each agent may have its own task and/or role. Agents and multi-agent systems are used as a metaphor to model complex distributed processes.

On one hand we considered the *SHARE-it* problem settings, an elder trying to live autonomously at his prefered environment/home burdened with a profile of disability be it cognitive, physical or a combination of both. On the other hand we have the *i-Walker* and other robotic platforms developed to assist these elders, and a specially designed intelligent environment equiped with sensors and ubiquitous communications tools to distribute the information gathered from them. In order to combine this set of sensing tools, process the information that they provide and the functionalities of the different platforms and actuators, we needed an intelligent and distributed approach. Thus, developing a multi-agent system to manage all this information and provide a sort of assistive services to the users, it is the decision we took considering the agent technology capabilities and background.

Rational agents have an explicit representation of their environment (sometimes called world model) and of the objectives they are trying to achieve. Rationality means that the agent will always perform the most promising actions (based on the knowledge about itself and the world) to achieve its objectives. As it usually does not know all of the effects of an action in advance, it has to deliberate about the available options. Regarding the theoretical foundation and the number of implemented and successfully applied systems, the most interesting and widespread agent architecture is the Belief-Desire-Intention (BDI) architecture, introduced by Bratman as a philosophical model for describing rational agents [2]. It consists of the concepts of belief, desire and intention as mental attitudes that generate human action. Beliefs capture informational attitudes, desires motivational attitudes, and intentions deliberative attitudes of agents. [23] have adopted this model and transformed it into a formal theory and an execution model for software agents, based on the notion of beliefs, goals, and plans. The agent development framework JADEX [21] has been our BDI model implementation choice to build the *SHARE-it* multi-agent system.

The *SHARE-it* agent layer architecture (see Fig. 3) focuses on delivering three main kind of services: monitorization, navigation support and cognitive support. This agent

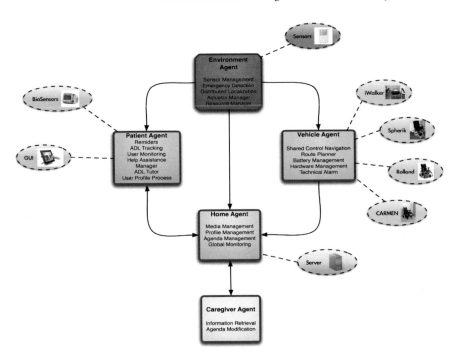

Fig. 3. *SHARE-it* Agent Architecture

system feeds of information gathered from the wide array of sensors included in the Ambient Intelligence environment and the rich positional, force and gait information that the *i-Walker* gets from the user. We will describe in detail the agent architecture along the rest of this section.

Environment Agent (*ea*) is the mechanism used to manage the Ambient Intelligence sensor network installed for the *SHARE-it* project. Its main role is to perform the autonomous data gathering and information extraction from the environment, as well as the interaction with the Ambient Intelligence devices that are included in the usual environment of the users. These sensors provide data, which has to be conveniently stored, filtered and delivered to the MAS, which will provide the autonomous decision and control tasks into *SHARE-it* . Just as an example of the set of Beliefs, Goals and Plans that each of these agents has we include table 1 that includes describes this set for *ea*. The final system ought to be intelligent enough to: (1) distinguish which data from all the available is significant for each one of the components of the system, and deliver them to those components, and (2) extract and infer information from the raw data retrieved from the environment and transform it into meaningful ontology concepts, so a better knowledge of the environment is acquired. Both capabilities will be achieved by means of the *ea*, which also is in charge of:

- Proactively take decisions about the rooms conditioning (e.g. domotic actuators)
- Provide services to the mobile entities (e.g. , localization)
- Process the sensor signals in order to extract meaningful qualitative information related to services tied to those sensors

Table 1. Environment Agent

Environment Agent		
Beliefs	Goals	Plans
Sensing Environmental Set	Sensors connection	Sensors Server
Acting environmental set	Check readings	Check sensor readings
Date	Add capabilities	Add capability
Alarm status	Remove Capability	Remove Capability
Localizations	Add sensor	Add sensor
	Remove Sensor	Remove Sensor
	Add interaction capability	Add interaction capability
	Monitor Status	Sensors connection
		Technical Alarm protocol

- Deploy a base to perform user activity tracking, in order to being able to record or recall user activities of daily living for adaptation and personalization.

Though some of the data presented by the environmental sensors is stored into the general database, the extraction and inference of information from the data provided by these environmental sensors is performed by the ea, which delivers it to the other Agents in the system when required. This information is also used for internal services of the ea, for instance detecting emergencies like a fire and starting up the security protocols defined. The ea also is capable of self-managing the infrastructure, detecting which components stop working and sending a technical alarm message to the administrators in charge, informing about the problem and the conflicting component.

The Patient Agent (pa) encases most of the cognitive support services oriented to the user. The GUI provides a window to access these services and exchange information with the pa. The pa cogntive services try to support memory and disorientation taking as starting point the user disability profile tailored for the MAS. In order to do that, not only a complex profiling work has to be done with each user, but also use the profile information to define which services to launch, and *how* to tune them to adapt to the user in terms of support offered. Moreover, the user's profile can change with time, and the services should adapt to those changes and even add new services to the pack in case the user needs them with his/her new state.

The pa is highly tied to the ea in order to perform activity tracking, follow the user's daily routine using the AmI sensors (*i.e.* presence sensors, detecting when the user access the fridge or the kitchenette, goes to the bathroom in the morning after getting up, etc). This activity tracking is used to enrich the Reminder service, that sends memory cues to the user in order to remind him of key activities that he has to perform along the day like taking the medication, preparing the food or going to the doctor to a programmed visit. This service distinguishes between mandatory activities like taking medication from others like attending an appointment with a friend. Mandatory activities are reminded a few times until a confirmation from the user is given, if that is not the case a SMS message is sent to the agreed caregiver to warn him about the situation. The Reminder service is feed by the Agenda service, that retrieves the programmed agenda from the Home Agent and shows it to the user. The representation of

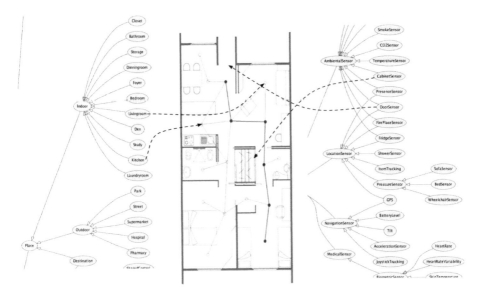

Fig. 4. Integration process in semantic map creation: merging topological maps with ontology concepts.

the agenda differs depending on the degree of cognitive disability of the user, showing less information and in a simpler way in case that disability is moderate or advanced and the probabilities of disorientation are higher. Even with assistive support, unexpected situations may arise in daily live, and when that happens is desirable that the elder user is able to get help when needed. Thus, there exists the Help Assistance service, that lets the user request for help using the interface, that triggers a SMS to the caregiver and provides the user a soothing message foretelling the incoming help. This service not only acts reactively, but also does it proactively for instance when the biometric sensors on the user provide readings under defined thresholds, an alarm SMS is also triggered.

Finally, the Tutorial service is conceived as a user assistant, guiding him/her on how to carry out daily activities such as housekeeping or cooking according to his impairment defined in the user profile of disability. Taking the profile as a point of start, we can determine which kind of activities need support for the user, and *how* this support should be shown to the user. Not all the users will be able to understand vocal intructions or understand icons/symbols. The tutorial service must be prepared to adapt itself the contents depending on the user and the user's evolution through time. We want the ADL tutoring service capable of adapting dynamically to the changing needs and performance of these users, providing them with the level of assistance they require on every situation.

The Vehicle Agent (*VA*) is located in the different robotic vehicle platforms developed for *SHARE-it* like the *i-Walker*. It is intended to keep track of different status indicators (stability, detection of falls, battery charge level, CPU usage of modules, hardware failures, . . .) and to offer several navigation services. Part of the monitorization tasks of the agent is to get feed from information supplied by the *ea* that keeps track of all the environmental sensorization including localization. *SHARE-it* assumes a known environment, so the *va* has available a semantic map of the world with tags (see Fig. 4). The *SHARE-it* agent layer relies on an Ontology for knowledge representation, which includes concepts related to space and contained objects among other facets of the *SHARE-it* system reality. All this relevant semantic information can be integrated with the topological maps in order to obtain a semantic map that the agents can use for higher level planning tasks. This high level information if used for Route planning service, where the user selects a place where it wants to go using room images and the *va* shows him instructions on how to reach there; although available, autonomous navigation is not recommended by doctors, as is does not foster user autonomy and could lead to capacity loses. The *va* also detects falls in the *i-Walker*, generating an alarm to the *pa* to request help to the caregivers just in case the user is hurt or can not get up. Like the *ea*, the *va* performs component monitoring and when some of the system part stop working, generates a *SMS* Technical alarm that is sent to the administrators to take care of it. The users navigation is also monitored, and depending on the users health status and profile, the agent will make decisions on the degree of control the user will have on navigation. The *va* can modulate the amount of force the user has to do on each handlebar or the amount of help he gets on them. Monitoring the user forces behaviour and merging that information with his updated disability profile, the agent can modulate the exervice or help granted to the user on every situation.

The Home Agent (*ha*) performs a global monitoring task, and stores all the media information needed for the personalized interface of the users or the media files used to build up the dynamic tutorials. The *ha* also stores the agenda or the user profiles that are sent to the *pa* regularly. The Caregiver Agent (*ca*) is a information frontend that allows the caregivers to watch whats going on with the elder user, if any alarms have been raised, which activities have been performed along the day or to access the user agenda and modify its entries.

Multi-agent systems have both the flexibility and the cognitive capabilities required in order to be able to support the needs of persons with different disability profiles and to complement the autonomy of the people with special needs in an adaptative way through the time. In some cases the disability is a consequence of a pathology, that may improve with some time and rehabilitation. An excess of support or lack of flexibility in the support can make this process more difficult, on the other hand an assistance adaptive to the daily state of the patient may be helpful in the rehabilitation process. Agents have proven their capacity of being flexible, adaptable and learn from experiences with the proper design.

Some patients may dislike an autonomous navigation system, or choosing among a set of maneuvers, they may prefer driving by themselves, to feel autonomous and in charge of the situation at all times. An intelligent agent with the necessary knowledge of a user's profile can supervise user's navigation and take part in some driving maneuvers, in a transparent way, in case the user needs some support (*e.g.* help crossing doorways, refining turning maneuvers, help keeping stable cruise navigation, ...).

In order to make this possible the user's agent must have to have deep knowledge of the user's disability profile and historical data about his/her driving behaviour, merge all this knowledge and translate it in control support and a set of assistive services. All this knowledge and information must be updated dynamically, since the user can progress in either good or bad way or just can have a good/bad day driving-wise. The knowledge learnt by each agent would be shared and distributed among other agents that have users with similar profiles so they can take advantage of the experiences traced by the first one. Agent's responsibility grows with the measure of his active intervention in the user's autonomy is exerted. This means a heavier charge of *obligations* regarding safety and soundness in the undertaken actions [8].

5   Generic Scenarios

Devices have been used to *assist* people with cognitive and/or physical disabilities to complete various tasks for almost 20 years. What represents a change and challenge are the abilities embedded in a new generation of tools that are able to cooperate with the user to complete a task. This implies that these new tools are context-aware and are able to learn from the interaction with the user.

Cooperation for problem solving between users and their *agent* and the cooperation between *agents* among themselves requires some kind of model which at least describes *what to expect from whom* in terms of questions, actions, *etc* and that uses previous experiences and trust.

Scenarios appear to be an easy and appropriate way to create partitions of the world and to relate them with time. Scenarios allow actions to be performed in a given time. For example, Mihailidis *et al.*, in [20], studied the *handwashing* scenario where a full instrumented environment was used to provide users with cues to support the completion of this task.

As in Mihalilidis' approach we are looking to support those tasks that are needed to perform the most important ADLs. In particular, those related with mobility but not only.

5.1   Scenarios in *SHARE-it*

A scenario is an example narrative description of typical interactions of the users with the system. There are several types of scenarios [5]:

— *As-is scenarios*, which describe the current situation.
— *Visionary scenarios*, which describe the future system. This is the main communication tool between the application and solution domain experts. In a sense, these scenarios are inexpensive prototypes.
— *Evaluation scenarios*, which are used to test if the system provides the desired functionality.

Scenarios are concrete, informal descriptions, and are not intended to describe all possible interactions [3]. In *SHARE-it* we defined 9 scenarios in here we will describe only a simplified version of them. For each scenario, we describe the following aspects:

Purpose of the scenario describes which aspects of the system and its interactions with the user are focused by the scenario.

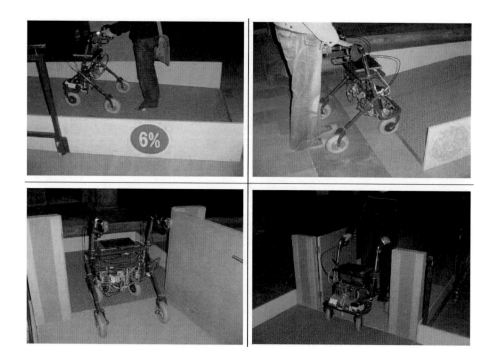

Fig. 5. *i-Walker* workbench

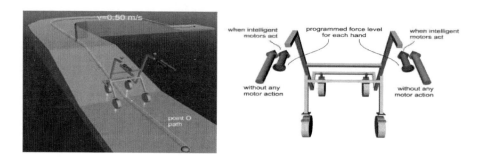

Fig. 6. Example of a real path that a user may need to follow with forces simulation

User Description a description of the typical user for the scenario. The actor represents the typical individual of a defined target population. Target population is described in §2.

Narrative Scenario the narrative that describes an example of the users interaction with the system. These descriptions can be used as evaluation scenarios to determine whether the intended functionality has been achieved.

Structure of the scenario this is a summary of the concepts present inside the scenario and is provided by the application domain experts. It describes the activities of the user, without the use of *SHARE-it* technology. Therefore, this part is the *as-is scenario.* At the same time, services provided by the *SHARE-it* system are anticipated (see table 2 as an example).

Roles of the Agents describes the interactions between the different agents and the technology they represent. The different interacting roles present are taken from the GAIA [30] specification of the *SHARE-it* Multi-Agent System and can be viewed as an abstract description of the agent's expected functions. The main agent types interacting in these scenarios are:

- Patient Agents (*pa*), which will run in PDAs or Ultra-Mobile PCs. An instantiation of this agent should provide all the available and permitted services to each user for instance security, mobility, monitoring and help services.
- The Vehicle Agents (*va*), allocated in the assistive hardware devices related to the project, be it the different wheelchair (CARMEN, Rolland, Spherik) or in the *i-Walker*. Most services will be related to mobility, monitoring and resource management.
- The Caregiver Agents (*cga*) will be situated in the computers belonging to the caregivers of *SHARE-it* target population as well as in their individual PDA. These agents will be in charge of managing all the user's help request messages, so they can be attended properly. Also, it will be notified if any anomalies are detected in the user's biometric signals.
- The Environment Agent (*ea*) will run in a network computer connected to all the environment network of sensors (*i.e.* AmI sensors). Its basic target is to distribute the information from all available sensors to all the agents interested.

Table 2. Structure of the Scenario

Disability	Degree	Disease	Device	Environment	Domain	Functional ADL	Services
Cognitive	Mild	Alzheimer	*i-Walker*	Indoor	Functional Activities	Take medication	Procedural Tutor
					Safety		Alarm

5.2 Scenario for the i-Walker: Pietro Goes to the Church

Purpose of the scenario. This scenario shows a typical interaction of one user moving from an indoor to an outdoor environment with the i-Walker. The scenario features procedural tutoring, reminder, navigation, and alarm services.

User Description. Pietro is an 80-year-old man who lives with an informal caregiver. He suffers from a **mild mixed disability after stroke** with a hemiparesis and impairment in the executive function. He uses as a support the i-Walker to walk.

Narrative scenario. Two years ago, Pietro suffered from a stroke. He recovered well and at moment he needs only a light support to walk, because he has left a mild decrease of strength in his left leg. Sometimes he is not confident enough in the sequence of actions needed to reach a goal. Today is Sunday and his caregiver has his day off. At eleven in the morning Pietro gets a reminder from the GUI that if he wants to go to church it is time to get ready. He is also reminded to put on his shoes, the overcoat, to turn off the lights, and to lock the door. He gets to the church, and while trying to open the churchs door, he gets hampered and falls on the pavement. The i-Walker detects the fall. It is also detected that Pietro is lying motionless. At the same time, the BCM detects stress. Pietros caregiver is informed via SMS of the alert. The SMS message includes Pietro's position information.

Structure of the scenario. (see table 3)

Table 3. Pietro goes to the church

Disability	Degree	Disease	Device	Environment	Domain	Functional ADL	Services
Mixed	Mild	Post Stroke hemiparesis	i-Walker	Home	Functional Activities	Dressing	Procedural Tutor
					Cognitiion		Reminder
				Outdoor	Functional Activities	Mobility	Navigation
					Safety		Alarm
					Emotional		Alarm

6   The i-Walker Benchmark

A generic training environment has horizontal and inclined surfaces over which the user can walk along. On inclined surfaces, the user may follow the maximum slope line or any other direction. In addition to this, it is useful to be able to know the absolute position of the O point and the orientation of the vehicle.

It is necessary to define a standard working path with the most common situations that a user will find when travelling with the i-Walker. To test the whole behaviour of the i-Walker, this path should include:

- A velocity change from 0 to a nominal value: to simulate the starting process.
- A velocity change from a certain value to a higher/lower value: to simulate positive or negative acceleration processes.
- Positive and negative slopes: to simulate inclined surfaces and the i-Walker going uphill and downhill.
- Orientation change segments: to simulate the necessity of avoiding obstacles.
- A velocity change from a certain value to zero: to simulate the stopping process. Examples of benchmarks can be seen in Figure 5, where different situations are tested. Figure 6 illustrates a complete simulated path with all the involved forces reflected as arrows, a previous step to live benchmarking.

In Figure 7 we show a comparison of the forces exerted by a real user while using the i-Walker downhill and uphill. In the left part of Figure 7 we show the forces exerted without any help given by the i-Walker, meanwhile in the right hand we show the same scenario with the i-Walker supporting the user. In the downhill case, without help, the figure shows how the user has to give an additional strength to support the weight of the walker down, while in the presence of i-Walker support the user has only lightly to push the walker. The first situation represent a very dangerous situation for user who suffers

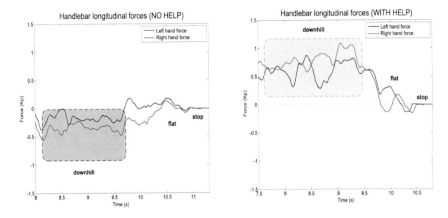

Fig. 7. Downhill experiment

from gait disturbances (like people who needs walker) because is forcing walking and balance. The risk of falls in this state is high and usually these routes are not advised for these users. However, when the system is working it assures safe conditions for the user in downhill path. Another crucial situation shown in the figure is represented by the transition between the downhill path and the flat. This moment require adequate balance and coordination to assure the transition to one posture to another and then can be considered as *a risk* situation. Thanks to the *i-Walker* it is possible to assure a smooth and safe movement.

We have the same comparison in Figure 8 when using the *i-Walker* uphill. In this second example the user clearly benefits from the system as he needs just to use the strength to walking uphill and not to push the walker while the *i-Walker* is helping in correct gait and balance. Besides, even if the user stops to rest up, he is not forced to to hold the walker and can use this freedom instead to rely on security.

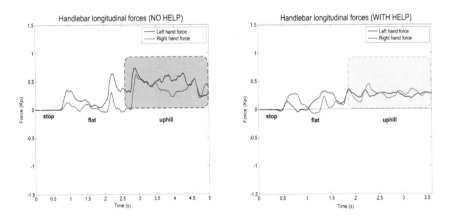

Fig. 8. Uphill experiment

Further research is needed to investigate the stability of the complete human user/*i-Walker* system and to infer the users stability.

An open topic is the acceptability of this technology. The work in *i-Walker* is important as after the cane is the most commonly used mobility device. Senior citizens facing some disabilities need to find this technology easy to learn to use as well as be confident with its usage in their preferred environment. This implies an effort to provide the appropriate infrastructure elsewhere. Also, it should be easy to adapt this technological solutions to different environments.

7   Conclusions and Future Work

The functionalities of the *i-Walker* are divided in three areas: analysis, support and navigation *i-Walker* (aid to move in a well-known environment). The *Analysis walker* consists in gathering, real time information coming from different sensors: forces in the handlebars and normal forces from the floor, feet relative position towards the walker, tilt information, speed of rear wheels, mainly. The analysis of this information will allow the study about: the gait, how the patient lays onto the walker and how much force exerts on the handlebars while following a predefined trajectory. The support walker consists in applying two strategies:

- A *helping strategy*. In the normal operation of the *i-Walker*, the user must apply pushing or pulling forces on the handlers to move around. The strategy of helping the user consists on relieving him from doing a determined percentage of the necessary forces.
- A *braking strategy*. It can oblige the patient to apply a forward pushing force in the handlers in a downhill situation instead of pulling force which can be less safe (see figure6).

The amount of helping percentage and braking force in each hand can both be determined by a doctor. Both strategies are not exclusive: we can have the user pushing the *i-Walker* going downhill and at the same time the *i-Walker* relieving him from part of the necessary pulling/pushing force to move around.

The *navigation walker* consists in connecting to a cognitive module that gives the appropriate commands to the platform in order to help a user to reach a desired destination indoors.

The *i-Walker* commands will consist in moderate braking for steering the *i-Walker* to the right direction. Other information will be shared with the cognitive module like: speed, operation mode. *etc*. The *i-Walker* platform can be used manually by a walking user, but it is also capable of performing autonomous moving. The platform can easily be adapted to accept commands to set a desired speed from a navigation module, when this is completed. Autonomous moving can be useful, for instance, to drive to a parking place for charging battery and returning to the side of patient when remotely called.

7.1   Future Work

The results obtained in our work suggested a new interesting scenario regarding rehabilitation. As a matter of fact many people use traditional walkers, not only as assistive devices, but also as rehabilitative devices during the rehabilitation program in order to recover functions as gait and balance. In this context, the possibility to detect, trough sensors, the performance of the user's hands and feet during gait, on smooth or uneven surface, could provide crucial information from the medical perspective. The opportunity to collect such information is decisive in the definition of different patterns of performance of different users in various scenarios; it could be also used - at an individual level - to modify and personalize the rehabilitation program and to follow changes. This project will be carried out at the Fondazione Santa Lucia facilities in Rome with the participation of inpatient volunteers.

There is a strong case for the use of the *i-Walker* inside the frame depicted by *SHARE-it* and, therefore, for the use of intelligent agents to support mobility and communication in senior citizens. Moreover, there is a clear evolutionary pathway that will take us from current AT to more widespread AmI where MAS will be kernel for interaction and support for decision-making.

The positive effects of assistive technologies on quality of life of elderly disabled people [11] have been largely argued and proven. The growing numbers of disabled people will increase the demand for adaptive assistive devices in the elderly population. As Prof. Pollack remarked in [22]:

> To be useful to older adults, assistive technology needs to be flexible and adaptive. Extensive customization for each user will be economically infeasible, and thus the systems we design need to be *self-tuning*. Advanced computational techniques, and in particular, Artificial Intelligence techniques, need to be developed to make these systems work.

We believe that passive robots combined with a MAS, as the *i-Walker* is, offer a decisive advantage to the elderly because they leave (almost always) final control in the hands of the user. Our work seeks to help people who can and want to walk. In our view the *user* should only be assisted according to his/her profile: not more, not less.

Acknowledgements

Authors would like to acknowledge support from the EC funded project *SHARE-it*: Supported Human Autonomy for Recovery and Enhancement of cognitive and motor abilities using information technologies (FP6-IST-045088). The views expressed in this paper are not necessarily those of the *SHARE-it* consortium. C. Barrué and U. Cortés like to acknowledge support from the Spanish funded project ASISTIR TEC2008-06734-C02-02.

References

1. Branch, L.G., Jette, A.M.: A prospective study of long-term care institutionalization among the aged. Am. J. Public Health 72, 1373–1379 (1992)
2. Bratman, M.E.: Intentions, Plans, and Practical Reason. Harvard University Press, Cambridge (1987)

3. Bruegge, B., Dutoit, A.H.: Object-Oriented Software Engineering: Using UML, Patterns and Java, 2nd edn. Prentice Hall, Upper Saddle River (2003)
4. Camarinha-Matos, L.M., Afasarmanesh, H.: Virtual communities and elderly support, pp. 279–284. WSES (2001)
5. Carroll, J.M. (ed.): Scenario-Based Design: Envisioning Work and Technology in System Development, 1st edn. Wiley, New York (1995)
6. Cortés, U., Annicchiarico, R., Vázquez-Salceda, J., Urdiales, C., Cañamero, L., López, M., Sànchez-Marrè, M., Caltagirone, C.: Assistive technologies for the disabled and for the new generation of senior citizens: the e-Tools architecture. AI Communications 16, 193–207 (2003)
7. Crews, D.E.: Artificial environments and an aging population: Designing for age-related functional losses. J. Physiol. Anthropol. Appl. Human Sc. 24(1), 103–109 (2005)
8. Fox, J., Das, S.: Safe and Sound: Artificial Intelligence in Hazardous Applications, 1st edn. AAAI Press/MIT Press (2000)
9. Espeland, M.A., Gill, T.M., Guralnik, J., et al.: Designing clinical trials of interventions for mobility disability: Results from the lifestyle interventions and independence for elders pilot (life-p) trial. J. Gerontol. A Biol. Sci. Med. Sci. 62(11), 1237–1243 (2007)
10. Glover, J., Holstius, D., Manojlovich, M., Montgomery, K., Powers, A., Wu, J., Kiesler, S., Matthews, J., Thrun, S.: A robotically-augmented walker for older adults. Technical Report CMU-CS-03-170, Carnegie Mellon University, Computer Science Department, Pittsburgh, PA (2003)
11. Guralnik, J.M.: The evolution of research on disability in old age. Aging Clin. Exp. Res. 17(3), 165–167 (2005)
12. Guralnik, J.M., LaCroix, A.Z., Abbot, R.D., et al.: Maintaining mobility in late life. demographic characteristics and chronic conditions. Am. J. Epidemiol. 137, 137 (1993)
13. Iezzoni, L., McCarthy, E., Davis, R., Siebens, H.: Mobility difficulties are not only a problem of old age. J. Gen. Intern. Med. 16(4), 235–243 (2001)
14. Lankenau, A., Röfer, T.: The role of shared control in service robots - the bremen autonomous wheelchair as an example. In: Service Robotics - Applications and Safety Issues in an Emerging Market. Workshop Notes, pp. 27–31 (2000)
15. Lankenau, A., Rofer, T.: A versatile and safe mobility assistant. IEEE Robotics & Automation Magazine 8(1), 29–37 (2001)
16. Mahoney, F.I., Barthel, D.W.: Functional evaluation: The barthel index. Md. State Med. J. 14, 61–65 (1965)
17. Mangina, E.: Review of software products for multi-agent systems (2002)
18. McCreadie, C., Tinker, A.: The acceptability of assistive technology to older people. Ageing and Society 25, 91–110 (2005)
19. McCreadie, C., Tinker, A.: The acceptability of assistive technology to older people. Ageing & Society (25), 91–110 (2005)
20. Mihailidis, A., Ferniea, G.R., Cleghornb, W.L.: The development of a computerized cueing device to help people with dementia to be more independent. Technology and Disability 13(1), 23–40 (2000)
21. Pokahr, A., Braubach, L.: Jadex User Guide
22. Polack, M.E.: Intelligent Technology for an Aging Population: The use of AI to assist elders with cognitive impairment. AI Magazine 26(2), 9–24 (2005)
23. Rao, A.S., Georgeff, M.P.: BDI agents: from theory to practice. In: Lesser, V. (ed.) Proceedings of the First International Conference on Multi-Agent Systems (ICMAS 1995), pp. 312–319. The MIT Press, Cambridge (1995)
24. Simpson, R.C.: Smart wheelchairs: A literature review. Journal of Rehabilitation Research & Development 42(4), 423–436 (2005)

25. Stephanidis, C., Vernardakis, N., Akoumianakis, D.: Critical aspects of demand in the assistive technology market in europe. Technical Report No. 109, ICS-FORTH, Heraklion, Crete, Greece

26. Urdiales, C., Poncela, A., Annicchiarico, R., Rizzi, F., Sandoval, F., Caltagirone, C.: A topological map for scheduled navigation in a hospital environment. In: e-Health: Application of Computing Science in Medicine and Health Care, pp. 228–243 (2003)

27. Vanhooydonck, D., Demeester, E., Nuttin, M., Van Brussel, H.: Shared control for intelligent wheelchairs: an implicit estimation of the user intention. In: Proceedings of the 1st International Workshop on Advances in Service Robotics 2003 (2003)

28. Virone, G., Alwan, M., Dalal, S., Kell, S.W., Turner, B., Stankovic, J.A., Felder, R.: Behavioral patterns of older adults in assisted living. IEEE Transactions on Information Technology in Biomedicine 12(3), 387–398 (2008)

29. Wasson, G., Sheth, P., Alwan, M., Huang, C., Ledoux, A.: User intent in a shared control framework for pedestrian mobility aids. In: IEEE/RSJ International Conference on Intelligent Robots and Systems (IROS), pp. 2962–2967. IEEE, Los Alamitos (2003)

30. Wooldridge, M., Jennings, N.R., Kinny, D.: The gaia methodology for agent-oriented analysis and design. Autonomous Agents and Multi-Agent Systems 3(3), 285–312 (2000)

Part III
Case-Based in Healthcare

Chapter 7
Case-Based Reasoning in the Health Sciences: Foundations and Research Directions

Isabelle Bichindaritz[1] and Cindy Marling[2]

[1] University of Washington, Tacoma, Institute of Technology
1900 Commerce Street,
Tacoma, Washington 98402, USA
ibichind@u.washington.edu
[2] School of Electrical Engineering and Computer Science,
Russ College of Engineering and Technology,
Ohio University,
Athens, Ohio 45701, USA
marling@ohio.edu

Abstract. Case-based reasoning (CBR) is an Artificial Intelligence (AI) approach with broad applicability to building intelligent systems in health sciences domains. It represents knowledge in the form of exemplary past experiences, or cases. It is especially well suited to health sciences domains, where experience plays a major role in acquiring knowledge and skill, and where case histories inform current practice. This chapter provides a broad overview of CBR in the Health Sciences, including its foundations and research directions. It begins with introductions to the CBR approach and to health sciences domains, and then explains their synergistic combination. It continues with a discussion of the relationship between CBR and statistical data analysis, and shows how CBR supports evidence-based practice. Next, it presents an in-depth analysis of current work in the field, classifying CBR in the Health Sciences systems in terms of their domains, purposes, memory and case management, reasoning, and system design. Finally, it places CBR with respect to other AI approaches used in health sciences domains, showing how CBR can complement these approaches in multimodal reasoning systems.

1 Introduction

Case-based reasoning (CBR) is an Artificial Intelligence (AI) approach with broad applicability to building intelligent systems in health sciences domains. Biomedical domains have provided fertile ground for AI research from the earliest days. Moreover, the healthcare domain is one of the leading industrial domains in which computer science is applied today. The value of CBR stems from capturing specific clinical experience and leveraging this contextual, instance-based, knowledge for solving clinical problems. CBR systems have already proven useful in clinical practice for decision support, explanation, and quality control [1].

I. Bichindaritz et al. (Eds.): Computational Intelligence in Healthcare 4, SCI 309, pp. 127–157.
springerlink.com   © Springer-Verlag Berlin Heidelberg 2010

Over the past decade, seven Workshops on CBR in the Health Sciences have been conducted at the International and European Conferences on Case-Based Reasoning, and four special journal issues have been published on the topic [2,3,4,5]. Today, CBR in the Health Sciences is a vibrant and rapidly growing field of research and development.

This chapter presents an overview of the field, including its foundations, current work, and research directions. The next section, Section 2, is an introduction to CBR, including an overview of the Retrieve, Reuse, Revise, Retain reasoning cycle [6], and a list of CBR resources. Section 3 describes health sciences domains and their significance for computer science. In Section 4, the intersection of CBR and the health sciences is discussed, including its rationale and historical roots. Section 5 describes the impact of CBR in the Health Sciences and considers the complementarity and synergies of CBR with statistics. In Section 6, research directions are presented. Here, tasks, domains, and research themes are considered in light of an extensive review and analysis of the CBR in the Health Sciences literature. Section 7 considers the role of AI as a whole in the health sciences, exploring CBR's synergies with data mining and knowledge discovery, and discussing CBR's role in multimodal reasoning architectures. Section 8 presents a summary and conclusion.

Resources. Several comprehensive overview articles have been published on CBR in the Health Sciences [1,7,8,9,10]. There have also been special journal issues devoted to this topic in *Applied Intelligence* [2], *Artificial Intelligence in Medicine* [3], and *Computational Intelligence* [4,5]. A series of seven Workshops on CBR in the Health Sciences was held between 2003 and 2009 at the International and European Conferences on CBR. Many of the workshop proceedings are available online at http://www.cbr-biomed.org/jspw/workshops/. CBR-BIOMED, http://www.cbr-biomed.org/, is a web site dedicated to CBR in biology and medicine.

2   Foundations of Case-Based Reasoning

CBR uses past experiences, or cases, to help in solving new problems or understanding unfamiliar situations. It is based on the premise that human knowledge and expertise is experiential in nature. Clearly, people are better able to accomplish tasks with which they have familiarity, whether in everyday life or in professional settings. For example, in driving to the home of a friend for the first time, you may need to consult a map, ask for directions, use a global positioning system, or otherwise attend to the route, to ensure that you arrive at the right place at the right time. If you are told that your friend lives a few blocks from some familiar landmark, like a favorite restaurant, the task becomes easier, because you already know most of the route. You do not expend much mental effort at all when driving a well-traveled route, such as between your home and office. Similarly, we expect professionals with greater relevant experience to perform complex tasks better than novices. For example, if a traveler contracts tick-borne encephalitis in the Vienna woods, an Austrian physician will more readily be able to recognize and treat the disease than the traveler's own physician in a tick-free part of the world.

CBR systems derive their power from capturing and recalling past experiences in much the same way as people do. Knowledge is stored in the form of individual cases, each of which represents some past problem or experience. For example, a case might contain a map from point A to point B, or the description of a patient's signs and symptoms with the treatment prescribed and the clinical outcome. The precise contents of a case depends upon the task that the system is meant to perform. To be useful for automated reasoning, a case must contain information pertinent to the task at hand. Often, this is the same information that a person would need to perform the task manually. If, for example, a physician was deciding whether or not to prescribe a neuroleptic drug for a patient with Alzheimer's disease, important factors would include medical history, physical state, emotional state, observed behaviors, cognitive status, caregiver support, and safety concerns. Some of this data might be available in the patient's chart or electronic health record, and some might be acquired during the office visit at which the decision is made. Each case in a CBR system built to support this decision making process would contain the specific details of these factors for an individual patient, along with a record of whether or not a neuroleptic drug was actually prescribed.

The knowledge base, then, is a collection of cases, known as a case library or case base. The case base is organized to facilitate retrieval of the most similar, or most useful, experiences when a new problem arises. When the system is given a new problem to solve, it searches its case base for applicable past cases. The solutions stored in past cases provide a starting point for solving the problem at hand. The reasoning process employed may be envisioned as a CBR cycle, as first described in the classic CBR overview by Aamodt and Plaza [6], and shown in Figure 1. Next, let us consider a simple example to illustrate the workings of this CBR cycle.

Suppose that a real estate agent needs to determine a fair selling price for a house. If the price is set too high, the house will not sell, but if the price is set too low, the agent will lose money. The agent, whether human or software, can use recent selling prices of similar past homes to assist with this task. Each past sale would constitute a case. A case would contain the selling price, plus a description of the house sold, including its address, school district, year of construction, living area, lot size, number of bedrooms, number of bathrooms, type of garage, and other amenities.

Reasoning begins when a new house comes on the market. The agent can ascertain its descriptive properties, but has not yet determined a selling price. The new house becomes a new case at the beginning of the CBR cycle. The new house is compared to the cases in the case base during the **Retrieve** phase. The most similar past case is retrieved, becoming the retrieved case shown in Figure 1. This retrieved case contains a selling price that can be considered for the new house. However, before finalizing the price, the agent would examine

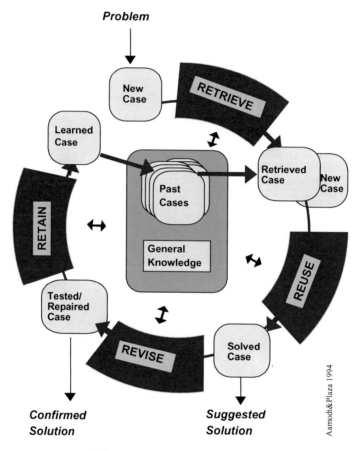

Fig. 1. The CBR cycle, from [6]

any differences between the old and new houses to see if price adjustments are in order. If the new house has one more bathroom than the old house, the price could be adjusted upwards. If the new house is in a less desirable school district, or has a smaller garage, the price could be adjusted downwards. Professional real estate agents have knowledge of the value added or subtracted by various features, and their adjustment mechanisms can be encoded for use in the **Reuse** phase of the CBR cycle. Once the price is adjusted accordingly, the agent has a solution, or a fair selling price for the house. Of course, if the house does not sell for this price, further adjustment may be needed during the **Revise** phase. Once the house is sold, the new case can be stored in the case base, along with its actual selling price, during the **Retain** phase. This last phase enables the system to grow and to learn by acquiring additional experiences that may be retrieved and reused in the future.

Resources. The definitive textbook for CBR remains Kolodner's *Case-Based Reasoning* [11]. An older book, *Inside Case-Based Reasoning* [12] gives insight into the very beginnings of the field. Good shorter overviews include Aamodt and Plaza's paper [6], which introduced the CBR cycle discussed above, and a tutorial introduction by Kolodner and Leake [13], which appears as a chapter in [14]. In 2005, the CBR research community collaboratively published a special issue of the Knowledge Engineering Review on CBR commentaries [15]. This issue catalogs important issues, trends, and techniques in CBR research and development, providing extensive bibliographic references to relevant work through that date. For the most up-to-date information on CBR as of this writing, consult the CBR Wiki maintained by the CBR research community at http://cbrwiki.fdi.ucm.es/wiki/. The latest advances in CBR research and development are presented each year at the International Conference on CBR, http://www.iccbr.org/.

3 Health Sciences Domains

The health sciences include medicine, nursing, and all other aspects of healthcare and health research, including human biology, genetics, proteomics, and phylogenetics. In terms of computer science, forecasts for the development of the profession confirm a general trend toward becoming increasingly influenced by application areas. Key influential application areas are health informatics and bioinformatics. For example, the National Workforce Center for Emerging Technologies (NWCET) lists healthcare informatics and global and public health informatics among such applications, as shown in Figure 2.

The predominant role played by health sciences sectors is confirmed by statistics from the U.S. Department of Labor. Predicted to have some of the highest increases in wage, salary and employment growth between 2006 and 2016 are healthcare practitioner offices (close second overall rank), private hospitals (sixth overall rank), residential care facilities (ninth overall), and home healthcare services (twelfth overall). By comparison, amusement, gambling, and recreational services rank only thirteenth [17].

The strength of health related industries is in response to a need for increased access to healthcare. This social need also fosters research funding and

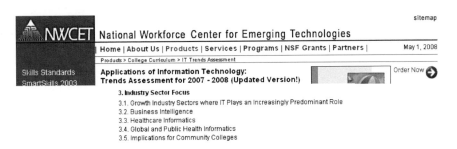

Fig. 2. Influential application areas for computer science identified by the NWCET, from [16]

Rank	Category (linked to category information)	Total Cites	Median Impact Factor	Aggregate Impact Factor	Aggregate Immediacy Index	Aggregate Cited Half-Life	# Journals	Articles
1	COMPUTER SCIENCE, ARTIFICIAL INTELLIGENCE	181386	1.405	2.011	0.300	7.3	94	6975
2	COMPUTER SCIENCE, CYBERNETICS	19396	1.103	1.128	0.336	7.5	17	1031
3	COMPUTER SCIENCE, HARDWARE & ARCHITECTURE	88293	1.244	1.488	0.190	8.4	45	3456
4	COMPUTER SCIENCE, INFORMATION SYSTEMS	139598	1.103	1.633	0.241	6.6	99	7035
5	COMPUTER SCIENCE, INTERDISCIPLINARY APPLICATIONS	149544	1.086	1.552	0.266	7.0	94	9008
6	COMPUTER SCIENCE, SOFTWARE ENGINEERING	101532	1.057	1.255	0.182	7.7	86	5756
7	COMPUTER SCIENCE, THEORY & METHODS	118433	0.994	1.341	0.210	8.8	84	4889

Fig. 3. Data supporting the importance of interdisciplinary applications, from the 2008 Journal Citation Reports in the ISI Web of Knowledge [18]

endeavors. It is notable that the Science Citation Index of the Institute for Scientific Information (ISI) Web of Knowledge lists among computer science categories a specialty called "Computer science, Interdisciplinary applications" [18]. Moreover, this area of computer science ranks highest in the discipline in terms of the number of articles published, and second highest in the number of total citations. These statistics, shown in Figure 3, support the other data pointing toward the importance of applications in computer science. Health sciences applications in particular, which are based on complex interdisciplinary work, represent a major specialization area in computer science.

4   CBR in Health Sciences Domains: Rationale and Roots

CBR has proven to be especially useful for problem solving and decision support applications in health sciences domains. Motivations for applying CBR to these domains have been present from the beginning, with the goal of improving public health. This application area has provided a rich experimental environment for evaluating and enhancing the CBR paradigm and for expanding CBR system development beyond the laboratory setting. There are many reasons why CBR is a good fit for health sciences applications, including:

- Case histories are established educational tools for health care professionals
- Health care professionals publish accounts of the treatments of individual patients in the medical literature
- Reasoning from examples comes naturally to health care professionals
- A complex biological system like the human body is hard to completely formalize, but there are many examples, or cases, of diseases, treatments and outcomes
- Many diseases are not well-enough understood for there to be cures or universally applicable specific treatments
- Cases can complement general treatment guidelines to support personalized medical care for individuals
- Extensive data stores are available, such as those in electronic health records, which may be mined for case examples

In this section, we describe early work in CBR in the Health Sciences. Current trends and research directions are discussed in the following sections. The earliest efforts in the field focused on modeling medical expertise, especially for diagnosis, treatment planning, and follow-up care. This was in line with the early AI goals of representing and utelizing the knowledge of human experts.

The first proof of concept that CBR could be used for health sciences applications is attributed to Janet Kolodner, who wrote the CBR textbook [11], and Robert Kolodner, a psychiatrist [19]. The two met by chance at a conference, where discovering that they shared the same last name, they began discussing their interests in computing and psychiatry. In [19], they proposed SHRINK, a case-based system to aid with psychiatric diagnosis and treatment. They aimed to establish a framework for clinical decision support systems that could also assist in the teaching of clinical reasoning. They presented actual psychiatric cases to demonstrate how these could be used to reason and to build expertise. While SHRINK was never fully implemented, many of its ideas were later implemented in MNAOMIA [20], a CBR system for diagnosing and treating psychiatric eating disorders.

MNAOMIA implemented the Retrieve, Reuse, Revise, Retain cycle shown in Figure 1, but added extensions to deal with challenges from the psychiatric domain. These extensions enabled the system to: reason from both episodal, or case, knowledge, and theoretical, or documentary, knowledge; assist with clinical tasks including diagnosis, treatment planning, follow-up care, and clinical research; use cases acquired by the system to inform clinical research; and reason over time to support patient follow-up. A psychiatrist involved in the MNAO-MIA project shared his vision of how a computer system could best support his clinical practice. He wanted an electronic repository for his patient records, storing details of medical history, environment, symptoms, diseases, treatments, tests, and procedures. He wanted online access to patient records of the other psychiatrists in his practice, as well. He envisioned being able to consult the system when he encountered a new patient or a new disease episode. The system would retrieve and display the most similar old patients or disease episodes, note similarities and differences to the current case, describe past successful treatments, and recommend diagnoses and treatments for the current situation. Completely realizing this vision of clinical decision support is still an important goal for CBR in the Health Sciences.

Many of the first CBR systems in health sciences domains were built for medical diagnosis. Two of the earliest and best-known diagnostic systems were PROTOS [21,22] and CASEY [23]. PROTOS diagnosed audiological, or hearing, disorders. Its case base contained approximately 200 cases for actual patients who had been diagnosed by an expert audiologist. A patient's disorder could be described by up to 58 distinct features, although, on average, values were known for only 11 features per patient. A patient's diagnosis was a categorical label, telling which of 15 pre-specified audiological disorders the patient had. Diagnosing a new patient, then, meant classifying the new patient into one of the 15 categories. PROTOS used reminding links to determine the most likely classification for a patient. If it found a past patient within that category that closely matched the new patient, it would extend the past patient's diagnostic label to the new patient. Otherwise, it would use difference links to suggest an alternate classification to try. Classification is a task for which other AI approaches, including neural networks and decision trees, are often used. Such techniques, however, work best when there are more exemplar cases, fewer descriptive features per case, and less missing data per case than PROTOS had to deal with. The case-based approach was effective given the nature of the data in the audiological disorders domain.

CASEY [23] diagnosed heart failure patients by comparing them to earlier cardiac patients with known diagnoses. The features of a case were the measures and states of the patient. Measures were quantitative clinical data, like heart rate, while states represented qualitative features, like high or low arterial pressure, or the presence or absence of a particular disease. A solution, or diagnosis, was the cause of the patient's heart failure. It was represented as a graph, showing the causality among the measures and states of the patient. In comparing past and present cases, CASEY determined how the cases differed, and how significant the differences were. For example, a new case might be missing a feature that was present in the old case; however, if some other feature could cause the same states as the missing feature, the cases could still match. A past diagnosis was adapted to fit a new case by modifying the graph with the new patient's data and causal relations.

CASEY was able to build upon and integrate an earlier model-based system, which diagnosed heart failures based on a physiological model of the heart. When it could not find a close enough match in its case base, CASEY would invoke the earlier system to produce a diagnosis. CASEY was originally cited for producing comparable diagnoses to the model-based system with an order of magnitude speed-up. It has since been recognized for its early integration of two different reasoning modalities. Today, applications of CBR in the Health Sciences are frequently integrated, not only with other AI approaches, but with other computer systems, such as health information management systems, and with laboratory and medical equipment.

Diagnosis and classification are tasks that have since been the focus of CBR systems in many different domains. The other types of tasks most commonly performed by CBR systems in the health sciences are therapy planning and education. An early therapy planning system was ICONS [24,25]. ICONS recommended antibiotic therapy for patients with bacterial infections in a hospital intensive care unit (ICU). Had it been possible to accurately and quickly diagnose the cause of an infection, selecting a treatment plan would have been a much easier task. However, it took two days for laboratory analysis to definitively identify the responsible bacterial pathogen, and delaying therapy for so long would endanger the patient.

Physicians would resort to calculated antibiotic therapy, in order to quickly prescribe the treatment most likely to combat the infection while taking into account any contraindications or side-effects. ICONS was built to provide decision support for physicians performing this task. Its case base contained experiences with ICU patients who received calculated antibiotic therapy. When a new infection would arise, ICONS would input information about the way in which the infection was acquired, the organ system affected, contraindications, and general patient data needed for dosage calculation. It would retrieve a similar actual or prototypical case from its case base, which would contain a solution set of potential antibiotics to prescribe. The solution set would be adapted, or refined, based on the needs of the current patient.

CBR has long been used for educational purposes [26]. Since CBR is predicated on the idea that knowledge is acquired through experience, it promotes the approach of teaching by providing meaningful experiences, or cases. Some CBR systems built for other purposes provide auxiliary educational benefit, as users learn from their interactions with the system or benefit from the examples stored in the case base. The nutritionist who served as domain expert for CAMP [27], which planned daily menus to meet individual nutrition requirements, believed that the case base was one of CAMP's most valuable contributions. The case base was a large repository of nutritionally sound daily menus, an educational resource for nutrition students that had been previously unavailable.

An early CBR-inspired system to educate the public about health was the Sickle Cell Counselor [28]. This system was built as an interactive video exhibit to teach museum visitors about sickle cell disease and the genetic inheritance of the sickle cell trait. Users were given simulated experiences as genetic counselors for virtual couples at risk of having children with sickle cell disease. Users could carry out simulated blood tests, calculate the probabilities of a baby being born with the disease, consult with videotaped experts, and counsel the couple as to the advisability of having children. A virtual year later, the couple told whether or not they had (a) taken the advice, (b) found the advice helpful, and (c) borne a child with sickle cell disease. Tests showed that system users learned more about sickle cell disease and genetic inheritance than control subjects given written instructional materials covering the same topics.

Since SHRINK was first proposed, many systems have been built for diagnosis, classification, treatment planning, education, and other tasks in a wide variety of health sciences domains. Some additional influential systems built before the turn of the century are noted here:

- MEDIC diagnosed pulmonary disease [29]
- BOLERO supported the diagnosis of pneumonia [30]
- FLORENCE assisted with nursing diagnosis, prognosis and prescription [31]
- ALEXIA planned assessment tests to determine a patient's hypertension etiology [32]
- T-IDDM supported insulin-dependent diabetes mellitus patient management [33]
- CARE-PARTNER supported long-term follow-up care of stem-cell transplantation patients [34]
- The Auguste project advised physicians about prescribing neuroleptic drugs for Alzheimer's patients [35]
- ROENTGEN helped to design radiation therapy plans for oncology patients [36]

- MacRad helped to interpret radiological images, supporting both diagnosis and education through its case base of reference images [37]
- CTS segmented CT-scans of the brain to assist in determining the degree of degenerative brain disease [38]
- SCINA interpreted myocardial perfusion scintigrams to detect coronary artery disease [39]
- ImageCreek interpreted abdominal CT images [40]
- PhylSyst mined phylogenetic classifications [41]
- CADI was a tutoring system designed to instruct medical students and residents in cardiac auscultation [42]

5   Impact of CBR in the Health Sciences

CBR in the Health Sciences is a particularly active area of research today. As health sciences sectors expand, advanced decision-support systems play an increasingly important role in the evolution of medicine towards a more standardized and computerized science. CBR decision-support systems base their recommendations on the most similar or most reusable experiences previously encountered. CBR is thus a methodology of choice for descriptive experimental sciences such as the natural and life sciences, especially biology and medicine.

5.1   Impact on CBR

CBR has found in biomedicine one if its most fruitful application areas, but also one of its most complex. The main reason for its achievements and for the interest of the biomedical community is that case-based reasoning capitalizes on the reuse of existing cases, or experiences. These abound in biology and medicine, where knowledge stems from the study of natural phenomena, patient problem situations, or other living beings and their sets of problems. In particular, the important variability in the natural and life sciences fosters the development of case-based approaches in areas where complete, causal models are not available to fully explain naturally occurring phenomena. Biomedicine is a domain where expertise beyond the novice level comes from learning by solving real and/or practice cases, which is precisely what case-based reasoning accomplishes. Prototypical models often describe biomedical knowledge better than other types of models, which also argues in favor of CBR [9].

One of the complexities of biomedicine is the high-dimensionality of cases, as found in bioinformatics [43,44,45] and also in long-term follow-up care [34]. Multimedia case representation and the development of suitable CBR methods for handling these represent another complexity, as in medical image interpretation [40,46,47,48], sensor data interpretation [49], and time series case features [50]. Other factors include: the co-occurrence of multiple diseases; overlapping diagnostic categories; the need to abstract features from time series representing temporal history [50], sensor signals [49], or other continuous input data; and the use of data mining techniques in addition to case-based reasoning [47,51].

Additional complexities arise in the medical domain when dealing with safety critical constraints, assisting the elderly and disabled [52], and providing useful explanations [53].

Recently, a major trend seems to be the broadening of CBR applications beyond the traditional diagnosis, treatment, or quality control types toward the *applicability of CBR to novel reasoning tasks*. An interesting example studies how cases can represent instances of non-compliance with clinical guidelines, eventually leading to expert refinement of these guidelines [54]. Another paper demonstrates the usefulness of CBR in configuring parameters for hemodialysis [50]. These papers open new fields of application for CBR, which will foster the spread of CBR in biomedical domains.

CBR in the Health Sciences papers address all aspects of the CBR methodology and attempt to advance basic research in CBR. For example, some research addresses retrieval questions [55], while others address adaptation [56,57]. Bichindaritz [55] shows how memory organization for CBR can bridge the gap between CBR and information retrieval systems. This article surveys the different memory organizations implemented in CBR systems, and the different approaches used by these systems to tackle the problem of efficient reasoning with large case bases. The author then proposes a memory organization to support case-based retrieval similar to the memory organization of information retrieval systems and particularly Internet search engines. This memory organization is based on an inverted index mapping case features with the cases in memory.

D'Aquin et al. provide principles and examples of adaptation knowledge acquisition in the context of their KASIMIR system for breast cancer decision support [56]. These authors have identified some key adaptation patterns, such as adaptation of an inapplicable decision, and adaptation based on the consequences of a decision. In addition, KASIMIR has also acquired retrieval knowledge to take into account missing data and the threshold effect. The paper broadens the discussion by proposing a sketch of a methodology for adaptation knowledge acquisition from experts. Several authors have focused on the importance of prototype-based knowledge representation for CBR in the Health Sciences [51,58], which encourages further research in this direction.

The impact on CBR is also seen in multimodal reasoning and synergism with other AI approaches and methodologies. The complementarity of CBR with AI as a whole is examined in depth in Section 7.

5.2   Impact on the Health Sciences

Several CBR in the Health Sciences systems have been tested successfully in clinical settings. However, it is a misperception that only clinical applications are pertinent to biomedical domains. Biomedical research support also lies within the purview of AI and CBR in the Health Sciences. For example, bioinformatics systems often aim to analyze data, as do data mining systems, which is more of value to biomedical researchers. Clinical CBR systems may remain in the realm of pilot testing or clinical trial rather than daily clinical use. However, the shift from CBR driven systems to application domain driven systems is currently occurring. Several systems under development aim at being placed in routine clinical use. One of the most interesting impacts of CBR on the health sciences lies in the position CBR must find with respect to statistics, which is routinely used for data analysis and processing in experimental sciences. This is a major trend in CBR in the Health Sciences research, as described next.

5.3   CBR versus Statistics in the Health Sciences

In health sciences domains, statistics is considered to be the scientific method of choice for data analysis. Therefore, CBR in the Health Sciences systems researchers have studied how to position CBR in these domains in relation to statistics. Biometry is "the application of statistical methods to the solution of biological problems" [59]. Statistics itself has several meanings. A classical definition of statistics is "the scientific study of data describing natural variation" [59]. Statistics is generally used to study populations or groups of individuals: it deals with collections of data, not with single data points. Thus, the measurement of a single animal or the response from a single biochemical test will generally not be of interest; unless a sample of animals is measured or several such tests are performed, statistics ordinarily can play no role [59]. Another main feature of statistics is that the data are generally numeric or quantifiable in some way. Statistics also refers to any computed or estimated statistical quantities such as the mean, mode, or standard deviation [59].

The origin of statistics can be traced back to the seventeenth century, and derives from two sources. One is related to political science and was created to quantitatively describe the various affairs of a government or state. This is the origin of the term "statistics." In order to deal with taxes and insurance data, problems of censuses, longevity, and mortality were studied in a quantitative manner [59]. The second source is probability theory, which was also developed in the seventeenth century, spurred by the popular interest in games of chance among upper society (Pascal, de Fermat, Bernouilli, de Moivre) [59]. The science of astronomy also fostered the development of statistics as a mathematical tool to build a coherent theory from individual observations (Laplace, Gauss). Applications of statistics to the life sciences emerged in the nineteenth century, when the concept of the "average man" was developed (Quetelet) along with the concepts of statistical distribution and variation [59]. Statistics researchers focus on summarizing data: "All these facts have been processed by that remarkable computer, the human brain, which furnishes an abstract" [59]. Statistics involves reducing and synthesizing data into figures representing trends or central tendencies.

There are actually two approaches in statistics, experimental and descriptive. The experimental approach, at the basis of any theory formation in experimental sciences, and in particular the life sciences, refers to a method aimed at identifying relations of cause to effect. A statistical experiment needs to follow a precise and controlled plan with the goal of observing the effect of the variation of one or more variables on the phenomenon under study, while eliminating any potential hidden effects. The statistician is responsible for the design of the experiment from the onset, to ensure that the data collected will be able to support or refute the stated research hypothesis given the laws of probability. Researchers gather data in very strict contexts such as randomized clinical trials in medicine. The subsequent statistical data analysis of collected data represents only a small part of the statistician's work. The descriptive approach deals with summarizing or representing a set of data in a meaningful way through primarily quantitative features, although qualitative variables are also considered. Statistical data analysis stems from the descriptive approach, but deals only with the data analysis part. This aspect of statistics, and in particular inferential statistics, is related to data mining, which builds data models to produce inferences from data. Here, data analysis has freed itself from the constraints of probability theory to analyze data *a posteriori*.

5.4   The Role of CBR in the Health Sciences

CBR brings to the life sciences a method for processing and reusing data without generalizing them, which statistics clearly considers outside of its scope. CBR, like statistics, promotes "the scientific study of data describing natural variation." CBR deals with natural variation in a novel manner, through analogical inference and similarity reasoning. Current computer capacity has made it feasible to study individual cases, because large numbers of cases can be efficiently processed without having to be summarized. Therefore, CBR can be seen as an advance in the scientific study of data made possible by progress in computer science. This study of how CBR can complement statistics has been a main focus of CBR in the Health Sciences research. This is also one of the most salient contributions CBR in the Health Sciences can make to CBR in general. Advances in this area will be useful in any application of CBR to experimental sciences.

Many of the tasks performed by CBR in the Health Sciences systems compete with corresponding statistical methods, particularly those of inferential statistics. For example, Schmidt et al. present a CBR system for the prediction of influenza waves for influenza surveillance [60]. The authors compare their method with classical prediction methods, which are statistical, and argue that CBR is more appropriate in this domain due to the irregular cyclicality of the spread of influenza. The rationale behind this is that statistical methods rely on laws of probability theory which are not always met in practice. In these circumstances, methods like CBR can be advantageous because they do not rely on these laws. Another interesting example demonstrates how CBR can be used to explain exceptions to statistical analysis [61] and particularly data summaries [62].

Some of the most interesting research in this area focuses on the role of CBR as an evidence gathering mechanism for medicine [34]. CBR can detect and represent how cases can illustrate contextual applications of guidelines, and spark the generation of new research hypotheses, such as how repeated exceptions to clinical guidelines can lead to modifications of the clinical guidelines [34,54].

More generally, one of the main motivations for the development of case-based reasoning systems in biomedicine is that cases, as traces of the clinical experience of the experts, play a unique and irreplaceable role for representing knowledge in

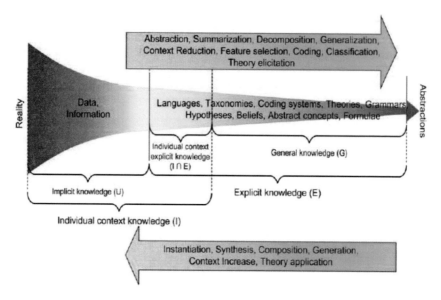

Fig. 4. The knowledge spectrum in biomedical informatics [63]

these domains [62]. Recent studies have worked at better formalizing this specific role. These studies explain that the gold standard for evaluating the quality of biomedical knowledge relies on the concept of evidence. Pantazi et al. propose an extension of the definition of *biomedical evidence* to include knowledge in individual cases, suggesting that the mere collection of individual case facts should be regarded as evidence gathering [62]. To support their proposal, they argue that the traditional, highly abstracted, hypothesis centric type of evidence that removes factual evidence present in individual cases, implies a strong *ontological commitment* to methodological and theoretical approaches, which is the source of the never-ending need for *current* and *best* evidence, while, at the same time, offering little provision for the reuse of knowledge disposed of as obsolete [62]. By contrast, the incremental factual evidence about individuals creates, once appropriately collected, a growing body of context-dependent evidence that can be reinterpreted and reused as many times as possible. See Figure 4, from [63] for a graphical representation of this knowledge spectrum.

Currently, the concept of evidence most often refers to an abstract proposition derived from multiple cases obtained in the context of a randomized controlled trial [62]. Hypothesis forming is the cornerstone of this kind of biomedical research. Hypotheses that pass an appropriately selected statistical test become evidence. However, the process of hypothesis forming also implies a commitment to certain purposes (e.g., research, teaching, etc.), and inherently postulates ontological and conceptual reductions, orderings and relationships. These result from the particular conceptualizations of a researcher who is influenced by experience, native language, background, etc. [62] This reduction process will always be prone to errors as long as uncertainties are present in our reality. In addition, even though a hypothesis may be successfully verified statistically, its applicability may be hindered by our inability to fully construe its complete meaning. This meaning is defined by the complete context in which the hypothesis was formed, which includes the data sources as well as the context of the researcher who formed the hypothesis [62].

These considerations led Pantazi et al. to propose extending the definition of the concept of evidence in biomedicine to align it with an intuitively appealing direction of research: CBR [62]. From this perspective, the concept of evidence evolves to a more complete, albeit more complex, construct which emerges naturally from the attempt to understand, explain and manage unique, individual cases. This new view of the concept of evidence is surprisingly congruent with the currently accepted idea of evidence in forensic science [62]. Here, evidence includes the recognition of any spatio-temporal form (i.e., pattern, regularity) in the context of a case (e.g., a hair, a fiber, a piece of clothing, a sign of struggle, ...) which may be relevant to the solution of that case. This new view, where a body of evidence is incremental in nature and accumulates dynamically in the form of facts about individual cases, is in striking contrast with traditional definitions of biomedical evidence. Using case data as evidence reduces sensitivity to the issues of *recency* (i.e., current evidence) and *validity* (i.e., best evidence) [62].

The evidence gathering mechanism enabled by CBR can lead to the design of new research hypotheses, and engender statistical experiments aimed at integrating new knowledge with theory, traditionally accomplished through the statistical approach. Therefore, CBR's evidence gathering role complements that of the statistical approach. As a matter of fact, CBR, by enabling the scientific study of individual and contextual data elements, fills a gap in the purpose of statistics, which is the scientific study of data.

6   Research Directions

To ascertain research directions, the first author conducted an extensive review and analysis of the literature in the field of CBR in the Health Sciences. Included were 117 papers from all International and European Conferences on Case-Based Reasoning until 2008, the first six Workshops on CBR in the Health Sciences, the two DARPA CBR workshops of 1989 and 1991, and the survey papers on CBR in the Health Sciences. A tiered classification scheme was developed, and the overall architecture is shown in Figure 5. Five distinct categories (domain, purpose, memory and case management, reasoning, and system design) are defined. In addition, a research theme is selected to characterize the main research hypothesis and findings of the paper. This work was first presented at the Seventh Workshop on CBR in the Health Sciences, which was held in 2009. This section includes excerpts from the workshop paper [64].

6.1   Classification System

Domain. The range of domains in the health sciences fields is vast and, as a result, it was chosen as the first level of classification. However, rather than

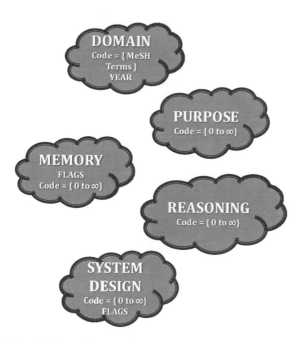

Fig. 5. The CBR in the Health Sciences tiered classification scheme

creating a new set of descriptors, it is proposed to use the MeSH descriptors, of which there are over 24,000 that cover just about every aspect of the health sciences. Along with the domain, another primary means of discriminating the relevance of an article is its publication date. Since the date plays no real role in classifying an article, the date has no field of its own, but instead is combined with the Domain.

Purpose. The purposes, or tasks, of CBR systems have been thoroughly discussed in many articles summarizing CBR in the Health Sciences. One of the first papers to survey the field in 2001, by Schmidt et al., used the purpose as the primary means to subdivide the different systems [7]. In their paper, Schmidt et al. specified four main purposes: diagnosis, classification, planning, and tutoring. Later, both Holt et al. [1] and Nilsson and Sollenborn [8] used the same four descriptors. In the early years, the majority of systems were diagnostic in nature, but in recent years more therapeutic and treatment systems have been developed [9].

Table 1 presents examples of purpose classifications. Planning has been replaced here by treatment since most of the time planning refers to treatment planning. However, planning tasks may involve not only treatment but also other aspects such as diagnosis assessment, which often consists of a series of exams and labs orchestrated in a plan. Planning is a classical major task performed by AI systems. Therefore, planning can be added to the treatment choice in the purpose dimension.

Table 1. Sample purpose classifications

Code	Purpose	Code	Purpose
10	Medical Purpose	20.2	Evaluation
10.1	Decision Support	20.2.1	System Level Testing
10.1.1	Diagnosis	20.2.2	Pilot Testing
10.1.2	Treatment/therapy	20.2.3	Clinical Trial
10.1.3	Prognosis	20.2.4	Routine Clinical Use
10.1.4	Follow-up	20.3	Concept
10.1.5	Classification	20.4	Method
10.2	Tutoring	20.5	Survey
10.3	Epidemiology	30	Bioinformatics Purpose
10.4	Research support	30.1	Proteomics
10.5	Image interpretation	30.2	Phylogenetics
20	Research Purpose	30.3	Genomics
20.1	Formalization	40	Research Theme

CBR systems generally support either medical clinical work, research, or bioinformatics. Therefore we have added these as top level purpose categories. In the clinic, decision support systems support mostly diagnosis, treatment, prognosis, follow-up, and/or classification, such as in image interpretation. Well known diagnostic systems include CARE-PARTNER [34]. Well known classification systems include PROTOS [22] and IMAGECREEK [40]. Well known treatment planning systems include T-IDDM [65] and Auguste [35]. Several systems provide multi-expertise, such as CARE-PARTNER [34], ensuring diagnosis and treatment planning. Well known tutoring systems include ICONS [66].

More recent articles require differentiation between the purpose of the system developed, which is generally a clinical purpose, and the purpose of the research paper, which can be, among others, a survey paper or a classification paper. Some papers focus on formalization such as KASIMIR [67]. Among these, the evaluation of a system can be performed more or less thoroughly. This is an important dimension to note about a research paper: whether the system was tested only at the system level, which is the most frequent, at the pilot testing level, at the clinical trial level, or finally whether the system is in routine clinical use.

Finally, a paper is generally identified by a research theme by its authors. By indexing a set of 117 papers currently in our database, we have identified major research themes, such as CBR and electronic medical records (EMR), knowledge morphing, CBR and clinical guidelines, or application of a generic CBR framework.

Memory and Case Management. This is a very broad category and could easily be subdivided. It encompasses both how the cases are represented and also

Table 2. Sample memory and case management classifications

Code	Memory Organization	Case Representation Flag	
10	Flat	T	Time Series
20	Hierarchical	A	Text
20.1	Decision Tree	M	Microarray
20.2	Concept Lattice	V	Attribute/Values
20.3	Conceptual Clustering Tree	N	Plans
30	Network	Memory Structures Flag	
40	Inverted Index	G	Ground Cases
Case Representation Flag		P	Prototypes
I	Images	L	Clusters
S	Signals	O	Concepts

how they are organized in memory for retrieval purposes and more (see Table 2). As a result, it is made up of more than one code. The first part of the code represents the format of the cases. The primary types are images, signals, mass spectrometry, microarray, time series data and regular attribute/value pairs, which are used by the majority of the systems. There are also flags that represent what kinds of memory structures the CBR system uses, such as ground cases (G), prototypical cases (P), clusters (L), or concepts (O). Lastly, when it comes to memory management, there are potentially an infinite number of possibilities, some of which may never have been used before. The main types, however, represent how the memory is organized, whether it is flat or hierarchical, what kind of hierarchical structure, such as decision tree, concept lattice, conceptual clustering tree, or others.

Reasoning. This category regroups the inferential aspects of the CBR. Classically, retrieve, reuse, revise, and retain have been described. Nevertheless, researchers have often added many more aspects to the inferences, such that it is best to keep this category open to important variations (see Table 3). Each of these parts of the reasoning cycle can be hierarchically refined so that a tree is formed here also.

System Design. The construction of the CBR system specifies what technologies it uses. This area of classification may not seem intuitive at first, but upon the examination of CBR systems it can be seen that many use a combination of technologies, not just case-based reasoning. The most common technology used in conjunction with CBR is rule-based reasoning; however some systems combine CBR with information retrieval, data mining, or other artificial intelligence methods. See Table 4 for an example of different possible construction classifications. If the construction of the system does use additional technologies, a flag should be appended to the end of the code to denote whether the case-based reasoning is executed separately. Also, an additional flag is used to designate CBR's role in the system, whether primary, secondary, or equivalent.

Table 3. Sample reasoning classifications

Code	Reasoning
10	Retrieve
10.1	Index
10.2	Similarity measure
20	Reuse
20.1	Adaptation
20.2	Interpretation
30	Revise
40	Retain
40.1	Maintenance

6.2 Research Evolution and Themes

Trend tracking comprises domains, purposes, memory, reasoning, and system design. First some figures are provided.

Statistics. The 117 selected papers were written by 132 different authors from all over the world. However, a grouping of papers by author clearly identifies a group of researchers contributing particularly actively to CBR in the Health Sciences research (see Figure 6). The average number of papers per author is 2.19, and the range 1 to 21.

Table 4. Sample design classifications

Code	Construction	Code	Construction
10	Pure CBR	60	Information Retrieval Combination
20	Rule Based Combination	70	Explanation Combination
30	Model Based Combination	CBR Role Flag	
40	Data Mining Combination	P	Primary Technology
40.1	Conceptual Clustering	S	Secondary Technology
40.2	Neural Networks	E	Equivalent Role Technology
40.3	Nearest Neighbor	CBR Additional Technology Flag	
40.4	Decision Tree	T	CBR is Separate
40.5	Bayesian Networks	F	CBR is Combined
50	Planning Combination		

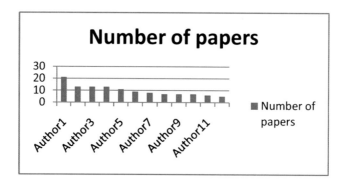

Fig. 6. The number of CBR Health Sciences papers by author

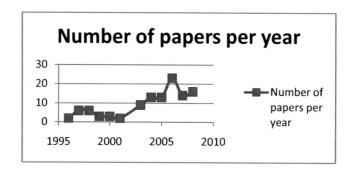

Fig. 7. CBR Health Sciences evolution of the number of papers per year

The number of papers by year has seen a rapid increase after 2003 – corresponding to the first Workshop on CBR in the Health Sciences (see Figure 6).

Domains. The 117 papers cover 41 domains all together. Although the domains of application all belong to the Health Sciences, some domains are more represented than the other ones. The most represented domain is medicine with 26 papers as a whole, which corresponds to either survey papers, or general frameworks and concepts applicable to any health sciences domains. Close second comes oncology (24 papers), then further come stress medicine (13 papers), transplantation (8 papers), diabetology (7 papers), fungi detection (6 papers), breast cancer (6 papers), nephrology (6 papers), genomics (5 papers), and infectious diseases (4 papers). All the other domains count less than 4 papers. Figure 8 shows the distribution of these domains. It is interesting to note in particular that cancer, being a very prominent disease, is studied by several CBR in the Health Sciences teams in the world.

Purpose. Among the 24 purposes listed for these papers, 30 papers propose treatments / therapies, 23 papers refer globally to decision support, 21 papers

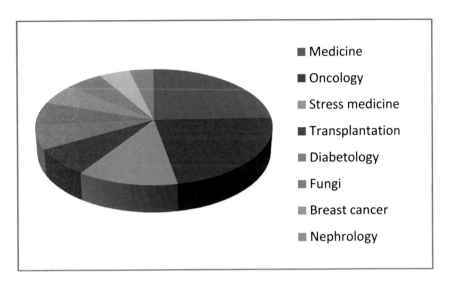

Fig. 8. CBR Health Sciences domains

describe diagnoses, 18 papers describe classification tasks, and 11 papers are survey papers. Image interpretation also accounts for 9 papers, and research support for 6 papers.

Memory. Memory structures and organization refers to 17 different concepts. The most represented is prototypes (24 papers), closely followed by time series (20 papers). Further come images (12 papers), text (6 papers), microarray data (5 papers), clusters (3 papers), generalized cases (3), inverted indexes (2 papers), networks (2 papers), and genomic sequences (2 papers). The other listed memory structures are graphs, multimedia data, plans, structured cases, and visio-spatial cases.

Reasoning. Surprisingly, for a methodology like CBR where research is very active in all reasoning cycle phases, in CBR in the Health Sciences the vast majority of systems refer to retrieval only (61 papers). Maintenance is also well represented (11 papers), and adaptation (8 papers). Further are represented: indexing (3 papers), retain (3 papers), similarity measures (2 papers), and revision (2 papers). However many systems also perform additional reasoning steps, even though the papers studied did not detail these steps, focusing on retrieval aspects instead.

System design. The main characteristics of developed systems include temporal abstraction (22 papers), knowledge-based systems combination (18 papers), prototype and generalized case mining (10 papers), temporal reasoning (7 papers), fuzzy logic (6 papers), information retrieval combination (6 papers), knowledge acquisition combination (5 papers), and in 3 papers: clinical guidelines integration, feature selection, distributed cases, neural networks combination, and planning combination. Thirty-eight different types of system design were identified, most of them dealing with some data mining / knowledge discovery combination, and as seen above temporal abstraction / temporal reasoning. However two categories are specific to medical domains: clinical guidelines integration, and electronic medical records integration.

Research themes. So far, the research themes are coded in free text format. More work remains to be done to categorize this part of each paper. One possibility to simplify the problem is to select one particular research focus among the dimensions of the paper: domain, purpose, memory, reasoning, and system design. With this simplification, the research themes are in majority oriented toward design (61 papers), purpose (38 papers), including 11 survey papers, and reasoning (14 papers). It is not surprising that no paper actually focuses exclusively on the application domain – this kind of publication would be better suited for a medical journal in a medical specialty. However it is surprising that so many papers focus on design aspects most of the time dealing with some combination with another methodology of AI (data mining, knowledge discovery, temporal reasoning and abstraction, knowledge based systems) or beyond, such as information retrieval and databases. Only 14 papers focus on some reasoning step – in practice only adaptation and retrieval – using methods intrinsic to CBR. The group of papers focusing on the paper purpose regroup such large subgroups as decision-support capability, classification, image understanding, survey papers, papers exploring different roles of CBR, and research support. The memory dimension is almost always connected with either some design aspect such as prototype learning, some reasoning aspect such as using prototypes to guide retrieval, or some purpose aspect, such as decision support. Indeed the memory needs to prove useful to the system in some way, since these papers are applied.

7   CBR versus AI in the Health Sciences

This section explores the research theme of synergies between CBR and other AI approaches. First is a look at the impact of the health sciences on AI and of AI on the health sciences. This is followed by a discussion of synergies with data mining and knowledge discovery and a look at multimodal reasoning architectures.

7.1   AI in the Health Sciences

History. Since the early days of AI, the health sciences have been a favorite area of application. The earliest systems were decision-support systems such as INTERNIST in 1970 [68] and MYCIN in 1976 [69]. INTERNIST was a rule-based expert system for the diagnosis of complex diseases. It was later commercialized as Quick Medical Reference (QMR) to support internists with diagnosis. MYCIN was also a rule-based expert system, for the diagnosis and treatment of blood infections. Created by Ted Shortliffe, this knowledge-based system mapped symptoms to diseases. It was clinically evaluated for effectiveness, and it led to the development of the expert system shell EMYCIN. New generations of AI systems in medicine expanded the range of AI methodologies in biomedical informatics. Newer applications include: implementing clinical practice guidelines in expert systems [70]; data mining to establish trends and associations among symptoms, genetic information, and diagnoses; medical image interpretation; and many more.

Impact on AI. Early researchers stressed the value of building systems for testing AI methodologies. These systems provided valuable feedback to AI researchers regarding the validity of their approaches. As reported by Shortliffe and Buchanan, "Artificial intelligence, or AI, is largely an experimental science – at least as much progress has been made by building and analyzing programs as by examining theoretical questions. MYCIN is one of several well-known programs that embody some intelligence and provide data on the extent to which intelligent behavior can be programmed. ... We believe that the whole field of AI will benefit from such attempts to take a detailed retrospective look at experiments, for in this way the scientific foundations of the field will gradually be defined" [71]. When evaluating the advances of AI systems in medicine, several levels of evaluation can be proposed, which can be roughly differentiated as computer system, user satisfaction, process variables, and domain outcomes levels:

1. The computer system level is how effectively the program performs its task. Measures include diagnosis accuracy for a decision-support system providing diagnostic recommendations, or precision and recall in an intelligent retrieval system for medical information. Measures can be integrated in the system programming.

2. The user satisfaction level involves assessing the user satisfaction with the system – the user can be either the physician or the patient, whether the patient uses the system or not. A questionnaire can be administered to the patients or physicians.

3. The process variables level works by measuring some variable connected in the clinical process, such as confidence in decision, pattern of care, adherence to protocol, cost of care, and adverse effects [72].

4. The domain outcomes level aims to measure clinical outcomes of the system. This requires conducting a randomized clinical trial to measure improvements in patient health or quality of life. For example, measures may involve the number of complications, or the cost of care, or even the survival duration.

Impact on the Health Sciences. Notably, critics of AI expressed concerns that the field had not been able to demonstrate actual clinical outcomes. AI researchers mostly showed satisfaction with computer system level evaluation results, some user satisfaction level results and a few process variables results.

One major step was to include AI systems in clinical practice. AI systems in use today are numerous. One of the first was NéoGanesh, developed to regulate the automatic ventilation system in the Intensive Care Unit (ICU), in use since 1995 [73]. Another example is Dxplain, a general expert system for the medical field, associating 4,500 clinical findings, including laboratory test results, with more than 2,000 diseases [74]. Some of these systems are available for routine purchase in medical supplies catalogues.

Several studies have shown the effectiveness of systems in clinical practice in terms of improving quality of care, safety, and efficiency [72]. One example is the study of a 1998 computer-based clinical reminder system that showed a particular clinical act – discussing advance directives with a patient – was performed significantly better with the clinical reminders than without them [75]. More generally, prescription decision-support systems (PDSS) and clinical reminder systems, often based on clinical guidelines implementation, have consistently shown clinical benefit in several studies [75]. However, clinical outcomes are rarely measured, while process variables and user satisfaction are more frequently measured. Obviously, computer system intrinsic measures are always reported.

The success of AI in the health sciences is explained by the shift of focus from centering the system success on the computational performance to the application domain performance. Indeed, successful systems provide a practical solution to a specific healthcare or health research problem. The systems with the largest impact, such as the clinical reminders, do not have to represent a challenging AI difficulty, but they do have to fit the clinical domain in which they are embedded. They are application domain driven rather than AI driven.

7.2   Synergies with Data Mining and Knowledge Discovery

These synergies may arise in different ways. They may involve using data mining as a separate pre-process for CBR, for example, to mine features from time series data [49]. Data mining may also be used for prototype mining [51], or during the CBR reasoning cycle, for example, to retrieve cases with temporal features [50], or for memory organization [47].

In the *decoupled synergy between knowledge discovery, data mining, and CBR*, Funk and Xiong present a case-based decision-support system for diagnosing stress related disorders [49]. This system deals with signal measurements such as breathing and heart rate expressed as physiological time series. The main components of the system are a signal-classifier and a pattern identifier. HR3Modul, the signal-classifier, uses a feature mining technique called wavelet extraction to learn features from the continuous signals. Being a case-based reasoning system, HR3Modul classifies the signals based on retrieving similar patterns to determine whether a patient may be suffering from a stress related disorder as well as the nature of the disorder. Advancing this research, Funk and Xiong argue that medical CBR systems incorporating time series data and patterns of events are fertile ground for knowledge discovery [49]. While CBR systems have traditionally learned from newly acquired individual cases, case bases as a whole are infrequently mined to discover more general knowledge. Such knowledge mining would not only improve the performance of CBR systems, but could turn case bases into valuable assets for clinical research.

The *integrated synergy between knowledge discovery, data mining, and CBR* is exemplified by Jänichen and Perner [47] who present a memory organization for efficient retrieval of images based on incremental conceptual clustering for case-based object recognition. These authors explain that case-based image interpretation in a biological domain, such as fungi spore detection, requires storing a series of cases corresponding to different variants of the object to be recognized in the case base. The conceptual clustering approach provides an answer to the question of how to group similar object shapes together and how to speed up the search through memory. Their system learns a hierarchy of prototypical cases representing structural shapes and measures the degree of generalization of each prototype [47].

Bichindaritz [51] explores automatically learning prototypical cases from the biomedical literature. The topic of case mining is an important recent trend in CBR, enabling CBR to capitalize on clinical databases, electronic patient records, and biomedical literature databases. This author explores how mined prototypical cases can guide the case-based reasoning of case-based decision-support systems and the different roles prototypical cases can play, particularly in aligning systems with recent biomedical findings [51].

7.3   Multimodal Reasoning Architectures

CBR is frequently used in conjunction with other AI approaches in order to capitalize on complementary strengths and synergies [76,77]. The first multimodal reasoning system in the health sciences was CASEY [23], which diagnosed heart failures, as described in Section 4. It integrated CBR with model-based reasoning, which it used when it did not have a sufficiently similar case in its case base to reach a satisfactory diagnosis. Rule-based reasoning (RBR) is the AI technique most commonly integrated with CBR. One example is the Auguste project, which combines CBR and RBR to recommend neuroleptic drugs for Alzheimer's patients with behavioral problems [35]. Here, CBR is used to determine whether or not a patient would benefit from a neuroleptic drug, and if so, RBR is used to determine the best choice of available neuroleptic drugs for the individual. Another example is the 4 Diabetes Support System [78], which helps to achieve and maintain good blood glucose control in patients with type 1 diabetes on insulin pump therapy. This system uses RBR to detect glucose control problems requiring changes in therapy and CBR to suggest the appropriate therapeutic changes. Researchers on the 4 Diabetes Support System have recently integrated a naive Bayes classifier to detect excessive glucose variability and are currently exploring the integration of other machine learning techniques for problem detection in continuous blood glucose data.

Several other AI methodologies and techniques have also been combined with CBR to advantage. Díaz et al. demonstrate the applicability of CBR to the classification of DNA microarray data and show that CBR can be applied successfully to domains struck by the "curse of dimensionality" [45]. This "curse," a well-known issue in bioinformatics, refers to the availability of a relatively small number of cases, each having thousands of features. In their Gene-CBR system, for cancer diagnosis, a case has 22,283 features, corresponding to genes. The authors have designed a hybrid architecture for Gene-CBR, which combines fuzzy case representation, a neural network to cluster the cases for genetically similar patients, and a set of if-then rules extracted from the case base to explain the classification results [45]. In other work, Montani explains how CBR can be used to configure the parameters upon which other AI methodologies rely [79]. McSherry presents a novel hypothetico-deductive CBR approach to minimize the number of tests required to confirm a diagnostic hypothesis [80]. Still other work capitalizes on the complementarity among knowledge bases, ontologies, and CBR [81].

8 Summary and Conclusion

Biomedical domains have long been a focus of AI research and development. CBR is an AI approach that is especially apropos, due to its leverage of experiential knowledge in the form of cases. Health sciences professionals reason naturally from cases, which they use, among other things, to inform practice, develop clinical guidelines, and educate future professionals. CBR is also highly synergistic with other AI approaches, which may be combined with CBR in multimodal reasoning systems. CBR in the Health Sciences systems have been built to support diagnosis, classification, treatment planning, and education, in areas as diverse as oncology, diabetology, psychiatry, and stress medicine. They support biomedical research and bioinformatics, as well as clinical practice. CBR in the Health Sciences researchers continue to branch out into new reasoning tasks and additional biomedical domains.

CBR and the health sciences impact each other in mutually beneficial and synergistic ways. The health sciences provide a rich and complex experimental field for evaluating CBR methodologies and extending the CBR approach. A complementarity with statistics allows CBR to support evidence gathering for biomedical research and evidence-based medical practice. As computer science becomes more application driven, and as the health sector continues to expand, this interdisciplinary field is expected to grow. CBR in the Health Sciences is poised today to push the state of the art in AI while contributing clinically useful systems that promote health and wellbeing.

References

1. Holt, A., Bichindaritz, I., Schmidt, R., Perner, P.: Medical applications in case-based reasoning. The Knowledge Engineering Review 20(3), 289–292 (2005)
2. Bichindaritz, I., Montani, S., Portinale, L. (eds.): Special issue on case-based reasoning in the health sciences. Applied Intelligence 28(3), 207–285 (2008)
3. Bichindaritz, I. (ed.): Special issue on case-based reasoning in the health sciences. Artificial Intelligence in Medicine 36(2), 121–192 (2006)

4. Bichindaritz, I., Marling, C. (eds.): Special issue on case-based reasoning in the health sciences. Computational Intelligence 22(3-4), 143–282 (2006)
5. Bichindaritz, I., Montani, S. (eds.): Special issue on case-based reasoning in the health sciences. Computational Intelligence 25(3), 161–263 (2009)
6. Aamodt, A., Plaza, E.: Case-based reasoning: Foundational issues, methodological variations, and system approaches. AI Communications 7(I), 39–59 (1994)
7. Schmidt, R., Montani, S., Bellazzi, R., Portinale, L., Gierl, L.: Case-based reasoning for medical knowledge-based systems. International Journal of Medical Informatics 64(2-3), 355–367 (2001)
8. Nilsson, M., Sollenborn, M.: Advancements and trends in medical case-based reasoning: An overview of systems and system development. In: Proceedings of the Seventeenth International Florida Artificial Intelligence Research Society Conference – Special Track on Case-Based Reasoning, pp. 178–183. AAAI Press, Menlo Park (2004)
9. Bichindaritz, I., Marling, C.: Case-based reasoning in the health sciences: What's next? Artificial Intelligence in Medicine 36(2), 127–135 (2006)
10. Bichindaritz, I.: Case-based reasoning in the health sciences: Why it matters for the health sciences and for CBR. In: Althoff, K.-D., Bergmann, R., Minor, M., Hanft, A. (eds.) ECCBR 2008. LNCS (LNAI), vol. 5239, pp. 1–17. Springer, Heidelberg (2008)
11. Kolodner, J.: Case-Based Reasoning. Morgan Kaufmann, San Francisco (1993)
12. Riesbeck, C.K., Schank, R.C.: Inside Case-Based Reasoning. Erlbaum, Hillsdale (1989)
13. Kolodner, J.L., Leake, D.B.: Chapter 2: A tutorial introduction to case-based reasoning. In: Leake, D.B. (ed.) Case-Based Reasoning: Experiences, Lessons & Future Directions. AAAI/MIT Press, Menlo Park (1996)
14. Leake, D.B. (ed.): Case-Based Reasoning: Experiences, Lessons & Future Directions. AAAI/MIT Press, Menlo Park (1996)
15. Aha, D.W., Marling, C.R. (eds.): Special issue on case-based reasoning commentaries. Knowledge Engineering Review 20(3), 201–328 (2005)
16. National Workforce Center for Emerging Technologies: Applications of information technology: Trends assessment for 2007-2008 (2007), http://www.nwcet.org/products/trends.asp (accessed April 2010)
17. Figueroa, E.B., Woods, R.A.: Industry output and employment projections to 2016. Monthly Labor Review (November 2007), http://www.bls.gov/opub/mlr/2007/11/art4full.pdf
18. ISI Web of Knowledge Journal Citation Reports: Subject category summary list (2008) http://admin-apps.isiknowledge.com/JCR/JCR (accessed April 2010)
19. Kolodner, J.L., Kolodner, R.M.: Using experience in clinical problem solving: Introduction and framework. IEEE Transactions on Systems, Man and Cybernetics 17(3), 420–431 (1987)
20. Bichindaritz, I.: MNAOMIA: Improving case-based reasoning for an application in psychiatry. In: Kohane, I., Patel, R., Shahar, Y., Szolovits, P., Uckun, S. (eds.) Artificial Intelligence in Medicine: Applications of Current Technologies, Working Notes of the AAAI 1996 Spring Symposium. AAAI Press, Menlo Park (1996)
21. Bareiss, R.: Exemplar-Based Knowledge Acquisition: A Unified Approach to Concept Representation, Classification, and Learning. Academic Press, San Diego (1989)
22. Bareiss, E., Porter, B., Wier, C.: PROTOS: An exemplar based learning apprentice. In: Proceedings of the Fourth International Workshop on Machine Learning, pp. 12–23. Morgan Kaufmann, Los Altos (1987)

23. Koton, P.: Reasoning about evidence in causal explanations. In: Mitchell, T.M., Smith, R.G. (eds.) Proceedings AAAI-88, pp. 256–261. AAAI Press, Menlo Park (1988)
24. Heindl, B., Schmidt, R., Schmidt, G., Haller, M., Pfaller, P., Gierl, L., Pollwein, B.: A case-based consilarius for therapy recommendation (ICONS): Computer-based advice for calculated antibiotic therapy in intensive care medicine. Computer Methods and Programs in Biomedicine 52, 117–127 (1997)
25. Schmidt, R., Pollwein, B., Gierl, L.: Case-based reasoning for antibiotics therapy advice. In: Althoff, K.-D., Bergmann, R., Branting, L.K. (eds.) ICCBR 1999. LNCS (LNAI), vol. 1650, pp. 550–559. Springer, Heidelberg (1999)
26. Kolodner, J.: Educational implications of analogy: A view from case-based reasoning. American Psychologist 52(1), 57–66 (1997)
27. Marling, C.R., Petot, G.J., Sterling, L.S.: Integrating case-based and rule-based reasoning to meet multiple design constraints. Computational Intelligence 15(3), 308–332 (1999)
28. Bell, B., Bareiss, R., Beckwith, R.: Sickle cell counselor: A prototype goal-based scenario for instruction in a museum environment. Technical Report 56, The Institute for the Learning Sciences, Evanston (1994)
29. Turner, R.M.: Using schemas for diagnosis. Computer Methods and Programs in Biomedicine 30, 199–208 (1989)
30. Lopez, B., Plaza, E.: Case-base planning for medical diagnosis. In: Komorowski, J., Raś, Z.W. (eds.) ISMIS 1993. LNCS, vol. 689, pp. 96–105. Springer, Heidelberg (1993)
31. Bradburn, C., Zeleznikow, J.: The application of case-based reasoning to the tasks of health care planning. In: Wess, S., Althoff, K.D., Richter, M.M. (eds.) EWCBR 1994. LNCS, vol. 984, pp. 365–378. Springer, Heidelberg (1995)
32. Bichindaritz, I., Séroussi, B.: Contraindre l'anologie par la causalité. Technique et Sciences Informatiques 11(4), 69–98 (1992)
33. Bellazzi, R., Montani, S., Portinale, L., Riva, A.: Integrating rule-based and case-based decision making in diabetic patient management. In: Althoff, K.-D., Bergmann, R., Branting, L.K. (eds.) ICCBR 1999. LNCS (LNAI), vol. 1650, pp. 386–400. Springer, Heidelberg (1999)
34. Bichindaritz, I., Kansu, E., Sullivan, K.M.: Case-based reasoning in CARE-PARTNER: Gathering evidence for evidence-based medical practice. In: Smyth, B., Cunningham, P. (eds.) EWCBR 1998. LNCS (LNAI), vol. 1488, pp. 334–345. Springer, Heidelberg (1998)
35. Marling, C., Whitehouse, P.: Case-based reasoning in the care of Alzheimer's disease patients. In: Aha, D.W., Watson, I. (eds.) ICCBR 2001. LNCS (LNAI), vol. 2080, pp. 702–715. Springer, Heidelberg (2001)
36. Berger, J.: Roentgen: Radiation therapy and case-based reasoning. In: Proceedings of the Tenth Conference on Artificial Intelligence for Applications, pp. 171–177. IEEE Computer Society Press, Los Alamitos (1994)
37. Macura, R.T., Macura, K.J.: MacRad: Radiology image resource with a case-based retrieval system. In: Veloso, M., Aamodt, A. (eds.) ICCBR 1995. LNCS, vol. 1010, pp. 43–54. Springer, Heidelberg (1995)
38. Perner, P.: An architecture for a CBR image segmentation system. Engineering Applications of Artificial Intelligence 12(6), 749–759 (1999)
39. Haddad, M., Adlassnig, K.P., Porenta, G.: Feasibility analysis of a case-based reasoning system for automated detection of coronary heart disease from myocardial scintigrams. Artificial Intelligence in Medicine 9(1), 61–78 (1997)

40. Grimnes, M., Aamodt, A.: A two layer case-based reasoning architecture for medical image understanding. In: Smith, I., Faltings, B.V. (eds.) EWCBR 1996. LNCS, vol. 1168, pp. 164–178. Springer, Heidelberg (1996)

41. Bichindaritz, I., Potter, S.: PhylSyst: un système d'intelligence artificielle pour l'analyse cladistique. Biosystema 12, 17–55 (1994)

42. Fenstermacher, K.D.: An application of case-based instruction in medical domains. In: Kohane, I., Patel, R., Shahar, Y., Szolovits, P., Uckun, S. (eds.) Artificial Intelligence in Medicine: Applications of Current Technologies, Working Notes of the AAAI 1996 Spring Symposium. AAAI Press, Menlo Park (1996)

43. Costello, E., Wilson, D.C.: A case-based approach to gene finding. In: McGinty, L. (ed.) Workshop Proceedings of the Fifth International Conference on Case-Based Reasoning, Trondheim, Norway (2003)

44. Davies, J., Glasgow, J., Kuo, T.: Visio-spatial case-based reasoning: A case study in prediction of protein structure. Computational Intelligence 22(3-4), 194–207 (2006)

45. Díaz, F., Fdez-Riverola, F., Corchado, J.M.: Gene-CBR: A case-based reasoning tool for cancer diagnosis using microarray datasets. Computational Intelligence 22(3-4), 254–268 (2006)

46. El Balaa, Z., Strauss, A., Uziel, P., Maximini, K., Traphoner, R.: FM-Ultranet: A decision support system using case-based reasoning applied to ultrasonography. In: McGinty, L. (ed.) Workshop Proceedings of the Fifth International Conference on Case-Based Reasoning, Trondheim, Norway (2003)

47. Jänichen, S., Perner, P.: Conceptual clustering and case generalization of 2-dimensional forms. Computational Intelligence 22(3-4), 177–193 (2006)

48. Perner, P.: Different learning strategies in a case-based reasoning system for image interpretation. In: Smyth, B., Cunningham, P. (eds.) EWCBR 1998. LNCS (LNAI), vol. 1488, pp. 334–345. Springer, Heidelberg (1998)

49. Funk, P., Xiong, N.: Case-based reasoning and knowledge discovery in medical applications with time series. Computational Intelligence 22(3-4), 238–253 (2006)

50. Montani, S., Portinale, L.: Accounting for the temporal dimension in case-based retrieval: A framework for medical applications. Computational Intelligence 22(3-4), 208–223 (2006)

51. Bichindaritz, I.: Prototypical cases for knowledge maintenance for biomedical CBR. In: Weber, R., Richter, M. (eds.) ICCBR 2007. LNCS (LNAI), vol. 4626, pp. 492–506. Springer, Heidelberg (2007)

52. Davis, G., Wiratunga, N., Taylor, B., Craw, S.: Matching SMARTHOUSE technology to needs of the elderly and disabled. In: McGinty, L. (ed.) Workshop Proceedings of the Fifth International Conference on Case-Based Reasoning, Trondheim, Norway (2003)

53. Doyle, D., Walsh, P.: An evaluation of the usefulness of explanation in a CBR system for decision support in bronchiolitis treatment. Computational Intelligence 22(3-4), 269–281 (2006)

54. Montani, S.: Case-based reasoning for managing non-compliance with clinical guidelines. In: Wilson, D.C., Khemani, D. (eds.) Workshop Proceedings of the Seventh International Conference on Case-Based Reasoning (ICCBR 2007), Belfast, Northern Ireland, pp. 325–336 (2007)

55. Bichindaritz, I.: Memory organization as the missing link between case-based reasoning and information retrieval in biomedicine. Computational Intelligence 22(3-4), 148–160 (2006)

56. d'Aquin, M., Lieber, J., Napoli, A.: Adaptation knowledge acquisition: A case study for case-based decision support in oncology. Computational Intelligence 22(3-4), 161–176 (2006)

57. Vorobieva, O., Gierl, L., Schmidt, R.: Adaptation methods in an endocrine therapy support system. In: McGinty, L. (ed.) Workshop Proceedings of the Fifth International Conference on Case-Based Reasoning, Trondheim, Norway (2003)
58. Schmidt, R., Waligora, T., Vorobieva, O.: Prototypes for medical case-based applications. In: Perner, P. (ed.) ICDM 2008. LNCS (LNAI), vol. 5077, pp. 1–15. Springer, Heidelberg (2008)
59. Sokal, R., Rohlf, F.: Biometry: The Principles and Practice of Statistics in Biological Research. W.H. Freeman, New York (2001)
60. Schmidt, R., Waligora, T., Gierl, L.: Predicting influenza waves with health insurance data. Computational Intelligence 22(3-4), 224–237 (2006)
61. Vorobieva, O., Rumyantsev, A., Schmidt, R.: ISOR-2: A case-based reasoning system to explain exceptional dialysis patients. In: Perner, P. (ed.) ICDM 2007. LNCS (LNAI), vol. 4597, pp. 173–183. Springer, Heidelberg (2007)
62. Pantazi, S., Bichindaritz, I., Moehr, J.: The case for context-dependent dynamic hierarchical representations of knowledge in medical informatics. In: Proceedings of the Conference on Information Technology and Communications in Health, ITCH 2007, Victoria, BC, pp. 123–134 (2007)
63. Pantazi, S., Arocha, J.: Case-based medical informatics. BMC Journal of Medical Informatics and Decision Making 4(1), 19–39 (2004)
64. Bichindaritz, I., Reed Jr., J.: Research trends in case-based reasoning in the health sciences. In: Delany, S. (ed.) Workshop Proceedings of the Eighth International Conference on Case-Based Reasoning (ICCBR 2009), Seattle, pp. 195–204 (2009)
65. Montani, S., Bellazzi, R., Portinale, L., Stefanelli, M.: A multi-modal reasoning methodology for managing IDDM patients. International Journal of Medical Informatics 58–59(1), 243–256 (2000)
66. Gierl, L.: ICONS: Cognitive functions in a case-based consultation system for intensive care. In: Andreassen, S., Engelbrecht, R., Wyatt, J. (eds.) Artificial Intelligence in Medicine: Proceedings of the 4th Conference on Artificial Intelligence in Medicine Europe, pp. 230–236. IOS Press, Amsterdam (1993)
67. Lieber, J., d'Aquin, M., Badra, F., Napoli, A.: Modeling adaptation of breast cancer treatment decision protocols in the KASIMIR project. Applied Intelligence 28(3), 261–274 (2008)
68. Miller, R., Pople Jr., H., Myers, J.: Internist-1, an experimental computer-based diagnostic consultant for general internal medicine. New England Journal of Medicine 307(8), 468–476 (1982)
69. Shortliffe, E.: Computer-Based Medical Consultations: MYCIN. Elsevier/North Holland, New York (1976)
70. Shahar, Y., Miksch, S., Johnson, P.: The Asgaard project: A task-specific framework for the application and critiquing of time-oriented clinical guidelines. Artificial Intelligence in Medicine 14(1), 29–51 (1998)
71. Shortliffe, E., Buchanan, B.: Rule-Based Expert Systems: The MYCIN Experiments of the Stanford Heuristic Programming Project. Addison-Wesley, Reading (1984)
72. Sinchenko, V., Westbrook, J., Tipper, S., Mathie, M., Coiera, E.: Electronic decision support activities in different healthcare settings in Australia. In: Electronic Decision Support for Australia's Health Sector, National Electronic Decision Support Taskforce, Commonwealth of Australia (2003), http://www.health.gov.au/healthonline/nedst.htm
73. Dojat, M., Brochard, L., Lemaire, F., Harf, A.: A knowledge-based system for assisted ventilation of patients in intensive care units. International Journal of Clinical Monitoring and Computing 9, 239–250 (1992)

74. Barnett, G., Cimino, J., Huppa, J.: Dxplain: an evolving diagnostic decision-support system. Journal of the American Medical Association 258, 69–76 (1987)
75. Dexter, P., Wolinsky, F., Gramelspacher, G.: Effectiveness of computer-generated reminders for increasing discussions about advance directives and completion of advance directive forms. Annals of Internal Medicine 128, 102–110 (1998)
76. Marling, C., Sqalli, M., Rissland, E., Muñoz-Avila, H., Aha, D.: Case-based reasoning integrations. AI Magazine 23(1), 69–86 (2002)
77. Marling, C., Rissland, E., Aamodt, A.: Integrations with case-based reasoning. The Knowledge Engineering Review 20(3), 241–245 (2005)
78. Marling, C., Shubrook, J., Schwartz, F.: Case-based decision support for patients with type 1 diabetes on insulin pump therapy. In: Althof, K.D., Bergmann, R., Minor, M., Hanft, A. (eds.) ECCBR 2008. LNCS (LNAI), vol. 5239, pp. 325–339. Springer, Heidelberg (2008)
79. Montani, S.: Exploring new roles for case-based reasoning in heterogeneous AI systems for medical decision support. Applied Intelligence 28(3), 275–285 (2008)
80. McSherry, D.: Hypothetico-deductive case-based reasoning. In: Wilson, D.C., Khemani, D. (eds.) Workshop Proceedings of the Seventh International Conference on Case-Based Reasoning (ICCBR 2007), Belfast, Northern Ireland, pp. 315–326 (2007)
81. Bichindaritz, I.: Mémoire: Case-based reasoning meets the semantic web in biology and medicine. In: Funk, P., González Calero, P. (eds.) ECCBR 2004. LNCS (LNAI), vol. 3155, pp. 47–61. Springer, Heidelberg (2004)

Chapter 8
Intelligent Signal Analysis Using Case-Based Reasoning for Decision Support in Stress Management

Shahina Begum, Mobyen Uddin Ahmed, Peter Funk, and Ning Xiong

School of Innovation, Design and Engineering, Mälardalen University,
PO Box 883 SE-721 23, Västerås, Sweden
Tel.: +46 21 10 14 53; Fax: +46 21 10 14 60
firstname.lastname@mdh.se

Abstract. Modern daily life triggers stress for many people in different every-day situations. Consequently many people live with increased stress levels under long durations. It is recognized that increased exposure to stress may cause serious health problems if undiagnosed and untreated. One of the physiological parameters for quantifying stress levels is finger temperature, which helps clinicians with the diagnosis and treatment of stress. However, in practice, the complex and varying nature of signals often makes it difficult and tedious for a clinician and particularly less experienced clinicians to understand, interpret and analyze complex and lengthy sequential measurements. There are very few experts who are able to diagnose and predict stress-related problems; hence a system that can help clinicians in diagnosing stress is important. In order to provide decision support in stress management using this complex data source, case-based reasoning (CBR) is applied as the main methodology to facilitate experience reuse and decision justification. Feature extraction methods which aim to yield compact representation of original signals into case indexes are investigated. A fuzzy technique is also incorporated into the system to perform matching between the features derived from signals to better accommodate vagueness and uncertainty inherently existing in clinicians reasoning as well as imprecision in case description. The validation of the approach is based on close collaboration with experts and measurements from twenty four people used as a reference. The system formulates a new problem case with 17 extracted features from finger temperature signal data. Every case contains fifteen minutes of data from 1800 samples. Thirty nine time series from 24 people have been used to evaluate the approach (matching algorithms) in which the system shows a level of performance close to an experienced expert. Consequently, the system can be used as an expert for a less experienced clinician or as a second option for an experienced clinician to supplement their decision making task in stress management.

1 Introduction

Today's increased use of computer-based systems in the medical domain requires computer processing of biomedical signals such as, ECG, EEG, EMG, heart rate etc. These are often obtaining from sensors, transducers, etc. and such signals contain

I. Bichindaritz et al. (Eds.): Computational Intelligence in Healthcare 4, SCI 309, pp. 159–189.

information, which is often hidden, about their underlying biological systems [1]. In manual processes, clinicians often make a diagnosis by looking at signal data but the level of complexity associated with manual analysis and interpretation of these biomedical signals is great even for experienced clinicians. So, signal processing to extract clinically significant information from these biomedical signals is valuable before the data is used by the clinician. Nilsson et al. [2] classify biomedical signals i.e. Respiratory Sinus Arrhythmia with CBR. Authors in [6], [7] deal with temporal abstraction by key sequences representing a pattern of signal changes in the medical domain. Ölmeza and Dokur [3] have applied artificial neural networks to classify heart sounds. Wavelet transformation is used in [4], [5] to characterize ECG signals.

Increased stress is a continuing problem today. Negative stress could particularly cause serious health problems if it remains undiagnosed/misdiagnosed and untreated. Different treatments and exercises can reduce this stress. Since one of the effects of stress is reduced bodily awareness, it is easy to miss signals such as high tension in the muscles, unnatural breathing, blood-sugar fluctuations and cardiovascular functionality etc. It may take many weeks or months to become aware of the increased stress level, and once it is noticed, the effects and misaligned processes, e.g. of metabolic processes, may need long and active behavioral treatment to revert to a normal state [8]. For patients with high blood pressure and heart problems high stress levels may be directly life-endangering. A system determining a person's stress profile and potential health problems would be valuable both in a clinical environment as a second opinion or in the home environment to be used as part of a stress management program.

During stress the sympathetic nervous system is activated causing a decrease in peripheral circulation which in turn decreases the skin temperature. However during relaxation, a reverse effect (i.e. activation of the parasympathetic nervous system) occurs resulting in the increase of skin temperature. In this way, the finger skin temperature responds to stress [69]. The pattern of variation within a finger temperature signal could help to determine stress-related disorders. Other conventional methods for measuring stress such as taking measurements of respiration (e.g. end-tidal carbon dioxide (ETCO2)), heart rate (e.g. calculating the respiratory sinus arrhythmia (RSA)) and heart rate variability (HRV) is often expensive and requires equipment (using many sensors) which is not suitable for use in non-clinical environments or without supervision of experienced clinical staff. Finger temperature measurements on the other hand can be collected using a sensor which is comparatively low in cost and can be used as a supplementary and convenient tool by general users to diagnose and control stress at home or at work. However, the characteristics of finger temperature (FT) is different for different individuals due to health factors, metabolic activity etc. In practice, it is difficult and tedious even for an experienced clinician to understand, interpret and analyze complex, lengthy sequential measurements in order to determine the stress levels. Since there are significant individual variations when looking at the FT, this is a worthy challenge to find a computational solution to apply it in a computer-based system.

Therefore, this chapter presents a general paradigm in which a case-based approach is used as a core technique to facilitate experience reuse based on signals to develop a computer-based stress diagnosis system that can be used by people who need to monitor their stress level during everyday situations e.g. at home and work for health reasons. Fuzzy similarity matching is incorporated into the CBR system to better accommodate the underlying uncertainty existing in the reasoning process.

1.1 Decision Support System and Case-Based Stress Diagnosis

The term Decision Support System (DSS) is defined by Little as a "model-based set of procedures for processing data and judgments to assist a manager in his decision making" [9]. Medical Decision Support Systems (DSS) have been defined by many people in many different ways. According to Shortliffe a medical DSS is "any computer program designed to help health professionals make clinical decisions [10]." The early AI systems for medical decision making emerged around the 1950's mainly built using decision trees or truth tables. After that, different methods or algorithms have been introduced to implement medical decision support systems such as, Bayesian statistics, decision-analytical models, symbolic reasoning, neural-networks, rule-based reasoning, fuzzy logic, case-based reasoning etc.

Since the implementation of MYCIN [11] many of the early AI systems attempted to apply rule-based systems in developing computer based diagnosis systems. However, for a broad and complex medical domain the effort of applying rule-based system has encountered several problems. Some of the preliminary criteria for implementing a rule-based system are that the problem domain should be well understood, constant over time and the domain theory should be strong i.e. well defined [12]. In psychophysiology, the diagnosis of stress is so difficult that even an experienced clinician might have difficulty in expressing his knowledge explicitly. Large individual variations and the absence of general rules make it difficult to diagnose stress and predict the risk of stress-related health problems. On the other hand, case-based reasoning (CBR) works well in such domains where the domain knowledge is not clear enough i.e. weak domain theory. Furthermore, CBR systems can learn automatically which is very important as the medical domain is evolving with time. Rule-based systems cannot learn automatically as new rules are usually inserted manually. Statistical techniques are also applied successfully in medical systems. But to apply statistical models a large amount of data is required to investigate a hypothesis which is also not available in our application domain.

Several motivations for applying CBR to stress diagnosis can be identified:

- CBR [12] [13] is inspired by the way humans reason i.e. to solve a new problem by applying previous experiences. This reasoning process is also medically accepted and the experts in diagnosing stress too rely heavily on their past memory to solve a new case. This is the prime reason why we prefer to use CBR.
- Knowledge elicitation is another problem in diagnosing stress, as human behaviour or our response to stress is not always predictable. Even an experienced clinician in this domain might have difficulty to articulate his knowledge explicitly. Sometimes experts make assumptions and predictions based on experiences or old cases. To overcome this knowledge elicitation bottleneck we use CBR because in CBR, this elicitation can be performed with the previous cases in the case base.

- For diagnosing stress we use finger temperature sensor signals. By analyzing this biomedical signal we identified large individual variations which make it difficult to define in a model or use a set of rules. Other AI systems such as, rule-based reasoning or model based reasoning is not appropriate in this context. CBR can be used when there are no sets of rules or a model [14].
- To implement a CBR system in this domain we need to identify features from the finger temperature sensor signal which would allow a clinician to identify features for the success or failure of a case. This would help to reduce the repetition of mistakes in the future.
- The knowledge in the domain is growing with time so it is important that the system can adapt and learn new knowledge. Many of the AI systems failed to continue because of the lack of this type of maintenance. CBR system can learn by adding new cases into the case base.
- The cases in the case base can be used for the follow up of treatment and also for training less experienced clinicians.

2   Background and Methods

2.1 Stress

The term 'stress' was first introduced by Hans Selye in the 1950s who noticed that patients suffer physically not only as a result of a disease or medical condition. He defined stress as a "non-specific response of the body to any demand" [15]. Stress is our body's response to any threat to defend it from potential harm. Another definition of stress by Lazarus is "stress occurs when an individual perceives that the demands of an external situation are beyond his or her perceived ability to cope with them" [16]. An individual's response to a situation/thing can be varied and depends on one's coping capability. For example, a person might take a huge workload without being worried and the same amount of work could make another person worried thinking how to cope with that situation. So, an individual's mental state and ability to appraise the stimulus determines whether stress occurs or not. In our everyday life we react to certain events or facts that may produce stress. Our body's nervous system activates and stress hormones are released to protect us. This is called the "fight-or-flight" reaction, or the stress response.

The human nervous system is divided into two main parts, the voluntary system and autonomic system. The automatic nervous system is divided into two parts: sympathetic and the parasympathetic nervous system. The sympathetic nervous system (SNS) works to protect our body against threats by stimulating the necessary glands (i.e. thyroid and adrenal glands) and organs. It decreases the blood flow to the digestive and eliminative organs (i.e. the intestine, liver, kidney etc.) and enhances the flow of blood to the brain and muscles. The thyroid and adrenal glands also supply extra energy. As a result it speeds up the heart rate, increases blood pressure, decreases digestion and constricts the blood vessels i.e. vasoconstriction which slows down the flow of blood etc. The SNS thus activates the body for the fight-or-flight response to stress. The parasympathetic nervous system counteracts the fight-or-flight response to return the body to its normal state. It stimulates digestion, the immune system and eliminative organs etc. to rebuild the body [17].

Physiology of the Stress Response. When our brain appraises stress, the sympathetic nervous system stimulates the hypothalamus, and prepares the brain to respond to stress (see Fig. 1). The SNS stimulates the adrenal gland to release the hormone Adrenaline into the blood supply. It also releases Noradrenalin to the nerve endings and activates various smooth muscles. These hormones decrease digestions, increase the heart rate, increase metabolic rate, dilates blood vessels in the heart and other muscles and constricts the skin blood vessels i.e. decreases skin temperature etc.

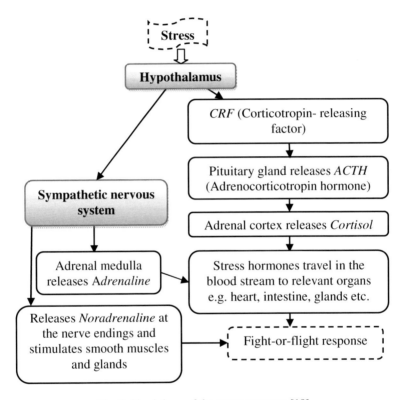

Fig. 1. Physiology of the stress response [18]

The Hypothalamus also releases Corticotropin-releasing hormone (CRH) which activates the pituitary gland to release the Adrenocorticotropin hormone (ACTH). ACTH then travels through the blood supply and stimulates the adrenal glands to release Cortisol into the blood supply. Thus the human body supplies energy and oxygen, and provides stimulation to the heart, muscles, brain and other organs to help the body response to stress [18]. When the brain receives the information that the stress situation is over, the parasympathetic nervous system helps to return the hormones to the baseline levels. Thus, the SNS activates during stress and helps to

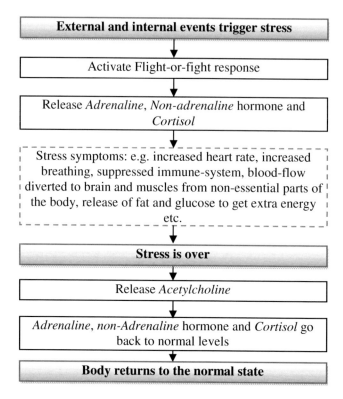

Fig. 2. General overview of the stress response

release the stored energy. On the other hand, the parasympathetic nervous system performs the opposite function i.e. returns the body to its normal state. So, due to a stress response the body releases large amount of energy immediately and this reaction to stress can affect many physiological mechanisms. To diagnose psychophysiological dysfunctions such as stress, clinicians often consider the balance between the activities in the sympathetic and parasympathetic nervous systems. A general overview of stress activity to our body is given in Fig. 2.

A small amount of stress is good for us. It can prepare us to meet difficult challenges in life. On the other hand, long-term exposure to stress i.e. when the emergency stress response is prolonged i.e. out of its functional context for most of the time, it may in the worst case cause severe mental and physical problems that are often related to psychosomatic disorders, coronary heart disease etc. Symptoms of stress can be experienced in different ways such as anxiety, muscle tensions/cramp, depression and other bodily symptoms which in turn can further influence our sympathetic nervous system. There are several stress management techniques, such as relaxation, exercise, and cognitive-behavioural stress management etc.

Psychophysiology. Psychophysiology is a branch of psychology. It addresses the relation between 'Psychology' and 'Physiology'. Andreassi [19] defined Psychophysiology as "the study of relations between psychological manipulations and resulting physiological responses, measured in the living organism, to promote under-standing of the relation between mental and bodily processes". There is an interaction between body and mind so for instance, a physical disease can be treated psychologi-cally or vice-versa. If a person is informed about this mind-body connection, he/she can utilize this knowledge and control psychophysiologic activity which could im-prove health [20]. Some physiological parameters that are commonly used include; skin conductance, skin temperature, respiration e.g. end-tidal carbon dioxide (ETCO2), electromyography (EMG), electrocardiography (ECG), heart rate e.g. cal-culating respiratory sinus arrhythmia (RSA), heart rate variability (HRV), electroe-ncephalography (EEG), brain imaging techniques, oculomotor and pupilometric measures etc. Stress medicine is a branch of Psychophysiology where the treatment of stress-related dysfunctions is studied. In stress medicine psychophysiologists investi-gate scientific ways to prevent stress-related dysfunctions. Skin temperature is one of the physiological parameters that can be used to measure stress. Also other parameters such as cardiovascular parameters i.e. heart rate, HRV can be used to quantify stress.

Biofeedback. Biofeedback training is an effective method for controlling stress. It is an area of growing interest in medicine and psychology and it has proven to be very efficient for a number of physical, psychological and psychophysical problems [21], [22].

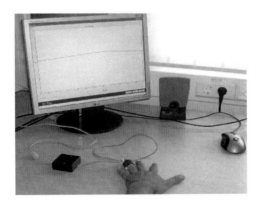

Fig. 3. Biofeedback training using finger temperature measurement

The basic purpose of biofeedback is that the patient can alter their physiological or psychological state while observing measurement changes, e.g. the changes in skin temperature on a graph. From prior education they are able to see how a positive or negative psycho-physiological change is represented on the graph and can behaviorally train the body and/or mind to change the biological response to improve the condition.

This finger temperature measurement was taken using a temperature sensor during different stress and relaxed conditions. It is possible to monitor temperature as an electronic signal on the computer screen as shown in Fig. 3. Thus the pattern of the finger temperature measurement observed from this signal can support biofeedback training for the management of stress-related dysfunctions. However, different patients with very different physical reactions to stress and relaxation make stress a complex area to apply biofeedback. A clinician normally supervises patients in the implementation of biofeedback in stress medicine, where the patient's individual profile is determined based on observed features and behavioral training is given.

2.2 Case-Based Reasoning (CBR)

Learning from the past and solving new problems based on previously solved cases is the main approach of CBR. This approach is inspired by humans and how they sometimes reason when solving problems. A case (an experience) normally contains a problem, a diagnosis/classification, a solution and its results. For a new problem case, a CBR system matches the problem part of the case against cases in the case library or case base and retrieves the solutions of the most similar cases after adapting it to the current situation.

CBR cycle. A case represents a piece of knowledge as experience and plays an important role in the reasoning process. The case comprises unique features to describe a problem. Cases can be presented in different ways [12]. To provide the solution of a new case, the cases can be represented using a problem and solution structure (Case structure A, Fig. 4). For the evaluation of a current case, cases can also contain the outcome/result (Case structure B, Fig. 4).

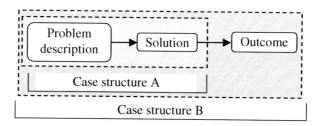

Fig. 4. Cases can contain a problem description and solution only or may include the result/outcome as a case structure in the medical domain [23]

Prior to the case representation many CBR systems depend on feature extraction because of the complex data format in some domains. In case retrieval, a major phase of CBR, matching of features between two cases plays a vital role. Cases with hidden key features may affect the retrieval performance in a CBR system. Therefore, the extraction of potential features to represent a case is highly recommended in developing a CBR system. However, feature extraction is becoming complicated in recent medical CBR systems due to complex data formats where data is coming from sensor signals and images or in the form of time series or free text [72]. A critical issue is therefore to identify relevant features to represent a case in such domains.

Aamodt and Plaza has introduced a life cycle of CBR [13] which is a four-step model with four Re-s, as shown in Fig. 5. The four Re-s: Retrieve, Reuse, Revise and Retain represent the key tasks to implement such a cognitive model. These steps will now be described here focusing on issues in medical CBR systems.

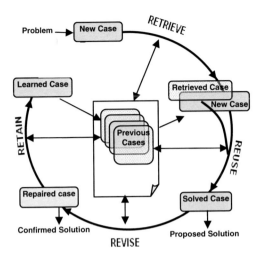

Fig. 5. Aamodt and Plaza's CBR cycle [13]

Retrieve: Case retrieval is a major phase in the CBR cycle where matching between two cases plays a vital role. The retrieval step is essential especially in medical applications since lack of similar cases may lead to a less informed decision. The reliability and accuracy of the diagnosis system depends on the storage of cases/experiences and on the retrieval of all relevant cases and their ranking. The retrieved cases are ranked on the basis of their similarity in matching the features of the new case and often the highest ranked case is proposed as the solution to the new case. In new areas of medical research such as diagnosis of stress related to psychophysiological issues, the domain knowledge is often not well understood. Therefore, retrieving a single matching case as a proposed solution may not be sufficient for the decision support system in this domain. The comparison of a new case with old cases from the case base could be carried out applying different similarity matching algorithms. One of the commonly used similarity measurement techniques is the Nearest-neighbour algorithm [12], [24]. A standard equation (shown in equation 1) for the nearest-neighbour is:

$$Similarity \ (C,S) = \sum_{f=1}^{n} w_f * sim (C_f, S_f) \qquad (1)$$

Where C is a current/target case, S is a stored case in the case base, w is the normalized weight, n is the number of the attributes/features in each case, f is the index for an individual attribute/feature and $sim(C_f, S_f)$ is the local similarity function. Generally there are two ways to specify the values of weights for individual features. One way is to define weights by experts in terms of the domain knowledge, while the other is to learn or optimize weights using the case library as an information source. The fuzzy similarity matching algorithm, which is another retrieval technique, is presented in section 5.

Reuse and revise: The retrieved cases are sent to the reuse step (see Fig. 5) where the solution of a past case can often be adapted to find a suitable solution for a new case. A user can adapt solutions e.g. a combination of two solutions from the list of

Table 1. CBR in medicine, examples of some systems and their application domain/context

No	Author/system	Application domain/context
1	De Paz/ExpressionCBR [46]	Cancer diagnosis
2	Perner/Fungi-PAD [47], [48]	Object recognition
3	Cordier/FrakaS [49]	Oncology
4	Corchado/GerAmi [50]	Alzheimer patients
5	Glez-Peña/geneCBR [51], [52]	Cancer classification
6	Perner/HEp2-PAD[53], [54], [55]	Image classifier
7	Schmidt/ISOR [56]	Endocrine
8	D'Aquin/KASIMIR [57]	Breast cancer
9	Bichindaritz/Mémoire [58]	Biology & medicine
10	Montani/RHENE [59]	Hemodialysis
11	Kwiatkowska/Somnus [60]	Obstructive sleep apnea
12	Lorenzi/SISAIH [61]	Fraud detection in health care
13	Ochoa /SIDSTOU [62]	Tourette syndrome
14	Brien/ADHD [63]	Neuropsychiatric
15	Doyle/Bronchiolitis [64]	Bronchiolitis
16	O'Sullivan/Dermatology [65]	Dermatology
17	Marling/Type-1diabetes [66]	Diabetes
18	Song/radiotherapy planning [67]	Prostate cancer

retrieved and ranked cases in order to develop a solution to the problem in a new case. The clinician/expert determines if it is a plausible solution to the problem and makes modifications to the solution. The case is then sent to the revision step where the solution is verified manually for correctness and is presented as a confirmed solution to the new problem case. In the medical system, there is not much adaptation, especially in a decision support system where the best cases are proposed to the clinician as suggestions of solutions and when the domain knowledge is not clear enough [12].

Retain: Finally, this new solved case is added to the case base functioning as a learning process in the CBR cycle and allows the user to solve a future problem by using this solved case. Retaining of a new solved case could be done manually based on the clinician or expert's decision.

CBR in Medicine. The origin of CBR stems from the work of Schank and Abelson in 1977 [25] at Yale University. According to Schank [26], "remembering is at the root of how we understand... at the root of how we learn." They have explored that new experiences reminds us of previous situations (i.e. cases) or the situation pattern. CYRUS [27], [28] developed by Janet Colodner, is the first CBR system. She employed knowledge as cases and used the indexed memory structure. Many of the early CBR systems such as CASEY [29], and MEDIATOR [30] were implemented based on CYRUS's work. The early works exploiting CBR in the medical domain were done by Konton [29], and Braeiss [31], [32] in the late 1980's.

CBR is suitable in the medical domain especially for its cognitively adequate model; a facility which integrates different types of knowledge with case representation which can be obtained from patients records [33]. In particular, diagnosis of a patient in the medical domain depends on experience. Historically, CBR diagnosis systems have most commonly been used in the medical domain. A clinician/physician may start their practice with some initial experience (solved cases), then try to utilize this past experience to solve a new problem while simultaneously increasing their experiences (i.e. case base). So, this reasoning process is gaining an increasing acceptance in the medical field since it has been found suitable for these kinds of decisions [34], [35], [36], [37], [38]. Some of the recent medical CBR systems with their application domain or context are summarized in table 1.

2.3 Fuzzy Logic

Fuzzy set theory has successfully been applied in handling uncertainties in various application domains [39] including the medical domain. Fuzzy logic was introduced by Lotfi Zadeh, a professor at the University of California at Berkley in 1965 [40]. The use of fuzzy logic in medical informatics began in the early 1970s. The concept of fuzzy logic has been formulated from the fact that human reasoning particularly, common sense reasoning is approximate in nature. So, it is possible to define inexact medical entities as fuzzy sets. Fuzzy logic is designed to handle partial truth i.e. truth values between completely true and completely false. For instance, Fuzzy logic allows a person to be classified as both young and old to be true at the same time. It explains fuzziness that exists in human thinking processes by using fuzzy values instead of using crisp or binary values. It is a superset of classical Boolean logic. In fuzzy logic, exact reasoning is treated as a special case of approximate reasoning. Everything in fuzzy logic appears as a matter of some degree i.e. degrees of membership function or degrees of truth. Using height classification as an example (Table 2), in Boolean logic if we draw a crisp boundary at 180 cm (Fig. 6), we find that Jerry, who is 179 cm, is small, while Monica is tall because her height is 181 cm. At the same time, using fuzzy logic all men are "tall", but their degrees of membership depend on their height.

Table 2. The classical 'tall men' example using Crisp and Fuzzy values

Name	Height, cm	Degree of membership	
		Boolean	Fuzzy
John	208	1	1.00
Monica	181	1	0.82
Jerry	179	0	0.78
Roger	167	0	0.15
Sofia	155	0	0.00

So for instance, if we consider Jerry is tall we can say the degree of truth of the statement 'Jerry is tall' is 0.78. A graph of this example interpreted as a degree of membership is given in Fig. 7.

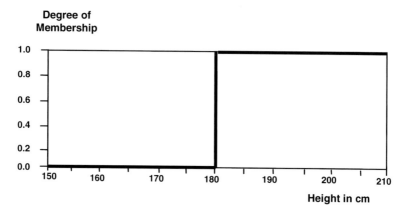

Fig. 6. Example presented in crisp set

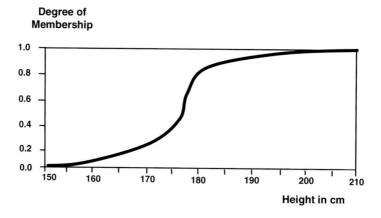

Fig. 7. Example presented in fuzzy set

Where, the X-axis is the universe of discourse which shows the range of all possible values for an input variable i.e. men's heights. The Y-axis represents the degree of membership function i.e. the fuzzy set of tall men height values mapped into corresponding membership values (Fig. 7).

Classical Set Theory. In classical set theory, a point x belongs to a set A if and only if it equals 1. i.e.

$$\varphi_A(x) = \begin{cases} 0, & x \notin A \\ 1, & x \in A \end{cases}$$

Where φ is a characteristic function, mapping from any universal set X to the binary set $\{0,1\}$.

Fuzzy Set Theory. A fuzzy set A is defined as any set that allows its members to have different degrees of membership i.e. membership function mapping from the universal set X to the interval [0, 1].

$$\mu_A(x): X \to \{0,1\},$$ Where, $\mu_A(x) = 1$; if x is totally in A

$$\mu_A(x) = 0 \text{ ; if x is not in A}$$

$$0 < \mu_A(x) < 1 \text{ ; if x is partially in A}$$

The characteristic function of a classical set $\varphi_A(x)$ is a special case of the membership function $\mu_A(x)$ of fuzzy set theory. Thus the fuzzy set is a generalization of the classical set theory.

The set operations (union, intersection, complement etc.) in terms of this membership function are:

Union: Union is the largest membership value of the element in either set (Fig. 8). The union of two fuzzy sets A and B on universe X can be given as:

$$\mu_{A\cup B}(x) = \max(\mu_A(x), \mu_B(x)) ,$$

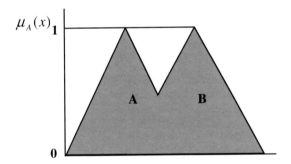

Fig. 8. Example of fuzzy union

Intersection: Intersection is the lower membership in both sets of each element (Fig. 9). The intersection of two fuzzy sets A and B on universe of discourse X can be given as: $\mu_{A\cap B}(x) = \min(\mu_A(x), \mu_B(x))$

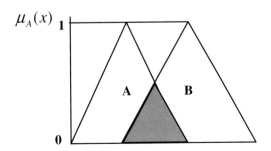

Fig. 9. Example of fuzzy intersection

Complement: The complement of a set is an opposite of that set (Fig. 10). For a fuzzy set A the complement is: $\mu_{notA}(x) = 1 - \mu_A(x)$

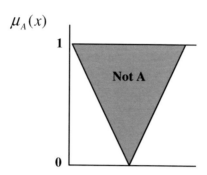

Fig. 10. Example of fuzzy complement

3   Calibration Phase and the System Overview

The system consists of a thermistor, sensing the finger temperature [41]. The sensor is attached to the finger of a subject and connected to an electronic circuit that is connected to the USB-port on a computer. Music is played to assist the subject to relax and instructions are given on how to control breathing.

Table 3. Measurement procedure used to create an individual stress profile

Test step	Observation time	Conditions	Finger temp	Notes
1.	3 min	Base Line		
2.	2 min	Deep Breath		
3.	2+2 min	Verbal Stress		
4.	2 min	Relax		
5.	2 min	Math stress		
6.	2 min	Relax		

A calibration phase [42] helps to establish an individual stress profile and is used as a standard protocol in the clinical environment. For calibration purposes the finger temperature is measured during different conditions in 6 steps (baseline, deep breath, verbal stress, relax, math stress, relax) as shown in Table 3. The baseline indicates the representative level for the individual when he/she is neither under intense stress nor in a relaxed state. The clinician asks the subject to read a neutral text during this step. The clinician not only identifies an individual's base finger temperature, but also notes fluctuations and other effects, e.g. disturbances in the environment or observes the subject's behavior. In the step 'Deep-breath', the subject breaths deeply which under guidance normally causes a relaxed state. How quickly changes in temperature occur during this step is relevant and recorded together with observed fluctuations.

The step 'Verbal-stress' is initiated by asking the subject to tell about some stressful event they experienced in life. During the second half of this step the subject thinks about some negative stressful events in their life. In the 'Relax step', the subject is instructed to think of something positive, either a moment in life when they were very happy or a future event they look forward to experiencing. The 'Math-stress' step tests the subject's reaction to directly induced stress by the clinician where the subject is requested to count backwards. Finally, the 'relaxation step' tests if and how quickly the subject recovers from stress. An example of the finger temperature measurement during the six different steps in the calibration phase is shown in Fig. 11.

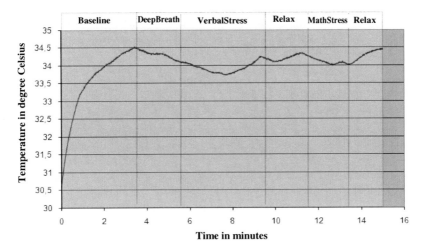

Fig. 11. An example of the finger temperature measurement during the six different steps in the calibration phase

The proposed CBR system works in several steps to diagnose individual sensitivity to stress as shown in Fig. 12.

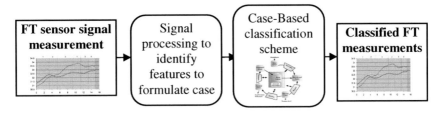

Fig. 12. Schematic diagram of the steps in stress diagnosis

The CBR system takes the finger temperature measurement as an input. Then, from this sensor signal, the system identifies the essential features and formulates a new problem case with the extracted features in a vector [71]. This new problem case is then fed into the CBR cycle to retrieve the most similar cases. The new case (feature vector extracted from the FT signal) in this system is then matched using different matching algorithms including modified distance function, similarity matrix and fuzzy similarity matching. Finally, as an output, the best matched case is presented i.e. a classification of the individual stress level which can be used to determine an individual's sensitivity to stress.

4 Finger Temperature Signal and Stress

In general, finger temperature decreases when a person is stressed and increases during relaxation or in a non-stressed situation. This relates to mainly sympathetic intervention of the alpha-receptor in the vascular bed. When relaxation occurs, activity of the sympathetic nervous system decreases as well as the intervention of the alpha receptors, which leads to increased dilation of the blood vessels which increases blood flow and temperature [8]. The reverse situation occurs during stress i.e. the sympathetic nervous system activates causing a decrease in peripheral circulation which leads to decreased skin temperature. Thus the blood flow in the finger temperature responds also to changes in emotional state. In clinical practice, the activities of the automatic nervous system (i.e. balance between the sympathetic and parasympathetic nervous systems) are monitored as a part of diagnosis of psychophysiological dysfunctions. Therefore, the rise and fall of finger temperature as illustrated in Fig. 3 can help to diagnose stress-related dysfunctions or dysfunctional behaviours; it is also an effective parameter for patients with Raynaud's syndrome [43]. Some conventional methods of diagnosing stress include measuring one or a combination of the following: respiration e.g. end-tidal carbon dioxide (ETCO2), heart rate e.g. calculating the respiratory sinus arrhythmia (RSA) and heart rate variability (HRV). One of the advantages of using FT in diagnosing stress is that the diagnosis and biofeedback training is often less expensive than using these other conventional measures, which require equipment not suitable for use in a non-clinical environment and cannot be used without experienced clinical staff. Since it is not always possible to provide clinical staff with laboratory facilities to measure many different parameters (often using many sensors) a supplementary convenient tool that can be used at any time and any place to diagnose and control stress for a general user is important. A temperature sensor can be used to collect finger temperature by attaching it to the finger. The FT signals from the sensor readings during different stress and relaxed conditions can be transmitted as an electronic signal to a computer screen. Thus it can serve as a convenient method to diagnose and treat stress i.e. give biofeedback to normalize stress-related dysfunctions at home and at work for general users. Also it can be used as an auxiliary medical system for clinical treatment.

4.1 Analysis of Finger Temperature Sensor Signal

Ideally the temperature is monitored repeatedly for short intervals during a longer period, i.e. a week, to determine the temperature consistency or pattern of the person. Some example signals are illustrated to show the individual variations. It has been observed from the measurements that different people have different representative temperatures, e.g. some may have representative temperature of $27°$ C as the lowest temperature while for other people $32°$ C may be the lowest. An example of different

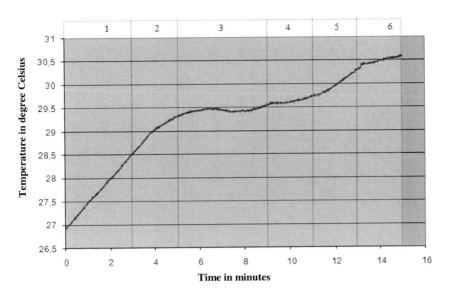

Fig. 13. Individual A. Variations of the representative temperature dependent on the individual.

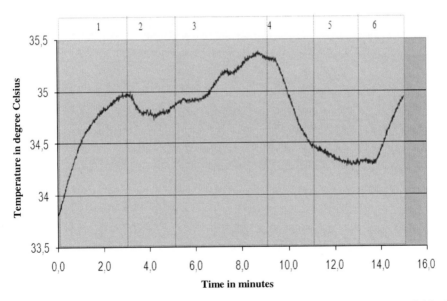

Fig. 14. Individual B. Variations of the representative temperature dependent on the individual.

representative temperature is illustrated in Fig. 13 and 14 for two different people (Individual A and Individual B).

Changes in temperature before and after meals can be pronounced in some individuals as shown in Fig. 15.

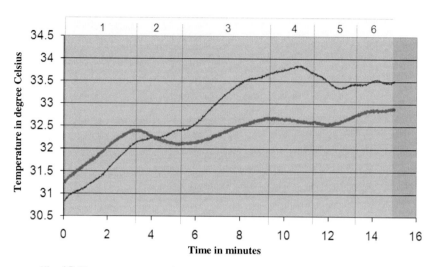

Fig. 15. Finger temperature for a person before (orange) and after lunch (blue).

Stress responses are different for different people and so are the coping capabilities. An individual's capability to cope with stress is also important to identify when measuring stress levels. A patient can be classified depending on their stress reaction and recovery capacity. Moreover, reaction time is also another important factor to make a proper individual treatment plan. For instance, in Fig. 16 the person was thinking of a stressful event in their life during stress conditions in step 3 and the finger temperature was decreasing. In step 4, the person had to relax but did not succeed in relaxing quickly.

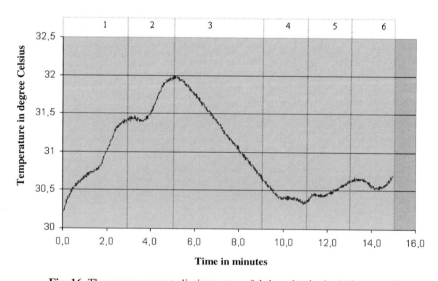

Fig. 16. The person cannot eliminate stressful thoughts in the 'relax stage'.

The finger temperature measurement in Fig. 17 is shown for a student before his master's thesis presentation. He explains that he was so stressed before the presentation that he could not recover from the stress in the next stages.

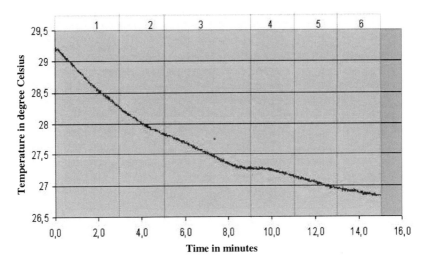

Fig. 17. A student before the thesis presentation.

Three situations have been observed while collecting the FT measurement: a. finger temperature decreases with increasing stress which is the most common situation, b. finger temperature increases with increasing stress i.e. paradoxical relation and c. little or no changes i.e. the temperature remains stable when a person is experiencing stress, this is exceptional but might happened for some people. In such cases clinical expertise is important. In general, finger temperature decreases when a person is stressed and increases during relaxation or in a non-stressed situation. So, the indication of a person's stress condition can be obtained from the individual temperature variations during the six phases.

4.2 Finger Temperature Sensor Signal Processing

After analyzing a number of finger temperature signals, we found large individual variations, but also a similarity in the pattern that temperature decreases during stress and increases during relaxation for most people. That is an important feature that needs to be identified by an automatic classification algorithm searching for "similar" patients. In CBR we need to extract important features from the sensor signal. Choice of the signal processing method depends mainly on the nature of the signal and the specific problem to be solved [44]. The following subsections provide a summary of the other traditional signal processing methods which have also been investigated before applying CBR to analyze the biomedical signal i.e. Finger temperature sensor signal.

Point-to-Point Matching. Finger temperature varies from person to person. FT lies for some people from 22^0 C to 23^0 C and for others from 34^0 C to 35^0 C. The variation of FT can be seen in Fig. 18 where 39 measurements are plotted in one chart. The indication of a person's stress might be found both from low or high temperatures. Point-to-point matching is not significant in identifying similarities or differences between two case features because: i) It needs to calculate the difference between all the measurement points of the two compared cases, which in our study means calculating the difference for 1800 samples contained in one case. The computational time is an important issue here, and with several hundred cases in a case library it would take too long to be of practical use. ii) It does not calculate similarity in patterns of two cases. Let's consider this example: one case with 15 minute sample data where finger temperature lies between 33^0 C and 35^0 C, with the same pattern compared with another case where the finger temperature lies between 24^0C and 28^0C and also follows a similar pattern. From a clinical viewpoint these two cases are similar since they follow a similar pattern; however Point-to-Point matching would classify them as not similar according to their different temperature values. iii) If the finger temperature for a new problem case lies at a higher level (e.g. 35^0C) then the system will never consider any cases where the finger temperature lies at a lower level (e.g. 23^0 C) and vice versa. iv) This similarity method does not consider any variation in FT when calculating the difference between two cases, whereas the change in the finger temperature is an important factor for classifying stress.

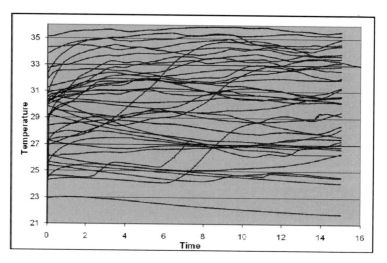

Fig. 18. Sample of FT measurements plotted for 39 sensor signals

Fourier Transform. Discrete Fourier Transform (DFT) and Fast Fourier Transform (FFT) are efficient and well known methods in Fourier analysis to compute a sequence of values into components of different frequencies. It is widely employed in signal processing to analyze the frequencies contained in a sampled signal such as human voice or speech sounds. However, for the finger temperature sensor signal the amplitude of the frequency components is not an indication of stress, rather the change in finger temperature signal can easily be captured by calculating the slopes for each step.

Calculating the Mean and Standard Deviation. Our opinion is that neither the mean value nor the standard deviation of the FT measurement was adequate indicators of stress. For instance, consider two signals: one is increasing from 20° C to 30° C, the other decreasing from 30° C to 20° C. Although both signals have the same mean/standard deviation value in the duration, however they indicate opposite stress levels. An example of such measurement is illustrated in Fig. 19.

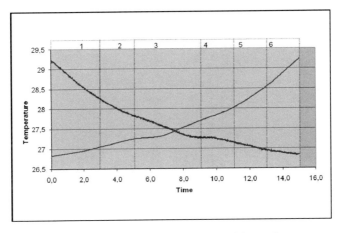

Fig. 19. Temperature is increasing and decreasing

From Fig. 19, it can be seen that temperature is increasing and decreasing from 27° C to 29° C, so one measurement might be classified as stress and other one as relaxation. If we consider the mean temperature or standard deviation for both the cases the value will be the same. Alternatively, the mean slope value might be a feasible feature to convey a relation with stress. If the mean slope value is sufficiently positive, it will be a clear indication that activity of the sympathetic nervous system is decreasing e.g. relaxation, otherwise an indication of stress. But if the mean slope is around zero, it shows a situation with greater uncertainty in diagnosing stress and a greater probability in making a poorly justified decision.

5 Feature Extraction and Case-Based System

It is often convenient to classify a signal if it can be simplified to a form that describes the characteristics of the signal i.e. extract features that represent the signal. During diagnosis, when performed manually, an experienced clinician often classifies FT signals without intentionally pointing out all the features used in the classification. However, extracting appropriate features is of great importance in performing accurate classification in a CBR system.

The decision support system shown in Fig. 20 assists in the case-based classification of FT sensor signals in stress management. It takes a finger temperature measurement during the calibration phase and identifies a number of individual parameters. Then, from this sensor signal, it identifies the essential features and formulates a new problem case with the extracted features in a vector. This new problem case is then fed into the CBR cycle to retrieve the most similar cases.

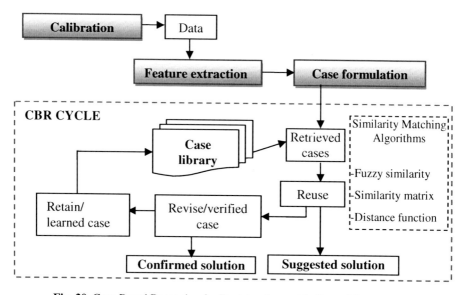

Fig. 20. Case-Based Reasoning for Decision Support in Stress Management

Classification of the FT measurement is done using case retrieval and matching based on the extracted features. Here, the k-Nearest Neighbour (kNN) algorithm is applied for the retrieval of similar cases. The new problem case is matched using different matching algorithms including *modified distance function, similarity matrix* and *fuzzy similarity matching*. A *modified distance* function uses Euclidean distance to calculate the distance between the features of two cases. Hence, all the symbolic features are converted into numeric values before calculating the distance. For example, for the feature 'gender', male is converted to one (1) and female is two (2). The function '*similarity matrix*' is represented as a table where the similarity value between two features is determined by the domain expert. For example, the similarity between same genders is defined as 1 otherwise 0.5.

In *fuzzy similarity,* a triangular membership function (*mf*) replaces the crisp value of the features for new and old cases with a membership grade of 1. In both cases, the width of the membership function is fuzzified by 50% on each side. For example, an attribute '*S*' of a current case and an old case have the values -6.3 and -10.9 respectively. If the weight of the membership function (*mf*) is fuzzified with 50 % on each side, which can be done using a trial and error process based on the problem domain, the input value for the current case -6.3 can be represented with a *mf* grade of 1 and the lower and upper bounds -9.45 and -3.15 can be represented with an *mf* of grade 0.

For the old case, the input -10.9 can be represented with an *mf* grade of 1 and the lower and upper bounds -16.35 and -5.45 with an *mf* grade of 0.

Fuzzy intersection is applied between the two fuzzy sets to get a new fuzzy set which represents the overlapping area between them. Similarity between the old case (S_f) and the new case (C_f) is now calculated using Equation 2:

$$sim(C_f, S_f) = s_f(m1, m2) = \max(om/m1, om/m2) \qquad (2)$$

where *m1*, *m2* and *om* are the area of the corresponding fuzzy sets. For instance, m_1=5.45 and m_2=3.15 where area is defined by the equation area=(1/2) x base x height. For *om*=0.92, height is defined from the intersection point of the two fuzzy membership functions. So from Equation 2, the calculated local similarity can be *min (0.17, 0.29)=0.17* and *max* is 0.29. If the *mfs* are considered as 100 % fuzzified then minimum local similarity will be 0.34 and maximum will be 0.58. Thus, a user can get the options both for tuning the *mfs* and choosing the min/max values for the similarity function based on their requirements. When the overlapping areas become bigger, then the similarity between the two features will also increase, and for completely matched features similarity will be 1.

The system can provide matching outcomes in a sorted list of best matching cases according to their similarity values in three circumstances: when a new problem case is matched with all the solved cases in a case base (between subject and class), within a class where the class information is provided by the user and also within a subject. Thus, the CBR system provides the classified FT measurement as an output for the diagnosis of individual sensitivity to stress.

5.1 Calculating the Degree of Changes and Extracting the Features

Together with clinicians we have agreed on a standardization of the slope to make changes visible and patients and situations easier to compare. The proposal is that the X axis displays minutes and the Y axis degrees Celsius, hence a change during 1 minute of 1 degree gives a "degree of change" of 45°. A low angle value, e.g. zero or close to zero indicates no change or a stable finger temperature.

A high positive angle value indicates rising finger temperature, while a negative angle, e.g. -20° indicates falling finger temperature. Usually, the purpose of step 1 (the baseline, shown in Table 3) is to stabilize the finger temperature before starting

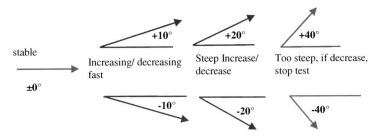

Fig. 21. Example of visualizations of temperature change, X-axis minutes, Y-axis in degree Celsius

the test, hence it has been agreed with the clinician that this step should not been considered. Classification of individual sensitivity to stress based on "degree of change" is shown in Fig. 21.

As seen in Fig. 22 each step of the calibration is divided into one minute time intervals (Step 3 is 4 minutes in duration and 4 features are extracted) while each feature contains 120 sample data (time, temperature).

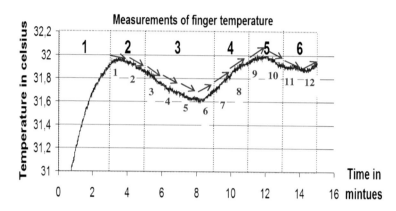

Fig. 22. Changes in FT data against time during different stress and non-stress conditions

Thus 12 features are extracted from 5 steps (step 2 to 6) and named as Step2_Part1, Step2_Part2, Step3_Part1 etc. First, a slope of the linear regression line has been calculated through the data points by using Equation 3 for each extracted feature from the measurement.

$$slope_f = \frac{\sum_{i=0}^{n}(x-\bar{x})(y-\bar{y})}{\sum_{i=0}^{n}(x-\bar{x})^2} \tag{3}$$

Where f denotes the number of features (1 to 12 see Fig. 22), i is the number of samples (1 to 120) and $\bar{x}, \bar{y}$ is the average of the samples. Then the slope value is converted to arctangent as a value of angle in radians ($-pi/2$ to $+pi/2$) and finally expressed arctangent values in degrees by multiplying *180/PI* where *PI* is 3.14 as a standard value. So these 12 features contain degree values comprising of 120 sample data (time, temperature). Instead of keeping the sample data, these degree values are used or represented as features. Five other features which have also been extracted from the sensor signal are: start temperature and end temperature from step2 to step6, minimum temperature of step3 and step5, maximum temperature of step4 and step6, and the difference between ceiling and floor. Finally, 17 (12+5) features are extracted (Table 4) automatically from the fifteen minutes (1800 samples) of FT sensor signal.

A new case is then formulated from these extracted features (Table 4). Finally, this new case is passed to the CBR cycle to use it in an automated classification scheme.

Table 4. List of features extracted from the FT sensor signal

No.	Features	No.	Features
1	Step2_part1	9	Step5_part1
2	Step2_part2	10	Step5_part2
3	Step3_part1	11	Step6_part1
4	Step3_part2	12	Step6_part2
5	Step3_part3	13	Start temperature
6	Step3_part4	14	End temperature
7	Step4_part1	15	Maximum_ temperature
8	Step4_part2	16	Minimum_ temperature
17	Difference between ceiling and floor temperature		

6 Result and Evaluation

To evaluate the use of FT measurements as a diagnostic tool for stress, a computer based prototype system has been built and tested.

A user can select different matching algorithms and see the detailed information for a new case compared to an old case. Fig. 23 displays a screen shot which shows similarity matching of a current case with the previous cases in a ranked list. The system identifies the current case with the reliability of 71.8% that the subject is under the state 'very_stressed'.

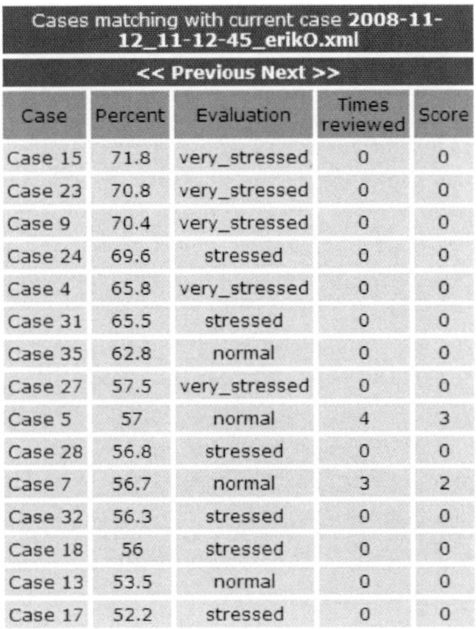

Cases matching with current case **2008-11-12_11-12-45_erikO.xml**

<< Previous Next >>

Case	Percent	Evaluation	Times reviewed	Score
Case 15	71.8	very_stressed	0	0
Case 23	70.8	very_stressed	0	0
Case 9	70.4	very_stressed	0	0
Case 24	69.6	stressed	0	0
Case 4	65.8	very_stressed	0	0
Case 31	65.5	stressed	0	0
Case 35	62.8	normal	0	0
Case 27	57.5	very_stressed	0	0
Case 5	57	normal	4	3
Case 28	56.8	stressed	0	0
Case 7	56.7	normal	3	2
Case 32	56.3	stressed	0	0
Case 18	56	stressed	0	0
Case 13	53.5	normal	0	0
Case 17	52.2	stressed	0	0

Fig. 23. Similarity matching of a current case with previous cases is presented in a ranked list of cases as solution.

The performance of the system in terms of accuracy has been compared with experts in the domain, where the main goal is to see how close the system could work compared to an expert. The evaluation in this chapter, considers several test data sets to illustrate the overall system performance compare to an expert.

The initial case base comprised of 39 FT measurements as reference cases from 24 subjects. Seven woman and seventeen men between the age ranges of 24 to 51 participated in this study. The cases, in their conditional or problem description part, contain a vector with the extracted features and the solution part comprised of expert's defined classification as diagnosis. The levels of stress are classified by the expert into five classes ranging from 1 to 5 where 1=VeryStressed, 2=Stressed, 3=Normal/Stable, 4=Relaxed and 5=VeryRelaxed.

The performance of the three matching algorithms: modified distance, similarity matrix, and fuzzy matching are evaluated where the test is done for the three test groups for three different query cases. Both in ranking and in similarity performance, fuzzy similarity matching algorithm shows better results than the other algorithms (i.e. distance function and similarity matrix) when compared with the expert's opinion [71].

For this experiment, 5 test groups consisting of various numbers of cases have been created (i.e. TG-A=5, TG-B=7, TG-C=9, TG-D=11 and TG-E=14) where cases are selected randomly and all the cases are classified by the expert. These formulated test cases were then used in the classification process by the CBR system using the fuzzy similarity matching algorithm. The main goal of this experimental work was to see how the CBR classification system supported the diagnosis of stress compared to an expert.

Table 5. Experimental results for the test groups

Test Group	Number of Cases	Goodness-of-fit (R^2)	Absolute mean Difference
TG-A	5	0.94	0.20
TG-B	7	0.92	0.14
TG-C	9	0.67	0.33
TG-D	11	0.78	0.30
TG-E	14	0.83	0.28
Average	9.2	0.83	0.25

The results of the experiment for each test group are illustrated in Table 5. As can be seen from Table 5, the first two columns present the name and the number of the cases for each test group. The classification of the cases in each group by the CBR system is then compared with the expert's classification. Goodness-of fit (R2) [45] and absolute mean difference (error) by the system for these five groups have been calculated and presented in Table 5. R2 values of all the sets are 0.94, 0.92, 0.67, 0.78 and 0.83; absolute mean differences of the five sets are 0.20, 0.14, 0.33, 0.30 and 0.28; so the average R2 and error values of these sets are 0.83 and 0.25, respectively.

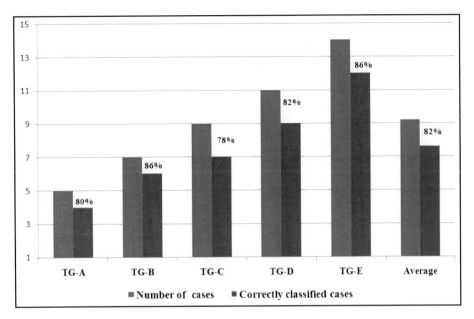

Fig. 24. Comparison results of the classification for the five test groups (i.e. TG-A, TG-B, TG-C, TG-D, TG-E and average of all the groups)

Fig. 24 illustrates a comparison for each group on the basis of the number of cases and correctly classified cases. In Fig. 24, the blue line represents the total number of the cases in a group and the red line shows the number of cases correctly classified by the system for the corresponding group. For each case in each test group, the CBR system correctly classifies 80%, 86%, 78%, 82%, 86% of the cases. So, from the experimental result, it can be observed that the classification system correctly classifies cases with an average accuracy of 82%.

7 Discussions and Conclusions

In this chapter, a combined approach based on a calibration phase and CBR to provide assistance in diagnosing stress is proposed using data analysis from finger temperature sensor readings. Finger temperature is an indirect measurement of stress and relaxation and as shown in this chapter. It contains information on changes to a person's stress level which can be measured using a low cost sensor. CBR is a method which enables the diagnosis of stress despite large variations between individuals. The calibration phase also helps to establish a number of individual parameters. Fuzzy logic incorporated into the CBR system for similarity matching between cases reduces the sharp distinction between cases and provides a more reliable solution.

From the experimental result, it is observed that the classification result on average is 82% for all the three sets of cases using the same feature sets. Fig. 24 suggests that using extracted features the CBR system can classify a promising number of cases and that only a few cases are misclassified out of the total number of the cases.

Therefore we have shown that it is possible to reach near expert level performance of a decision support system based on CBR for diagnosing stress. It is crucial to understand what features an expert uses to see similarity between subjects. The development of the approach has also lead to experts more clearly seeing what features they use for classification which may lead to a standard procedure for diagnosis in the future. This also provides important information to the clinician to make a decision about individual treatment plans.

The CBR system with rather simple and intelligent analysis of sensor signals, allows the use of finger temperature measurements in an autonomous system. This enables the treatment of individuals to be carried out at home or in the work environment. This system can be valuable for decision support for non-experts or as a second opinion for experts in stress management.

References

1. Northrop, R.B.: Signals and systems in biomedical engineering. CRC Press, New York (2003)
2. Nilsson, M., Funk, P.: A case-based classification of respiratory sinus arrhythmia. In: Funk, P., González Calero, P.A. (eds.) ECCBR 2004. LNCS (LNAI), vol. 3155, pp. 673–685. Springer, Heidelberg (2004)
3. Ölmeza, T., Dokur, Z.: Classification of heart sounds using an artificial neural network. Pattern Recognition Letters 24(1-3), 617–629 (2003)
4. Sahambi, J.S., Tandon, S.N., Bhatt, R.K.P.: Using wavelet transforms for ECG characterization. An on-line digital signal processing system. Engineering in Medicine and Biology Magazine 16(1), 77–83 (1997)
5. Kalayci, T., Ozdamar, O.: Wavelet preprocessing for automated neural network detection of EEG spikes. Engineering in Medicine and Biology Magazine 14(2), 160–166 (1995)
6. Funk, P., Xiong, N.: Case-based reasoning and knowledge discovery in medical applications with time series. Computational Intelligence 22(3-4), 238–253 (2006)
7. Xiong, N., Funk, P.: Concise case indexing of time series in health science by means of key sequence discovery. Applied Intelligence 28(3), 247–260 (2008)
8. Von Schéele, B.H.C., von Schéele, I.A.M.: The Measurement of Respiratory and Metabolic Parameters of Patients and Controls Before and After Incremental Exercise on Bicycle: Supporting the Effort Syndrome Hypothesis. Applied Psychophysiology and Biofeedback 24(3), 167–177 (1999)
9. Turban, E., Aronson, E.J.: Decision support systems and intelligent systems, 6th edn. Prentice Hall, Englewood Cliffs (2001)
10. Bemmel, J.H.V., Musen, M.A.: Handbook of Medical informatics. Springer, Heidelberg (1997)
11. Shortliffe, E.: Computer-based medical consultations: MYCIN. Elsevier North Holland, New York (1976)
12. Watson, I.: Applying Case-Based Reasoning: Techniques for Enterprise Systems. Morgan Kaufmann Publishers Inc., San Francisco (1997)
13. Aamodt, A., Plaza, E.: Case-based reasoning: Foundational issues, methodological variations, and system approaches. AI Communications 7, 39–59 (1994)
14. Hinkle, D., Toomey, C.: Applying Case-Based Reasoning to Manufacturing. AI Magazine 16(1), 65–73 (1995)
15. Selye, H.: The Stress of Life. McGraw Hill, New York (1956); Rev. ed. (1976)

16. Lazarus, R.S.: Psychological stress and the coping process. McGraw-Hill, New York (1966)
17. http://www.drlwilson.com/Articles/NERVOUS%20SYSTEM.htm (last referred March 2010)
18. http://www.s-cool.co.uk/alevel/psychology/stress/what-is-stress.html (last referred March 2010)
19. Andreassi, J.L.: Psychophysiology: Human Behavior and Physiological Response, 3rd edn. Erlbaum, Hillsdale (1995)
20. John, T.C., Louis, G.T., Gary, G.B.: Handbook of Psychophysiology. Cambridge University Press, Cambridge (2000)
21. AAPB.: The Association for Applied Psychophysiology and Biofeedback, http://www.aapb.org/i4a/pages/index.cfm?pageid=336 (last referred March 2010)
22. Lehrer, M.P., Smetankin, A., Potapova, T.: Respiratory Sinus Arrytmia Biofeedback Therapy for Asthma: A report of 20 Unmediated Pediatric Cases Using the Smetaniknnnn Method. Applied Psychophysiology and Biofeedback 25(3), 193–200 (2000)
23. https://www.cs.tcd.ie/medilink/index.htm?href=components/CBR.htm (last referred March 2010)
24. Kang, S.H., Lau, S.K.: Intelligent Knowledge Acquisition with Case-Based Reasoning Techniques. Technical report, University of Wollongong, NSW, Australia, pp. 1–8 (2002)
25. Schank, R.C., Abelson, R.P.: Scripts, Plans, Goals and Understanding. Erlbaum, Hillsdale (1977)
26. Schank, R.: Dynamic memory: a theory of reminding and learning in computers and people. Cambridge University Press, Cambridge (1982)
27. Kolodner, J.L.: Maintaining Organization in a Dynamic Long-Term Memory. Cognitive Science 7(4), 243–280 (1983)
28. Kolodner, J.L.: Reconstructive Memory: A Computer Model. Cognitive Science 7(4), 281–285 (1983)
29. Koton, P.: Using experience in learning and problem solving. Massachusetts Institute of Technology, Laboratory of Computer Science, Ph.D. Thesis MIT/LCS/TR-441 (1989)
30. Simpson, R.L.: A Computer Model of Case-Based Reasoning in Problem Solving: An Investigation in the Domain of Dispute Mediation. Technical Report GIT-ICS-85/18, Georgia Institute of Technology, School of Information and Computer Science, Atlanta USA (1985)
31. Bareiss, E.: RPROTOS: A Unified Approach to Concept Representation, Classification, and learning. Ph.D. thesis, Department of Computer Science, University of Texas (1988)
32. Bareiss, E.: Examplar-based Knowledge Acquisition: A unified Approach to Concept, Classification and learning. PHD thesis, 300 North Zeeb Road, Ann Arbor, AI 48106–1346 (1989)
33. Gierl, L., Schmidt, R.: CBR in Medicine. In: Lenz, M., Bartsch-Spörl, B., Burkhard, H.-D., Wess, S. (eds.) Case-Based Reasoning Technology. LNCS (LNAI), vol. 1400, pp. 273–298. Springer, Heidelberg (1998)
34. Ahmed, M.U., Begum, S., Funk, P., Xiong, N.: Fuzzy Rule-Based Classification to Build Initial Case Library for Case-Based Stress Diagnosis. In: 9th International conference on Artificial Intelligence and Applications, Austria, pp. 225–230 (2009)
35. Ahmed, M.U., Begum, S., Funk, P., Xiong, N., von Schéele, B.: A Multi-Module Case Based Biofeedback System for Stress Treatment. Artificial Intelligence in Medicine (in press, 2010)
36. Bichindaritz, I., Marling, C.: Case-based reasoning in the health sciences: What's next? Artificial Intelligence in Medicine 36(2), 127–135 (2006)

37. Bichindaritz, I.: Mémoire: A framework for semantic interoperability of case-based reasoning systems in biology and medicine. Artificial Intelligence in Medicine, Special Issue on Case-based Reasoning in the Health Sciences 36(2), 177–192 (2006)
38. Begum, S., Ahmed, M.U., Funk, P., Xiong, N., Folke, M.: Case-Based Reasoning Systems in the Health Sciences: A Survey on Recent Trends and Developments. Accepted in IEEE Transactions on Systems, Man, and Cybernetics–Part C: Applications and Reviews (2010)
39. Jang, J.S.R., Sun, C.T., Mizutani, E.: Neuro-fuzzy and Soft Computing. A computional approach to learning and machine intelligence. Prentice Hall, NJ (1997)
40. Zadeh, L.: Fuzzy sets. Information and Control 8(3), 338–353 (1965)
41. http://www.pbmsystems.se/system2/ft.asp (last referred March 2010)
42. Begum, S., Ahmed, M.U., Funk, P., Xiong, N., Scheele, B.V.: Using calibration and fuzzification of cases for improved diagnosis and treatment of stress. In: 8th European Workshop on Case-based Reasoning, pp. 113–122 (2006)
43. Caramaschi, P., Biasi, D., Carletto, A., Manzo, T., Randon, M., Zeminian, S., Bambara, L.M.: Finger skin temperature in patients affected by Raynaud's phenomenon with or without anticentromere antibody positivity. Journal of the Rheumatology International 15, 217–220 (1996)
44. Northrop, R.B.: Signals and systems in biomedical engineering. CRC Press, New York (2003)
45. Carol, C.H.: Goodness-Of-Fit Tests and Model Validity. Birkhäuser, Basel (2002)
46. De Paz, F.J., Rodriguez, S., Bajo, J., Corchao, M.J.: Case-based reasoning as a decision support system for cancer diagnosis: A case study. International Journal of Hybrid Intelligent Systems, 97–110 (2008)
47. Perner, P., Bühring, A.: Case-Based Object Recognition. In: Funk, P., González Calero, P.A. (eds.) ECCBR 2004. LNCS (LNAI), vol. 3155, pp. 375–388. Springer, Heidelberg (2004)
48. Perner, P., Perner, H., Jänichen, S.: Recognition of Airborne Fungi Spores in Digital Microscopic Images. Journal of Artificial Intelligence in Medicine 36(2), 137–157 (2006)
49. Cordier, A., Fuchs, B., Lieber, J.: Mille A. On-Line Domain Knowledge Management for Case-Based Medical Recommendation. In: Workshop on CBR in the Health Sciences, pp. 285–294 (2007)
50. Corchado, J.M., Bajo, J., Abraham, A.: GERAmI: Improving the delivery of health care. Journal of IEEE Intelligent Systems, Special Issue on Ambient Intelligence 3(2), 19–25 (2008)
51. Glez-Peña, D., Glez-Bedia, M., Díaz, F., Fdez-Riverola, F.: Multiple-microarray analysis and Internet gathering information with application for aiding diagnosis in cancer research, vol. 49, pp. 112–117. Springer, Heidelberg (2009)
52. Díaz, F., Fdez-Riverola, F., Corchado, J.M.: GENE-CBR: a Case-Based Reasoning Tool for Cancer Diagnosis using Microarray Datasets. Computational Intelligence 22(3-4), 254–268 (2006)
53. Plata, C., Perner, H., Spaeth, S., Lackner, K.J., von Landenberg, P.: Automated classification of immunofluorescence patterns of HEp-2 cells in clinical routine diagnostics. International Journal of Transactions on Mass-Data Analysis of Images and Signals 1(2), 147–159 (2009)
54. Perner, P.: Flexible High-Content Analysis: Automatic Image Analysis and Image Interpretation of Cell Pattern. International Journal of Transactions on Mass-Data Analysis of Images and Signals 1(2), 113–131 (2009)
55. Perner, P.: An Architeture for a CBR Image Segmentation System. Journal on Engineering Application in Artificial Intelligence, Engineering Applications of Artificial Intelligence 12(6), 749–759 (1999)
56. Schmidt, R., Vorobieva, O.: Case-based reasoning investigation of therapy inefficacy. Journal Knowledge-Based Systems 19(5), 333–340 (2006)

57. D'Aquin, M., Lieber, J.: Napoli A. Adaptation knowledge acquisition: a case study for case-based decision support in oncology. Computational Intelligence 22(3-4), 161–176 (2006)
58. Bichindaritz, I.: Semantic Interoperability of Case Bases in Biology and Medicine. Artificial Intelligence in Medicine, Special Issue on Case-based Reasoning in the Health Sciences 36(2), 177–192 (2006)
59. Montani, S., Portinale, L., Leonardi, G., Bellazzi, R., Bellazzi, R.: Case-based retrieval to support the treatment of end stage renal failure patients. Artificial Intelligence in Medicine 37(1), 31–42 (2006)
60. Montani, S., Portinale, L.: Accounting for the temporal dimension in case-based retrieval: a framework for medical applications. Computational Intelligence 22(3-4), 208–223 (2006)
61. Kwiatkowska, M., Atkins, M.S.: Case Representation and Retrieval in the Diagnosis and Treatment of Obstructive Sleep Apnea: A Semio-fuzzy Approach. In: Funk, P., González Calero, P.A. (eds.) ECCBR 2004. LNCS (LNAI), vol. 3155, pp. 25–35. Springer, Heidelberg (2004)
62. Lorenzi, F., Abel, M., Ricci, F.: SISAIH: a Case-Based Reasoning Tool for Hospital Admission Authorization Management. In: Workshop on CBR in the Health Sciences, pp. 33–42 (2004)
63. Ochoa, A., Meza, M., González, S., Padilla, A., Damiè, M., Torre, D.L.J., Jiménez-Vielma, F.: An Intelligent Tutor based on Case-based Reasoning to Medical Use. In: Sidorov, G., et al. (eds.) Advances in Computer Science and Engineering. Research in Computing Science, vol. 34, pp. 187–194 (2008)
64. Brien, D., Glasgow, I.J., Munoz, D.: The Application of a Case-Based Reasoning System to Attention-Deficit Hyperactivity Disorder. In: Muñoz-Ávila, H., Ricci, F. (eds.) ICCBR 2005. LNCS (LNAI), vol. 3620, pp. 122–136. Springer, Heidelberg (2005)
65. Doyle, D., Cunningham, P., Walsh, P.: An Evaluation of the Usefulness of Explanation in a CBR System for Decision Support in Bronchiolitis Treatment. Computational Intelligence 22(3-4), 269–281 (2006)
66. O'Sullivan, D., Bertolotto, M., Wilson, D., McLoghlin, E.: Fusing Mobile Case-Based Decision Support with Intelligent Patient Knowledge Management. In: Workshop on CBR in the Health Sciences, pp. 151–160 (2006)
67. Marling, C., Shubrook, J., Schwartz, F.: Case-Based Decision Support for Patients with Type 1 Diabetes on Insulin Pump Therapy. In: Althoff, K.-D., Bergmann, R., Minor, M., Hanft, A. (eds.) ECCBR 2008. LNCS (LNAI), vol. 5239, pp. 325–339. Springer, Heidelberg (2008)
68. Song, X., Petrovic, S., Sundar, S.: A Case-based reasoning approach to dose planning in Radiotherapy. In: Workshop Proceedings, 7th International Conference on Case-Based Reasoning, Belfast, Northern Ireland, pp. 348–357 (2007)
69. http://www.iworx.com/LabExercises/lockedexercises/LockedSkin TempNL.pdf (last referred March 2010)
70. Begum, S., Ahmed, M.U., Funk, P., Xiong, N., Schéele, B.V.: A case-based decision support system for individual stress diagnosis using fuzzy similarity matching. Computational Intelligence 25(3), 180–195 (2009)
71. Begum, S.: Sensor signal processing to extract features from finger temperature in a case-based stress classification scheme. In: 6th IEEE International Symposium on Intelligent Signal Processing (Special Session on Signal Processing in Bioengineering), Budapest, Hungary, pp. 193–198 (2009)

Chapter 9
Case-Based Reasoning in a Travel Medicine Application

Kerstin Bach, Meike Reichle, and Klaus-Dieter Althoff

Intelligent Information Systems Lab
University of Hildesheim
Marienburger Platz 22, 31141 Hildesheim, Germany
lastname@iis.uni-hildesheim.de
http://www.iis.uni-hildesheim.de

Abstract. This chapter focuses on knowledge management for complex application domains using Collaborative Multi-Expert-Systems. We explain how different knowledge sources can be described and organized in order to be used in collaborative knowledge-based systems. We present the docQuery system and the application domain travel medicine to exemplify the knowledge modularization and how the distributed knowledge sources can be dynamically accessed and finally reassembled. Further on we present a set of properties for the classification of knowledge sources and in which way these properties can be assessed.

1 Introduction

This chapter will give an introduction how Case-Based Reasoning (CBR) can be used, among other methodologies from the field of Artificial Intelligence (AI), to build a travel medical application. There are a high variety of AI methods and we focus on how these methods can be combined, coordinated and further developed to meet the requirements of an intelligent information system. We will use Information Extraction techniques to analyze text, we have multi-agent technologies to coordinate the different methods that are executing the retrieval and in the following to combine the result sets. Further on we have to deal with rules and constraints that insure correct results and since we are accessing different kinds of knowledge sources we use XML and RDF as description languages. Within our application CBR will be the main underlying methodology. We will explain how travel medical case bases can be structured, how the required knowledge can be acquired, formalized and provided, as well as how that knowledge can be maintained.

The chapter will begin by describing Aamodt's and Plaza's 4R cycle [1] from the travel medical point of view. Then it will explain how the CBR methodology fits in the travel medical application domain. For this purpose we will present an intelligent information system on travel medicine, called docQuery, which is based on CBR and will serve as a running example throughout the whole chapter.

I. Bichindaritz et al. (Eds.): Computational Intelligence in Healthcare 4, SCI 309, pp. 191–210.
springerlink.com   © Springer-Verlag Berlin Heidelberg 2010

Following the definition and motivation of travel medicine as an application domain, we will introduce a novel approach to CBR using a number of heterogeneous case bases of which each one will cover one individual field within the general application domain. Each case base provides information that is required to compute a travel medical information leaflet and we will describe how we manage the case bases and use them to compose such information leaflets with regard to given constraints.

Moreover we will point out how we keep our case bases up-to-date using a web-based community as source of information. We will further describe the technologies we use to extract information, knowledge and experiences from the community, formalize them and use a Case Factory for its maintenance. Additionally we describe how and in which way techniques from Machine Learning and Information Extraction can be applied to extend a case base. The chapter will close up with a discussion of related topics followed by a short summary and future developments in this area.

2   Requirements of Travel Medicine as an Application Domain

Today the World Wide Web is a widely accepted platform for communication and the exchange of information. It does not matter where people live, to which culture they belong or of which background they are - web communities can be used from anywhere and by anyone. Especially in discussion forums a lot of topics are reviewed and experiences are shared. Unfortunately, much information gets lost in discussion boards or web pages caused by the quantity and variety of different web communities. Hence it is hard to find detailed information, since the topic of a discussion is often not clear and a wide range of expressions are used. Furthermore the users do not know enough about the authors and their background to ensure a high quality of information.

2.1   Motivation

Nowadays it is easier than ever to travel to different places, experience new cultures and get to know new people. In preparation for a healthy journey it is important to get a high quality and reliable answer on travel medicine issues. Both layman and experts should get information they need and, in particular, they understand. For that reason the idea of docQuery - a medical information system for travelers - has been developed.

docQuery provides information for travelers and physicians (those who are no experts in the field of travel medicine) by travel medicine experts and also gives an opportunity to share information and ensures a high quality because it is maintained by experts. Furthermore it will rise to the challenge of advancing the community alongside their users. User can obtain detailed information for their journey by providing the key data on their journey (like travel period, destination, age(s) of traveler(s), activities, etc.) and the docQuery system will prepare an information leaflet the traveler can take to his general practitioner to discuss the planned journey. The leaflet will contain all the information needed to be prepared and provide detailed information if they are required. In the event that docQuery cannot answer the traveler's question, the request will be sent to experts who will answer it. Further on, those information will not only be provided to the user, it will also be included in the docQuery case base so it will be available for future requests.

The information contained in docQuery will be processed using several methods from the field of artificial intelligence, especially CBR. Both existing knowledge about countries, diseases, prevention, etc. and experiences of travelers and physicians will be integrated and aid in further advancing docQuery's knowledge base. docQuery will provide information for travel medicine prevention work and can be used by:

- Physicians, who are advising their patients
- Physicians, who provide their knowledge
- Travelers who plan a journey and look for information about their destination

Because of docQuery's individual query processing and information leaflet assembling, the system is able to adapt to different target audiences.

2.2   Travel Medicine

Travel medicine is an interdisciplinary medical field that covers many medical areas and combines them with further information about the destination, the activities planned and additional conditions which also have to be considered when giving medical advise to a traveler. Travel medicine starts when a person moves from one place to another by any mode of transportation and stops after returning home without diseases or infections. In case a traveler gets sick after a journey a travel medicine consultation might also be required. A typical travel medical application could be a German family who wants to spend their Easter holidays diving in Alor to dive and afterward they will travel around Bali by car. In case a traveler gets sick after a journey a travel medicine consultation might also be required. First of all we will focus on prevention work, followed by information provision during a journey and information for diseased returnees. Since there are currently no sources on medical information on the World Wide Web that are authorized by physicians and/or experts, we aim at filling this gap by providing trustworthy travel medical information for everybody.

mediScon[1] is a team of certified doctors of medicine from European countries with a strong background in tourism related medicine, e.g. tropical medicine, and will support docQuery by providing travel medical information and assisting the modeling of the information. It is self-supporting and independent, and all information is scientifically proven and free of advertising. docQuery will provide all the information existing on mediScon and its sub domains. Hence the community can be used to provide new information and give feedback on given

---

[1] http://www.mediscon.com/

advices to ensure a high quality of information. Any information in docQuery is maintained by experts so users can trust the system.

docQuery will aim at providing high quality travel medicine information on demand. The system will not provide a huge amount of data that the traveler has to go through - instead, it focuses on the information the traveler already has and extend it with the required information required to travel healthily. Furthermore we will integrate the users of docQuery in its development. On the one hand, experts will take part in the community by exchanging and discussing topics with colleagues, and on the other hand, the travelers will share their experiences.

The research project is a collaborative multi-expert system (CoMES) using subsymbolic learning algorithms and offering travel medicine prevention work for any traveler. Each request will be processed individually, although the system will not substitute consulting a general practitioner. The leaflet should inform travelers and enable them to ask the right questions. Furthermore, the information given should help them to travel healthily and enjoy their stay. In developing docQuery the following requirements set our goal:

- Providing reliable, scientifically proven, up-to-date and understandable Information
- Giving independent information (no affinity to any pharmaceutical company)
- Informing any travelers without charging them
- Intuitional usability of the Front-End (accessible with a common web browser via WWW)
- Universally available
- Offering a communication platform for experts and travelers
- Enabling a multilingual and multicultural communication
- Applying new technologies and focusing on social problems to further their solution

docQuery is support travelers giving trustworthy information based on key data like destination, travel period, previous knowledge, planned activities and language. The information on the leaflets will cover the following issues:

- Medical travel prevention: vaccination, clarification of threats, information about medicaments
- Each information is tailored especially for the travelers and their needs - especially country-specific information as well as outbreaks or natural disasters (e.g. hurricanes, tsunamis, earthquakes)
- Information about local hospitals at the destination - especially hospitals where the native language of the traveler is spoken
- Outbreaks of diseases and regional epidemics
- Governmental travel advice
- General information and guidelines like "What to Do if..." in case of earthquakes, volcanic eruptions, flooding, etc.

docQuery is the core application and supports establishing a community to exchange experiences. Furthermore the users are involved in advancing the knowledge provided by docQuery and influence which issues are raised by sending requests, giving feedback and sharing experiences. docQuery is supposed to be a non-profit project and will provide travel medical information, prevention and preparation free of charge.

3   4R Cycle from the Travel Medical Point of View

CBR is a methodology based on Schank's theory [2] on the transfer of the function of human behavior onto computational intelligence. The main idea describes how people's experiences (or parts of the experiences) are remembered and later reconsidered when facing new and similar problems, reusing or adapting the previous solution in order to solve new problems. In CBR a case is described as a problem and its according solution.

In comparison to other methodologies like logical programming, CBR can deal with incomplete information and the domain does not have to be completely covered by a knowledge model before a system can be built. The integrated learning process allows a CBR system to learn while it is used. Based on Schank's ideas Aamodt and Plaza [1] introduced the Retrieve-Reuse-Revise-Retain (4R) process cycle that is until today the reference model for CBR applications.

Today there are three major types of CBR systems: Textual CBR systems [3] that basically deals with textual cases and combine Natural Language Processing Techniques with the CBR approach. Conversational CBR applications with are characterized by subsequent retrieval steps that narrow down the possible solution by iteratively setting attributes and the most often applied approach of Structural CBR which features a strict case representation and various retrieval techniques. Today many applications combine those approaches according to the given system requirements. A more detailed description of the CBR approaches and their application domains is discussed by Bergmann [4].

Although not all applications implement each process, most CBR systems are based on this model. To describe the 4R cycle, we will again use the travel medicine example presented in section 2.2 and illustrate the 4R example in Figure 1.

The current situation is a family plans that to spend their Easter holidays in Alor and Bali. This is the problem description that has to be transfered in the problem representation to initiate a *retrieval* request. Within this example we are only looking for vaccination suggestions. To enable an efficient retrieval different case base indexing structures have been developed and each of them addresses special features of a CBR type. Before a retrieval can be executed the problem has to be analyzed so an similarity-based retrieval within the case base can be executed.

The case base or knowledge base contains previous cases as well as background knowledge, this can be *rules* to either complete requests (enriched with tags) or modify solutions, or *similarity measures* to compute the similarity between two

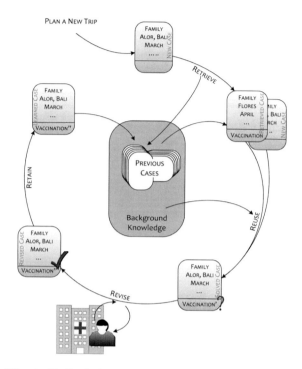

Fig. 1. 4R Cycle from the Travel Medical Point of View

cases or *vocabulary* to recognize keywords. The so called knowledge containers are described in more detail by Richter [5].

The background knowledge is required to find similar cases during the retrieval process and if necessary adapt solutions. After the retrieval process has been executed a CBR system has an ordered set of possible solutions, which usually do not match perfectly. Hence they need some modification and the *reuse* process is initiated. Within this process the system uses background knowledge, mostly adaptation rules, to change the solution in order to exactly (or as close as possible) fit to the problem description. In our example we can exchange the month April through March because the background knowledge, i.e. a rule, says that both months are in the rainy season and though can be handled equally. Also we can substitute Flores through Alor and Bali because this are all Indonesian islands with very similar properties (geographical location, climate, etc.).

Figure 2 exemplifies one type of knowledge representation for geographic regions. Based on continents, regions and countries we have developed a taxonomy that can be used to find similar countries. Knowledge models like taxonomies or light ontologies provide different types of knowledge in terms of knowledge containers: the names of the nodes and leafs are representing *vocabulary knowledge*. Since those terms are ordered in a taxonomy, *similarities* between countries, here regarding their geographic position. Also *adaptation knowledge* can be acquired

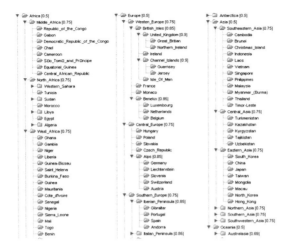

Fig. 2. Knowledge model representing the geographical location of countries

from taxonomies, because countries that share a node also might have features in common that can be applied completing incomplete case as described in Bach et. al. [6]. Along with taxonomies, similarity measures for symbolic representations can also be realized using tables, ontologies or individually defined data strucutres.

After the adaptation process has been executed the new case has to be revised. The *revision* can either be realized using again background knowledge or external feedback. In our example we send our solution to an expert who revises the case manually and gives feedback. Afterwards we have a new revised problem-solution pair (case) that can be included in the case base. In this way the case base and thus the whole CBR system is able to learn and to adapt to different circumstances.

4   Underlying Architecture

docQuery will be an intelligent information system based on experts which are distributed all over the world and use the platform giving information to travelers and colleagues. The implementation will pursue an approach mainly based on software agents and CBR. Both software agent and CBR have already been used to implement experience based systems [7,4,8]. docQuery will use different knowledge sources (diseases, medications, outbreaks, guidelines, etc.) which are created in cooperation with experts, provided in databases and maintained by the users of docQuery. However, medicine cannot deal with vague information how they might occur in extractions of community knowledge. Therefore we also integrated data bases as knowledge sources in case exact matches are required.

Collaborative Multi-Expert-Systems (CoMES) are a new approach presented of Althoff et. al.[9] which presents a continuation of combining established techniques and the application of the product line concept (known from software engineering) creating knowledge lines. Furthermore this concept describes the collaboration of distributed knowledge sources which makes this approach adequate for an application scenario like docQuery. The system will follow the CoMES-architecture, called SEASALT (Sharing Experience using an Agent-based System Architecture LayouT), as it can be seen in Figure 3 and is explained in detail in Reichle et. al.[10].

The SEASALT architecture provides an application-independent architecture that features knowledge acquisition from a web-community, knowledge modularization, and agent-based knowledge maintenance. It consists of five main components which will be presented in the remaining of this section.

The SEASALT architecture is especially suited for the acquisition, handling and provision of experiential knowledge as it is provided by communities of practice and represented within Web 2.0 platforms [11]. The *Knowledge Provision* in SEASALT is based on the *Knowledge Formalization* that has been extracted from WWW *Knowledge Sources*. Knowledge Sources can be wikis, blogs or web forums in which users, in case of docQuery travel medicine experts, provide different kinds of information. They can for instance discuss topics in web forums which are broadly established WWW communication medium and provide a low entry barrier even to only occasional WWW users. Enabling an analysis of the discussed topics, we enhanced the forum with agents for different purposes. Additionally its contents can be easily accessed using the underlying data base. The forum itself might serve as a communication and collaboration platform for the travel medicine community, which consists of professionals such as scientists and physicians who specialize in travel medicine and local experts from the health sector and private persons such as frequent travelers and globetrotters. The community uses the platform for sharing experiences, asking questions and general networking. The forum is enhanced with agents that offer content-based services such as the identification of experts, similar discussion topics, etc. and communicate by posting relevant links directly into the respective threads [12].

The community platform is monitored by a second type of agents, the so called Collector Agents. These agents are individually assigned to a specific Topic Agent, their task is to collect all contributions that are relevant with regard to their assigned Topic Agent's topic. The Collector Agents pass these contributions on to the Knowledge Engineer and can in return receive feedback on the delivered contribution's relevance. Our Collector Agents use information extraction tools, like GATE [13] or TextMarker [14] to judge the relevance of a contribution. The Knowledge Engineer reviews each Collector Agent's collected contributions and realizes his or her feedback by directly adjusting the agents' rule base.

The SEASALT architecture is also able to include external knowledge sources by equipping individual Collector agents with data base or web service protocols or HTML crawling capabilities. This allows us to include additional knowledge sources such as the web pages of the Department of Foreign Affairs or the WHO.

In order for the collected knowledge to be easily usable within the Knowledge Line the collected contributions have to be formalized from their textual

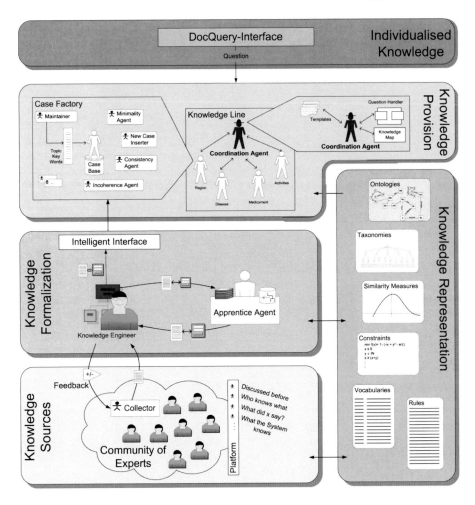

Fig. 3. SEASALT Architecture

representation into a more modular, structured representation. This task is mainly carried out by the Knowledge Engineer. In the docQuery project the role of the Knowledge Engineer is carried out by several human experts, who execute the Knowledge Engineer's tasks together. The Knowledge Engineer is the link between the community and the Topic Agents. He or she receives posts from the Collectors that are relevant with regard to one of the fields, represented by the Topic Agents, and formalizes them for insertion in the Topic Agents' knowledge bases using the Intelligent Interface. In the future the Knowledge Engineer will be additionally supported by the Apprentice Agent. The Intelligent Interface serves as the Knowledge Engineer's case authoring work bench for formalizing textual knowledge into structured CBR cases. It has been developed analogous to [15] and offers a graphical user interface that presents options for searching, browsing and editing cases and a controlled vocabulary.

The Apprentice Agent is meant to support the Knowledge Engineer in formalizing relevant posts for insertion in the Topic Agents' knowledge bases. It is trained by the Knowledge Engineer with community posts and their formalizations. The apprentice agent is currently being developed using GATE [13] and RapidMiner [16]. We use a combined classification/extraction approach that first classifies the contributions with regard to the knowledge available within the individual contributions using term-doc-matrix representations of the contributions and RapidMiner then attempts to extract the included entities and their exact relations using GATE. Considering docQuery's sensitive medical application domain we only use the Apprentice Agent for preprocessing. All its formalizations will have to be reviewed by the Knowledge Engineer, but we still expect a significantly reduced workload for the Knowledge engineer(s).

Although CoMES is a very new approach, the used techniques, like the Experience Factory[7], Case-Based Reasoning or Software Agents are well known. docQuery will integrate those techniques in a web community and creating an intelligent information system which is based on the knowledge of experts, experiences discussed on discussion boards and novelties presented by travel medicines that are a part of the community. Sharing knowledge at this level furthers the web 2.0 approach and allows us to develop new techniques.

5   Combination of Heterogeneous Knowledge Sources

When dealing with complex application domains it is easier to maintain a number of heterogeneous knowledge sources than one monolithic knowledge source. The knowledge modularization within SEASALT is organized in the Knowledge Line that is based on the principle of product lines as it is known from software engineering [17] and we apply it to the knowledge in knowledge-based systems, thus splitting rather complex knowledge in smaller, reusable units (knowledge sources). Moreover, the knowledge sources contain different kinds of information as well as there can also be multiple knowledge sources for the same purpose. Therefore each source has to be described in order to be integrated in a retrieval process which uses a various number of knowledge sources (see the third layer (Knowledge Line) in Figure 3).

The approach presented in this work does not aim at distributing knowledge for performance reasons, instead we are planning to specifically extract information for the respective knowledge sources from WWW communities or to have experts maintaining one knowledge base. Hence, we are creating knowledge sources, especially CBR systems, that are accessed dynamically according to the utility and accessibility to answer a given question. Each retrieval result of a query is a part of the combined information as it is described in the CoMES approach [18].

For each specific issue a case or data base will be created to ensure a high quality of knowledge. The data structure of each issue is different and so is the case format and domain model. Creating high quality "local knowledge bases" will guarantee the high quality of the systems knowledge.

5.1   Knowledge Sources

Considering knowledge sources, different characteristics, and aspects on which to assess knowledge source properties come to mind. The possible properties can refer to content (e.g. quality or topicality) as well as meta-information (e.g. answer speed or access limits). These properties do not only describe the individual sources but are also used for optimizing the query path. When working with distributed and – most importantly – external sources it is of high importance to be able to assess, store and utilize their characteristics in order to achieve optimal retrieval results. In detail we have identified the meta and content properties for knowledge sources (see Table 1, a more detailed description can be found in Reichle et. al. [19]).

Table 1. Knowledge source properties

Meta Property	Content Property
Access Limits	Content
Answer Speed	Expiry
Economic Cost	Up-to-dateness
Syntax	Coverage
Format	Completeness
Structure	
Cardinality	
Trust or Provenance	

Not all of the properties identified are fully unrelated. Properties like syntax, format, structure and cardinality for instance are partially related which allows for some basic sanity checks of their assigned values; also some of the properties such as answer speed, language or structure can be automatically assessed. Apart from these possibilities for automation the knowledge source properties currently have to be assessed and maintained manually by a Knowledge Engineer who assigns values to the properties and keeps them up to date. Adapting the properties' values based on feedback is only partially possible since feedback is mostly given on the final, combined result and it is thus difficult to propagate back to the respective knowledge sources. Also the more differentiated feedback is needed (in order to be mapped to the respective properties) the less feedback is given, so a good balance has to be found in this regard. Despite these difficulties the inclusion of feedback should not be ruled out completely. Even if good knowledge sources are affected by bad general feedback and the other way around the mean feedback should still provide a basic assessment of a knowledge source's content and can for instance be included in a combined quality measure. Depending on the respective properties we have defined possible values. Although there are not all properties usable for routing optimization, there are some properties like format, syntax, structure or content that cannot be used in the routing process since no valency can be assigned to them, that is one possible value cannot be judged as better or worse as the other. The computation

of the routes with regard to defined properties is carried as described in Reichle
et. al. [19].

docQuery will initially consist of the several heterogeneous knowledge sources
and each type of knowledge source will cover on specific topic. Each knowledge
source is accessible by the application and will be used to process the requests
given by the user. Furthermore the knowledge sources will be able to be extended
by more knowledge bases in future as well as maintenance processes can be
defined for each knowledge base.

Region: For any country specific information consisting of "Before the journey",
"During the journey" and "After the journey" will be provided. The country
information includes required vaccinations and guides for a healthy journey.
Further on this case base contains information on how to behave in various
situations, which are explained to the users if necessary.

Disease: This knowledge base holds more than 100 diseases considered in travel
medicine. They are described in detail and linked to medicaments, region, etc.
It focuses on diseases that might affect a traveler on a journey, for instance
Malaria, Avian Influenza, or Dengue. A disease in this case base is characterized
by general information on the disease, how to avoid the disease, how to behave
if one has had the disease before, and how to protect oneself.

Medicament: Details about medicaments and its area of application (diseases,
vaccinations, age, etc.) used in the system are contained in this knowledge base.
Basically it contains information about active pharmaceutical ingredients, effectiveness, therapeutic field, contraindication and interdependences.

Dates/Seasons: For each country we will cover dates and seasons. This information is used to assign the season to a request and subsequently only retrieve
information that is necessary.

Vaccinations: If there are vaccinations recommended this database contains
vaccination periods and types of vaccines. Further on it lists contraindications
of each vaccination and experiences of users with the vaccinations in similar
situations.

Activity: This case base will contain safety advice for intended activities when
planning a journey. For travelers, activities are the major part of their journey,
but they may involve certain risks for which safety advice is needed and furthermore when asked for their plans travelers will usually describe their activities
which we can use to provide better guidance. Examples of such activities are
diving, hill-climbing or even swimming.

Health Risk: This knowledge base contains information about health risks that
might occur at a certain place under certain previously defined circumstances
including medical details on prevention, symptoms and consequences. Further
on it contains safety advice and the type of person who might be affected.

Description: Any information given in the system can be described in different ways. This knowledge base contains different descriptions which can be given to the user: there will be a specific and detailed description (e.g. for physicians), detailed descriptions for travelers (who are no physicians) and brief information (for experienced travelers as reminders, etc.).

Guidelines: This knowledge source will contain the "How to"-descriptions to help travelers to put the given information in practice. This case base is especially for travelers.

Experience: According to the motivation we will integrate the users experience to the system. This knowledge base will contain experiences and feedback given by travelers.

Template: This database contains templates to display the result created during the processing of the request. The templates will be used to ensure a structured and printable output.

Profile: This database contains user profiles of experts who edit data, administers or regular users who want to create a profile to get faster access to their required information.

5.2   Combination of Information Retrieved from Knowledge Sources

The flexible knowledge provision based on distributed, heterogeneous knowledge sources can be accessed in different ways. We combine retrieval results of several CBR systems embedded in a multi-agent system. The novelty of our approach is the use of heterogeneous case bases for representing a modularized complex knowledge domain. There have been other approaches using partitioned and/or distributed case bases, but still differ from our approach. In SEASALT the knowledge provision task is carried out by a so called Knowledge Line that contains a Coordination Agent and a number of Topic Agents that each covers one homogeneous area of expertise. In terms of SEASALT we use the modularization aspect to combine knowledge based on numerous different and homogeneous knowledge sources implemented as CBR software agents. The Coordination Agent is the center of the Knowledge Line and orchestrates the Topic Agents to enable the combination of the retrieval results. The implementation of the Coordination Agent followed a set of requirements that were derived from the SEASALT architecture description itself and from the implementation and testing of the Topic Agents.

During the design phase of the Coordination Agent the following requirements were identified:

  – The case representations of the Topic Agents differ from each other as well as the agents' respective location might vary. This requires flexible access methods that are able to deal with distributed locations, different kinds of result sets and possibly also different access protocols.

- Some Topic Agents require another Topic Agent's output as their input and thus need to be queried successively, others can be queried at any time. In order for the Coordination Agent to be able to obey these dependencies they need to be indicated in the Knowledge Map in an easily comprehensible way.
- Based on the dependencies denoted in the Knowledge Map the agent needs to be able to develop a request strategy on demand. This request strategy should also be improvable with regard to different criteria such as the Topic Agents' response speed, the quality of their information, the possible economic cost of a request to a commercial information source and also possible access limits.
- In order to guarantee the quality of the final result of the incremental retrieval process there needs to be a possibility to control what portion of the result set is passed on to the subsequent Topic Agent. This portion should be describable based on different criteria such as the number of cases or their similarity.
- In order to allow for higher flexibility and a seamless inclusion in the SEASALT architecture the functionalities need to be implemented in an agent framework.

Firstly, in order for the Coordination Agent to be able to navigate the different knowledge sources a format for the Knowledge Map had to be designed and implemented. Since the dependencies between Topic Agents can take any form, we decided to implement the Knowledge Map as a graph where each Topic Agent is represented by a node and directed edges denote the dependencies. The case attributes that serve as the next Topic Agent's input are associated with the respective edges. The optimization criteria are indicated by a number between 0 (worst) and 100 (best) and are represented as node weights. In order to be able to limit the portion of the result that is passed on to the next node we implemented four possible thresholds, namely the total number of cases to be passed on, the relative percentage of cases to be passed on, the minimum similarity of cases to be passed on, the placement with regard to similarity of the cases to be passed on (For instance the best and second best cases). An example graph from the docQuery application can be seen in Fig. 4.

According to our example introduced in the beginning of this chapter the region agent would return a case including the information that Alor and Bali are Indonesian islands. Based on this information (i.e. Country = Indonesia) queries for general safety information about this country, diseases that can be contracted in the country, and certified (international standard) hospitals at the destination are initiated. In this example there are two agents offering that information: a free one[2] with information of lesser quality and a commercial one[3] with information of higher quality. The retrieved diseases (Malaria, Yellow Fever, Diphtheria, Tetanus, Hepatitis A, Typhoid Fever, etc.) are then subsequently used to query the medicaments agent for recommendable vaccinations

---

[2] The cost 100 denotes a minimal price, that is 0,-.

[3] The price is medium high, thus the cost value is 50, an agent with a higher cost would have an even lower cost value.

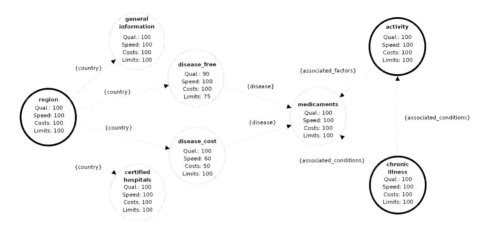

Fig. 4. Example graph based on the docQuery application

and medicaments that can be taken at the location. This query returns an initial list of recommendable medicament candidates. Further on, the information given by the user (Activities = "diving" and "road trip") is used to request information from the activity agent defining constraints for medicament recommendations (e.g. Activity = "Diving" ⇒ Associated_factors = "high sun exposure") which are then again used to query the medicaments agent. In this example a query for Counter_Indication = "high sun exposure" would return, among others, the Malaria prophylaxis Doxycyclin Monohydrat, which would then be removed from the initial list of recommended medicaments. Also, if specified, the influences of chronic illnesses on recommended medicaments and planned activities are queried. The combined information from all Topic Agents is compiled into an information leaflet using ready prepared templates. ("*When traveling to Indonesia, please consider the following general information: ... Certified hospitals can be found in the following places: ... A journey to Indonesia carries the following risks: ... We recommend the following medicaments: ... These medicaments are not recommended because of the following reasons ...*") The Knowledge Map itself is stored as an XML document. We use RDF as the wrapper format and describe the individual nodes with a name space of our own. Based on the knowledge map we then use a modified Dijkstra algorithm [20] to determine an optimal route over the graph. The algorithm is modified in such a way that it optimizes its route by trying to maximize the arithmetic mean of all queried nodes. In the case of a tie between two possible routes the one with the lesser variance is chosen.

5.3   Maintenance of Knowledge Sources

docQuery deals with different kinds of data and each kind has to be maintained differently. We will define maintaining processes for each source focusing on exact, up-to-date and reliable data. Furthermore each source will have its own maintainer in case old or erroneous data has to be removed or corrected. To follow this goal the maintenance processes has to be created along with the data models regarding the interfaces and the applications built upon them.

To ensure up-to-date data the system has to be checked by experts regularly, and by integrating a web community new topics will have to be identified and new cases will have to be entered in the knowledge sources. For that purpose processes for updating (inserting, maintaining, deleting, extending, etc.) have to be implemented and established. For instance, we assume that a group of experts takes care of new entries in docQuery: In this case we are assigning topics with the expert's field of expertise to each of them and if there is a new discussion in the respective area detected, this is e-mailed to the expert so he oder she can follow this discussion. Further on, when the system extracted and processed information the complete set which should be inserted is sent to the expert and has to be approved before it can be inserted in the according case base. This proceeding is not for any application domain necessary, but since we deal with medical information we have to make sure that correct information are provided, although we are only giving information that do not substitute a medical consultation.

Even if we have different kinds of Topic Agents and their according Case Factories, the behavior of some Case Factory agents (like the new case inserter) can be reused in other Case Factories of the same Knowledge Line. We differentiate between agents that handle general aspects and are contained in any Case Factory and agents that are topic-specific and have to be implemented individually. General Case Factory agents usually focus on the performance or regular tasks like insertion, deletion, merging of cases. Topic specific Case Factory agents are for example agents that transfer knowledge between the knowledge containers [5] or define certain constraints and usually they have to be implemented for an individual topic considering its specifications or fulfilling domain dependent tasks. The Knowledge Line retrieves its information, which is formalized by a Knowledge Engineer and/or machine learning algorithms, from knowledge sources like databases, web services, RSS-feeds, or other kinds of community services and provides the information as a web service, in an information portal, or as a part of a business work flow. The flexible structure of the knowledge line allows designing applications incrementally by starting out with one or two Topic Agents and enlarging the knowledge line, for example with more detailed or additional topics, as soon as they are available or accessible.

6   Related Work

The approach of distributed sources has been a research topic in Information Retrieval since the mid-nineties. An example is the Carrot II project [21], which also uses a multi-agent-system to co-ordinate the document sources. However, most of our knowledge sources are CBR-systems, which is the reason why we concentrate on CBR-approaches. The issue of differentiating case bases in order to be more suitable for its application domain has been discussed before. Weber et al. [22] introduce the horizontal case representation, a two case base approach in which one contains the problem and the other one the solutions. They motivate splitting up the case bases for a more precise case representation, vocabulary and a simplified knowledge acquisition.

Retrieval strategies have been discussed in the context of Multi-Case-Base Reasoning in [23]. Leake and Sooriamurthi explain how distributed cases can be retrieved, ranked and adapted. Although they are dealing with the same type of case representations of the distributed case bases, both approaches have to determine whether a solution or part of solution is selected or not. The strategy of Multi-Case-Base Reasoning is to either dispatch cases if a case-base cannot provide a suitable solution or to use cases of more than one case base and initiate an adaptation process in order to create one solution.

Collaborating case bases have been introduced by Ontañón and Plaza [24] who use a multi-agent system to provide a reliable solution. The multi-agent system focuses on learning which case base provides the best results, but they do not combine or adapt solutions of different case bases. Instead their approach focuses on the automatic detection of the best knowledge source for a certain question.

Combining parts of cases in order to adapt given solutions to a new problem has been introduced by Redmond in [25] in which he describes how snippets of different cases can be retrieved and merged into other cases, but in comparison to our approach, Redmond uses similar case representations from which he extracts parts of cases in order to combine them. His approach and the knowledge provision in SEASALT have in common that both deal with information snippets and put them together in order to have a valid solution. Further on, Redmond mostly concentrates on adaptation while we combine information based on a retrieval and routing strategy.

Our notion of knowledge source properties is comparable to and thus benefits from advances in the respective field in CBR like the recent work of Briggs and Smyth [26], who also assign properties, but to individual cases. On the other hand the graph-like representation of the knowledge sources and its use in the composition of the final results do not have a direct equivalent in CBR. It depends on the cases' separation by topic and a clear dependency structure of the topics (e.g. *the country determines the possible diseases, the diseases determine the respective vaccinations and precautions, etc.*) which is not necessarily given in traditional CBR.

7   Conclusion and Final Remarks

The SEASALT architecture offers several features, namely knowledge acquisition from web 2.0 communities, modularized knowledge storage and processing and agent-based knowledge maintenance. SEASALT's first application within the docQuery project yielded very satisfactory results, however, in order to further develop the architecture we are planning to improve it in several areas. One of these are the Collector Agents working on the community platform, which we plan to advance from a rule-based approach to a classification method that is able to learn from feedback, so more workload is taken off the Knowledge Engineer.

docQuery is the first instantiation of SEASALT and has a strong focus on the knowledge modularization and reassembly with the goal to provide an information leaflet for a traveler. Moreover, docQuery shows how various AI methodologies can be used to realize an intelligent information system that provides complete and reliable information for individual journeys considering all aspects a travel medicine physician would do. We also introduced how various heterogeneous knowledge sources can be queried as well as we provided a web-based maintenance strategy that enables an intelligent system to use Web 2.0 platforms like web forums to extend its case base.

Travel medicine is for sure a specific application domain that cannot compared to any other application because the information we deal with are health related and we have to make sure that only correct and understandable are produced. We are confident that the techniques along with the SEASALT architecture can be used within different application domains that cover a combination of topics.

References

1. Aamodt, A., Plaza, E.: Case-based reasoning: Foundational issues, methodological variations, and system approaches. AI Communications 1(7) (March 1994)
2. Schank, R.C.: Dynamic Memory: A Theory of Reminding and Learning in Computers and People. Cambridge University Press, New York (1983)
3. Wilson, D.C., Bradshaw, S.: Cbr textuality. In: Brüninghaus, S. (ed.) Proceedings of the Fourth UK Case-Based Reasoning Workshop, University of Salford, pp. 67–80 (1999)
4. Bergmann, R., Althoff, K.D., Breen, S., Göker, M., Manago, M., Traphöner, R., Wess, S.: Developing industrial case-based reasoning applications: The INRECA methodology. In: Bergmann, R., Althoff, K.-D., Breen, S., Göker, M.H., Manago, M., Traphöner, R., Wess, S. (eds.) Developing Industrial Case-Based Reasoning Applications, 2nd edn. LNCS (LNAI), vol. 1612. Springer, Heidelberg (2003)
5. Richter, M.M.: Introduction. In: Lenz, M., Bartsch-Spörl, B., Burkhard, H.D., Wess, S. (eds.) Case-Based Reasoning Technology. LNCS (LNAI), vol. 1400, p. 1. Springer, Heidelberg (1998)
6. Bach, K., Reichle, M., Althoff, K.D.: A value supplementation method for case bases with incomplete information. In: McGinty, L., Wilson, D.C. (eds.) Case-Based Reasoning Research and Development. LNCS (LNAI), vol. 5650, pp. 389–402. Springer, Heidelberg (2009)
7. Althoff, K.D., Pfahl, D.: Making software engineering competence development sustained through systematic experience management. Managing Software Engineering Knowledge (2003)
8. Minor, M.: Erfahrungsmanagement mit fallbasierten Assistenzsystemen. PhD thesis, Humboldt-Universität zu Berlin (Mai 2006)

9. Althoff, K.D., Bach, K., Deutsch, J.O., Hanft, A., Mänz, J., Müller, T., Newo, R., Reichle, M., Schaaf, M., Weis, K.H.: Collaborative multi-expert-systems – realizing knowlegde-product-lines with case factories and distributed learning systems. In: Baumeister, J., Seipel, D. (eds.) Workshop Proceedings on the 3rd Workshop on Knowledge Engineering and Software Engineering (KESE 2007), Osnabrück (September 2007)
10. Reichle, M., Bach, K., Althoff, K.D.: The seasalt architecture and its realization within the docquery project. In: Mertsching, B., Hund, M., Aziz, Z. (eds.) KI 2009. LNCS, vol. 5803, pp. 556–563. Springer, Heidelberg (2009)
11. Plaza, E.: Semantics and experience in the future web. In: Althoff, K.-D., Bergmann, R., Minor, M., Hanft, A. (eds.) ECCBR 2008. LNCS (LNAI), vol. 5239, pp. 44–58. Springer, Heidelberg (2008)
12. Feng, D., Shaw, E., Kim, J., Hovy, E.: An intelligent discussion-bot for answering student queries in threaded discussions. In: IUI 2006: Proc. of the 11th Intl. Conference on Intelligent user interfaces, pp. 171–177. ACM Press, New York (2006)
13. Cunningham, H., Maynard, D., Bontcheva, K., Tablan, V.: Gate: A framework and graphical development environment for robust nlp tools and applications. In: Proceedings of the 40th Anniversary Meeting of the Association for Computational Linguistics, ACL 2002 (2002)
14. Klügl, P., Atzmüller, M., Puppe, F.: Test-driven development of complex information extraction systems using textmarker. In: Nalepa, G.J., Baumeister, J. (eds.) Algebraic Logic and Universal Algebra in Computer Science. CEUR Workshop Proceedings, vol. 425 (2008), CEUR-WS.org
15. Bach, K.: Domänenmodellierung im textuellen fallbasierten schließen. Master's thesis, Institute of Computer Science, University of Hildesheim (2007)
16. Mierswa, I., Wurst, M., Klinkenberg, R., Scholz, M., Euler, T.: Yale: Rapid prototyping for complex data mining tasks. In: Ungar, L., Craven, M., Gunopulos, D., Eliassi-Rad, T. (eds.) KDD 2006: Proc. of the 12th ACM SIGKDD international conference on Knowledge discovery and data mining, August 2006, pp. 935–940. ACM, New York (2006)
17. van der Linden, F., Schmid, K., Rommes, E.: Software Product Lines in Action - The Best Industrial Practice in Product Line Engineering. Springer, Heidelberg (2007)
18. Althoff, K.-D., Reichle, M., Bach, K., Hanft, A., Newo, R.: Agent based maintenance for modularised case bases in collaborative multi-expert systems. In: Proceedings of AI 2007, 12th UK Workshop on Case-Based Reasoning, December 2007, pp. 7–18 (2007)
19. Reichle, M., Bach, K., Reichle-Schmehl, A., Althoff, K.D.: Management of distributed knowledge sources for complex application domains. In: Hinkelmann, K., Wache, H. (eds.) Proceedings of the 5th Conference on Professional Knowledge Manegement - Experiences and Visions (WM 2009), March 2009. Lecture Notes in Informatics, pp. 128–138 (2009)
20. Dijkstra, E.W.: A note on two problems in connexion with graphs. Numerische Mathematik 1, 269–271 (1959)
21. Cost, R.S., Kallurkar, S., Majithia, H., Nicholas, C., Shi, Y.: Integrating distributed information sources with carrot ii. In: Klusch, M., Ossowski, S., Shehory, O. (eds.) CIA 2002. LNCS (LNAI), vol. 2446, p. 194. Springer, Heidelberg (2002)
22. Weber, R., Gunawardena, S., MacDonald, C.: Horizontal case representation. In: Althoff, K.D., Bergmann, R., Minor, M., Hanft, A. (eds.) ECCBR 2008. LNCS (LNAI), vol. 5239, pp. 548–561. Springer, Heidelberg (2008)

23. Leake, D.B., Sooriamurthi, R.: Automatically selecting strategies for multi-case-base reasoning. In: Craw, S., Preece, A.D. (eds.) ECCBR 2002. LNCS (LNAI), vol. 2416, pp. 204–233. Springer, Heidelberg (2002)
24. Ontañón, S., Plaza, E.: Learning when to collaborate among learning agents. In: Flach, P.A., De Raedt, L. (eds.) ECML 2001. LNCS (LNAI), vol. 2167, pp. 394–405. Springer, Heidelberg (2001)
25. Redmond, M.: Distributed cases for case-based reasoning: Facilitating use of multiple cases. In: AAAI, pp. 304–309 (1990)
26. Briggs, P., Smyth, B.: Provenance, trust, and sharing in peer-to-peer case-based web search. In: Althoff, K.D., Bergmann, R., Minor, M., Hanft, A. (eds.) ECCBR 2008. LNCS (LNAI), vol. 5239, pp. 89–103. Springer, Heidelberg (2008)

Chapter 10
Providing Case-Based Retrieval as a Decision Support Strategy in Time Dependent Medical Domains

Stefania Montani

Dipartimento di Informatica, Università del Piemonte Orientale, Alessandria, Italy

Abstract. Case-based Reasoning (CBR), and more specifically case-based retrieval, is recently being recognized as a valuable decision support methodology in "time dependent" medical domains, i.e. in all domains in which the observed phenomenon dynamics have to be dealt with. However, adopting CBR in these applications is non trivial, since the need for describing the process dynamics impacts both on case representation and on the retrieval activity itself.

The aim of this chapter is the one of analysing the different methodologies introduced in the literature in order to implement time dependent medical CBR applications, with a particular emphasis on *time series* representation and retrieval.

Among the others, a novel approach, which relies on Temporal Abstractions for time series dimensionality reduction, is analysed in depth, and illustrated by means of a case study in haemodialysis.

1 Introduction

Several real world applications require to capture the evolution of the observed phenomenon over time, in order to describe its behaviour, and to exploit this information for future problem solving.

This issue is particularly relevant in medical applications, where the physician typically needs to recall the clinical history that led the patient to the current condition, before prescribing a therapy; actually, the pattern of the patient's changes is often more important than her/his final state [24]. The need for capturing the phenomenon's temporal evolution emerges even more strongly when a continuous monitoring of the patient's health indicators is required, such as in chronic diseases [5], or when control instruments that automatically sample and record biological signals are adopted, such as in the Intensive Care Unit [39], haemodialysis, or instrumental diagnostic procedures [33]. In these applications, (many) process features are naturally collected in the form of **time series**, either automatically generated and stored by the control instruments (as e.g. in Intensive Care Unit monitoring), or obtained by listing single values extracted from temporally consecutive situations (as e.g. the series of glycated haemoglobin values, measured on a diabetic patient once every two months).

I. Bichindaritz et al. (Eds.): Computational Intelligence in Healthcare 4, SCI 309, pp. 211–228.
springerlink.com   © Springer-Verlag Berlin Heidelberg 2010

Analysing long and complex time series of measurements at a screen or on paper can be tedious and prone to errors. Physicians may be asked to recognize small or rare irregularities in the signal, whose identification may be extremely relevant for an accurate diagnosis or for the patient monitoring activity. A manual identification of these irregularities requires a certain amount of expertise in the specific field [37]; an automated decision support strategy is therefore strongly needed in these domains.

Case-based Reasoning (CBR) [1], a reasoning paradigm that exploits the knowledge collected on previously experienced situations, known as *cases*, is recently being recognized as a valuable knowledge management and decision support methodology in time dependent applications (see e.g. [32]).

In CBR, problem solving experience is explicitly taken into account by storing past cases in a library (called the *case base*), and by suitably retrieving them when a new problem has to be tackled.

CBR can be summarized by the following four basic steps, known as the *CBR cycle*, or as the four *"res"* [1]:

- *retrieve* the most similar case(s) with respect to the input situation from the case base;
- *reuse* them, and more precisely their solutions, to solve the new problem;
- *revise* the proposed new solution (if needed);
- *retain* the current case for future problem solving.

However, in many application domains it is common to find CBR tools able to extract relevant knowledge, but that leave to the user the responsibility of providing its interpretation and of formulating the final decision: reuse and revise are therefore not implemented. Nevertheless, even retrieval alone may significantly support the human decision making process [54].

This consideration especially holds for the medical domain, where automated revision/adaptation strategies can hardly be identified [29], while experiential knowledge representation as cases and case-based retrieval can be particularly helpful, for the following reasons:

- *case retrieval resembles* human reasoning in general, and *medical decision making* in particular. As a matter of fact, physicians are used to reason by recalling past situations similar to the current one. The process is often biased by the tendency to recall only more recent or difficult cases, or only the positively solved ones. Case-based retrieval can enable to store and recall older, simpler or negative examples as well. Storing and recalling practical cases comes out to be very useful also for sharing other clinicians' skills, and for training un-experienced personnel, which are key objectives of every health care organization;
- *cases allow unformalized knowledge storage and maintenance.* Properly maintaining knowledge is a relevant issue to be addressed in the medical domain, where large amounts of operative and unformalized information are generally available. Every past case *implicitly* embeds an amount of domain knowledge (i.e. the problem-action pattern adopted on that occasion), which

can be represented without the need of making it *explicit* in a more generalized form, thus mitigating the well known knowledge acquisition bottleneck that affects other methodologies (such as Rule-based or Model-based Reasoning). Proper maintenance policies [25] can then be implemented in order to control the case base growth while preserving its problem solving competence;

- *cases allow to integrate different knowledge types.* When generalized domain knowledge is available, extracted from textbooks or physicians committees expertise, and formalized by means of rules, ontologies, or computerized guidelines, its integration with experiential and unformalized knowledge may represent a significant advantage. Cases can be quite naturally adopted to complement formalized knowledge, and to make it operational in a real setting, as testified e.g. by the wide number of multi-modal reasoning systems proposed in the literature [29].

Various Case-based Reasoning/retrieval works dealing with cases with time series features have been recently published, in the medical domain (see sections 2 and 3), as well as in different ones (e.g. robot control [42], process forecast [34,43], process supervision [13], pest management [9], prediction of faulty situations [19]). Moreover, general (e.g. logic-based) frameworks for case representation in time dependent domains have been proposed [32,18,27,8].

However, adopting case-based retrieval can be non trivial in time dependent applications, since the need for describing the process dynamics impacts both on case representation and on retrieval itself, as analysed in [32]. As a matter of fact, in classical CBR, a case consists of a *problem description* able to summarize the problem at hand, and of a *case solution*, describing the solution adopted for solving the corresponding problem. The problem description is typically represented as a collection of $\langle feature, value \rangle$ pairs. However, for intrinsically data intensive applications, where data come in the form of time series, data themselves cannot be simply stored as feature values "as they are". Pre-processing techniques are required in these situations, in order to simplify feature mining and knowledge representation, and to optimize the retrieval activity.

Most of the approaches proposed in the literature to this end are founded on the common premise of **dimensionality reduction**, which allows to reduce memory occupancy and to simplify time series representation, still capturing the most important characteristics of the time series itself.

Dimensionality is typically reduced by means of a **mathematical transform**, able to preserve the distance between two time series (or to underestimate it). Widely used transforms are the Discrete Fourier Transform (DFT) [2], and the Discrete Wavelet Transform (DWT) [10]. Another well known mathematical methodology is Piecewise Constant Approximation (PCA) [22,23]. Retrieval then works in the transformed time series space, and, in many cases, operates in a black-box fashion with respect to the end users: they just input the query, and collect the retrieved cases, but usually do not see (and might not understand the meaning of) the transformed time series themselves. Details of mathematical methods for dimensionality reduction and time series retrieval will be presented in section 2, which will also describe some CBR contributions in the medical field relying on these techniques.

On the other hand, our research group has recently proposed [32,31] to exploit a different technique for dimensionality reduction, namely **Temporal Abstractions** (TA) [46,6,40,30]. TA is an Artificial Intelligence (AI) methodology, which, among the other things, has been employed for:

- supporting a flexible description of phenomena at different levels of time granularity (e.g. hours, minutes, seconds);
- providing a knowledge-based interpretation of temporal data.

On the other hand, rather interestingly, TA have been scarcely explored for reducing time series dimensionality, especially in the CBR literature. Instead we have observed that, through TA, huge amounts of temporal information, like the one embedded in a time series, can be effectively mapped to a compact representation, that not only summarizes the original longitudinal data, but also abstracts meaningful behaviours in the data themselves, which can be interpreted by end users as well (in an easier way if compared to mathematical methods outputs). TA-based dimensionality reduction appears to be well suited for several application domains, and in particular for medical ones. TA for time series dimensionality reduction and retrieval in a CBR context will be presented in section 3. The section will also introduce a framework we are developing, which relies on TA both for dimensionality reduction and for supporting *multi-level* abstraction and retrieval, as well as flexible query answering. The approach will be illustrated by means of a case study in haemodialysis.

Finally, section 4 will address conclusions and future work.

2   Mathematical Methods for Dimensionality Reduction in Time Dependent Medical Domains

In this section, we will provide details of mathematical methods employed for time series dimensionality reduction, and will describe a set of significant applications of these techniques in a CBR context.

2.1   Theoretical Background

A wide literature exists about similarity-based retrieval of time series. Several different approaches have been proposed (see the survey in [17]), typically based on the common premise of dimensionality reduction. As a matter of fact, a (discretized) time series can always be seen as vector in an n-dimensional space (with n typically extremely large). Simple algorithms for retrieving similar time series take polynomial time in n. Multidimensional spatial indexing (e.g. resorting to R-trees [16]) is a promising technique, that allows sub-linear retrieval; nevertheless, these tree structures are not adequate for indexing high-dimensional data sets [7].

One obvious solution is thus to reduce the time series dimensionality, adopting a transform that preserves the distance between two time series (or underestimates it: in this case a post-processing step will be required, to filter out the so-called "false alarms"; the requirement is never to overestimate the distance, so that no "false dismissals" can exist [17]). Widely used transforms are the Discrete Fourier Transform (DFT) [2], and the Discrete Wavelet Transform (DWT) [10].

DFT maps time series to the frequency domain. DFT application for dimensionality reduction stems from the observation that, for the majority of real-world time series, the first (1-3) Fourier coefficients carry the most meaningful information, and the remaining ones can be safely discarded. Moreover, Parseval's theorem [38] guarantees that the distance in the frequency domain is the same as in the time domain, when resorting to any similarity measure that can be expressed as the Euclidean distance between feature vectors in the feature space. In particular, resorting only to the first Fourier coefficients can underestimate the real distance, but never overestimates it. The definition of similarity can also be extended with invariance under a group of transformations, like amplitude scaling and shift (see [15,41]).

In DFT, comparison is based on low frequency components, where most energy is presumed to be concentrated on. DFT is good for detecting irregularities in signals, but it looses the temporal aspects, i.e., when in time the irregularities occur. An interesting way of detecting these temporal attributes is to transform the time series into time-frequencies, i.e. to retain both temporal and frequency aspects of the signals. This can be reached exploiting DWT, since wavelets, which are basis functions used to represent other functions, are local both in time and in frequency. DWT can be repeatedly applied to the data: each application brings out a higher resolution of the data, while at the same time it smoothes the remaining data. The output of the DWT consists of the remaining smooth components and of all the accumulated detail components. DWT, like any orthonormal transform, preserves the Euclidean distance as the DFT does. Moreover, Chan & Fu [10] have obtained through experiments that the application of the Haar wavelet outperforms DFT in similarity-based time series retrieval. The number of wavelet coefficients to be kept, although lower than the original data dimensionality, is higher than in the case of DFT application. Since R-trees and variants perform well with 5 dimensions at most [7], other index structures, such as the X-tree [7], and the TV-tree [50], have to be adopted if resorting to DWT.

A different approach to dimensionality reduction is Piecewise Constant Approximation (PCA) (see e.g. [22,23]): it consists in dividing a time series into k segments, and in using their average values as a k-dimensional feature vector (where obviously $k << n$, the original data dimensionality). The best value of k can also be estimated. PCA is robust to various transformations, such as scaling and offset translation, and its calculation is claimed to be fast.

The choice of the most cost-effective transformation to apply should be done on the basis of the application at hand. Examples in the medical domain will be illustrated in the following subsection.

2.2   Mathematical Transforms in Medical CBR

Case-based retrieval is recently being proposed as a well suited decision support methodology in time dependent medical domains, where (some) case features are in the form of time series; in these works, time series dimensionality reduction is often performed relying on mathematical transforms. Two significant examples of mathematical transforms exploitation in medical CBR are illustrated below.

DFT in haemodialysis. Dimensionality reduction in medical CBR by resorting to DFT has been proposed in [33], where the application domain is the one of haemodialysis. Haemodialysis is the most widely used treatment for severe chronic renal diseases, and relies on a device, called haemodialyzer, which clears the patient's blood from catabolites, to re-establish acid-base equilibrium and to remove water in excess. During each single haemodialysis treatment (session), which lasts 3-4 hours on average, the haemodialyzer collects several variables, most of which are in the form of time series (while a few are "static", i.e. single-valued). Considering a case as a haemodialysis session, the system in [33] retrieves past cases, belonging to the same patient or to different ones, in which the collected variables had a similar behaviour: in this way the physician can derive indications about the patient at hand's current metabolic condition, or

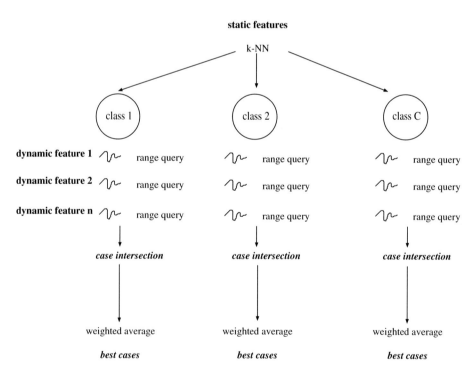

Fig. 1. The retrieval process in [33] (the picture is taken from [33]).

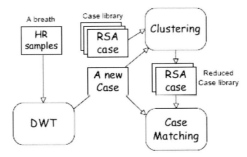

Fig. 2. The retrieval process in [37]. Time series of heart rate (HR) samples, which correspond to a breath, are matched for similarity with clusters of time series (the picture is taken from [37]).

be supported on how to solve current problems similar to those occurred in the past. In [33] time series are transformed by means of DFT, and only the first coefficients are kept for similarity calculation. Retrieval is implemented as a multi-step procedure, as described in figure 1. In particular, a first classification step exploits k-Nearest Neighbour in the static features space, in order to focus retrieval on a limited portion of the case base. Intra-class retrieval in the most similar class with respect to the input situation is then implemented. In particular, the most similar cases with respect to each one of the time series features, considered individually, are first extracted. To guarantee that retrieved cases have the required level of similarity on each time series feature, the intersection of the sets of returned cases is then computed. On the result set, global distance is finally calculated, by computing a weighted average; returned cases are ordered in terms of overall distance.

DWT in Respiratory Sinus Arrhythmia. A significant application of DWT-based dimensionality reduction in medical CBR can be found in [35,37]. The tool is able to classify Respiratory Sinus Arrhythmia (RSA), i.e. the respirations affecting the heart rate: persons do sometimes have physiological or psychological (e.g. stress-related) disorders, that appear as dysfunctions in the RSA patterns. The system uses CBR as the method for classification of dysfunctional patterns within the RSA. CBR is a very suitable methodology, because the domain is not fully understood. In the system, RSA time series are first dimensionally reduced by means of DWT; then the most similar clusters of previous cases are retrieved from the case base, in order to support disorder classification. The system architecture is described in figure 2. In particular the authors rely on Daubechies D4 DWT, which prove to be very well suited for biomedical time series retrieval, since they allow to detect a specific form of oscillating sequences. The authors were also able to compare the use of DWT to the one of DFT, since they originally applied DFT to the same domain in [36]; in RSA classification, they have obtained an increased retrieval rate when resorting to wavelets.

3   Temporal Abstractions for Dimensionality Reduction in Time Dependent Medical Domains

Mathematical methods for time series retrieval are widely accepted in the scientific community, and have been experimentally tested in several domains. Nevertheless, they have a number of limitations. For instance, they can be computationally complex, and their output is often not easily interpretable by end users (e.g. physicians). Moreover, they often require additional pre-processing steps, such as mean averaging and zero padding (see e.g. [37] for details). Finally, they work well with signals with relatively simple dynamics, but they can fail to characterize more complex patterns [11].

The study of an alternative way to deal with time series retrieval is therefore well justified.

The idea of relying on Temporal Abstractions (TA) methods for time series dimensionality reduction and retrieval support, originally introduced by our reserch group [32], starts to be reported in the literature, especially dealing with medical applications (see e.g. [14,31]).

Actually, we believe that TA represent a valuable alternative to more classical methods, in particular when:

- a more *qualitative* abstraction of the time series values is sufficient;
- a clear mapping between raw and transformed data has to be made available;
- the mapping itself needs to be easily interpreted by end users.

Details on the TA methodology and on an application of TA-based retrieval in a CBR context will be provided in the next sections.

3.1   Theoretical Background

TA is an Artificial Intelligence methodology able to solve a *data interpretation task* [46], the goal of which is to derive high level concepts from time stamped data. Operatively, the basic principle of TA methods is to move from a *point-based* to an *interval-based* representation of the data [6], where:

- the input points (*events* henceforth) are the elements of the discretized time series;
- the output intervals (*episodes* henceforth) aggregate adjacent events sharing a common behavior, persistent over time.

More precisely, the method described above should be referred to as *basic* TA [6].

Basic abstractions can be further subdivided into *state* TA and *trend* TA. *State* TA are used to extract episodes associated with *qualitative levels* of the monitored feature, e.g. low, normal, high values; *trend* TA are exploited to detect specific *patterns*, such as increase, decrease or stationary behaviour, from the time series. The output results of a basic TA depend on the value assigned to specific parameters, such as the granularity (the maximum temporal gap between two events allowed for aggregating them into the same episode) and the minimum extent (the minimum time extent for considering an episode relevant) for state TA, and the slope (the minimum allowed rate of change in an episode) for trend TA.

Complex TA [6] can be defined as well: instead of aggregating events into episodes, complex TA aggregate two series of episodes into a set of higher level episodes (i.e., they abstract output intervals over precalculated input intervals). In particular, complex abstractions search for specific *temporal* relationships between episodes that can be generated from a basic abstraction or from other complex abstractions. The relation between intervals can be any of the temporal relations defined by Allen [3]. This kind of TA can be exploited to extract patterns that depend on the course of several features, or to detect patterns of complex shapes (e.g. a peak) in a single feature.

If the time series has been pre-processed through TA, similarity based retrieval can benefit from the use of pattern matching techniques. Sequence matching can in fact be performed by a number of well-established methods [49] like dynamic programming based on the edit distance approach [52], suffix tree-based approaches [53], or general formal transformations of patterns [20]. For example the framework in [20] defines similarity between a pattern A and a pattern B (in a formal pattern language P) as a function of the transformations (defined on a transformation language T) needed to reduce B to A (or vice versa). The approach allows one to answer also queries such as "find all patterns similar to some pattern A, but not similar to pattern B". With symbolic time series it is also easier to apply data mining and knowledge discovery methods, which can be helpful to find non trivial knowledge patterns in the abstracted data [14].

Observe that TA are not the only methodology for transforming a time series into a sequence of symbols. Actually a wide number of symbolic representations of time series have been introduced in the past decades (see [11] for a survey). However, some of them require a strong domain knowledge, since they a priori partition the signal into intervals, naturally provided by the underlying system dynamics, which divide the overall time period into distinct physical phases (e.g. respiration cycles in [14]; see also [21]). Many other approaches to symbolizations are weakened by other relevant issues, i.e.: even if distance measures can be defined on symbolic representations, these distance measures have little correlation with distance measures defined over the original time series; moreover, the conversion to symbolic representation requires to have access to all the data since the beginning, thus making it not exploitable in a context of data streaming.

Rather interestingly, Lin [26] has introduced an alternative to TA, capable to deal with the issues above, in which intervals are first obtained through PCA, and subsequently labeled with proper symbols. In particular this contribution allows distance measures to be defined on the symbolic approach that lower bound the corresponding distance measures defined on the original data. Such a feature permits to run some well known data mining algorithms on the transformed data, obtaining identical results with respect to operating on the original data, while gaining in efficiency.

Despite these advantages, the approach in [26] is not as simple as TA, which allow a very clear interpretation of the qualitative description of the data provided by the abstraction process itself. As a matter of fact, such description is closer to the language of clinicians [48], and easily adapts to a domain where data values that are considered as normal at one time, or in a given context, may become dangerously abnormal in a different situation (e.g. due to disease progression or to treatments obsolescence). The ease at which knowledge can be adapted and understood by experts is an aspect that impacts upon the suitability and the usefulness of intelligent data analysis systems in clinical practice. Due to these characteristics, TA have been largely exploited to support intelligent data analysis in different medical application areas (from diabetes mellitus [47,5,45], to artificial ventilation of intensive care units patients [28,4,12]; see also the survey in [51]). However, TA have been typically adopted with the aim to solve a *data interpretation task* [46], and not as a retrieval support facility. For instance, TA have been adopted to study the co-occurrence of certain episodes in a set of clinical time series, which may justify a given diagnosis. Indeed, in [44] TA have been exploited in for time series retrieval, but basically for data pre-processing as a noise filtering tool.

Therefore, our proposal to rely on TA for time series dimensionality reduction and retrieval appears to be significantly innovative in the recent medical informatics literature panorama.

In the next section, we will introduce a flexible TA-based time series retrieval approach, in which orthogonal index structures optimize the response time. An example application to the field of haemodyalisis will be provided as well.

It is also worth noting that TA series can be considered as an input to a further knowledge discovery process, able to extract key symbol sequences in the symbolic series themselves. These key sequences might, for instance, highlight significant transitional patterns between symbols, which can be more important than static symbols within single intervals, especially in medical diagnosis support. Such key sequences are also able to further reduce the data dimensionality,

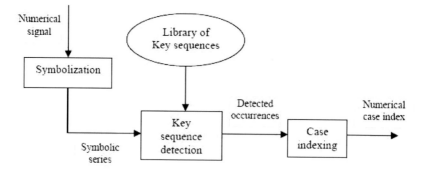

Fig. 3. Detection of key sequences in symbolic (e.g. TA) series in [14] (the picture is taken from [14]).

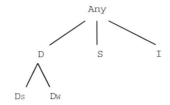

Fig. 4. An example taxonomy of symbols

since their number is usually much smaller than the number of symbol in a
TA series. Such a process has been proposed in a CBR context in [14], and is
illustrated in figure 3.

3.2   TA-Based Retrieval in Medical CBR

Our research group is currently working at the definition of a time series retrieval
framework, which exploits TA for dimensionality reduction in medical domains.

In particular, our framework allows for *multi-level abstractions*, according to
two *dimensions*, namely a taxonomy of (trend or state) TA symbols, and a
variety of time granularities.

Actually, TA symbols can be organized in a conventional *is-a* taxonomy, in
order to provide different levels of detail in the description of episodes. An example taxonomy of symbols for trend TA is the one illustrated in figure 4, in which
the symbol *Any* is specialized into D (decrease), S (stationary) and I (increase),
and D is further specialized into D_S (strong decrease) and D_W (weak decrease),
according to the slope.

On the other hand, time granularities allow one to describe episodes at increasingly more abstract levels of temporal aggregation (see figure 5). Obviously,
the number of levels in the time granularities taxonomy and in the symbol taxonomy, as well as the dimension of granules, can be differently set depending on
the application domain. However it is worth noting that our approach is applicable in absence of domain knowledge as well (in the worst case, by resorting
to flat taxonomies). Observe that the time dimension requires that aggregation is "homogeneous" at every given level, in the sense that each granule at a
given level must be an aggregation of exactly the same number of consecutive
granules at the lower level (while this number may vary from level to level; for
instance, two 1-hour-long granules compose a 2-hours-long granule, while three
20-minutes-long granules compose a 1-hour-long granule). Such an "homogeneity" restriction is motivated by the fact that, in such a way, the duration of
each episode is (implicitly) represented in the sequence of symbols. For example,
at the time granularity level of 20 minutes, the string $DDDS$ may represent a
1-hour episode of D followed by 20 minutes of S.

Although the use of a symbol taxonomy and/or of a temporal granularity
taxonomy has been already advocated in other works (e.g. in a data warehouse
context, see [55]), to the best of our knowledge we are proposing the first approach attempting to fully exploit the advantages of taxonomical knowledge in

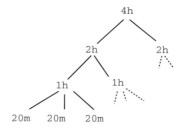

Fig. 5. An example taxonomy of time granularities

flexible case retrieval. In particular our framework takes advantage of a forest of *multi-dimensional orthogonal index structures*, allowing for early pruning and focusing during the retrieval process, each of which orthogonally spans both the time and the symbol taxonomy dimensions. Currently, we have chosen time as the leading dimension (but dimension roles can be switched, depending on the application domain).

The root node of each index structure is represented by a string of symbols, defined at the highest level in the symbol taxonomy (i.e. the children of *Any*, see figure 4) and in the time granularity taxonomy. Potentially, a complete index can stem from each root, describing each possible refinement along the symbol and/or time granularity dimension. An example, taking as a root the D symbol, is provided in figure 6. Here, the root node D is refined along the time dimension from the 4 hours to the 2 hours granularity, so that the nodes DD, DS and SD stem from it (provided that DS and SD generalize to D when switching to a coarser time granularity level, see figure 6). Orthogonally, each node can be specialized in the symbol taxonomy dimension; for instance, DD can be specialized into $D_W D_W$ (weak decrease, weak decrease), $D_W D_S$ (weak decrease, strong decrease), etc.

Moreover, each node in each index structure is itself an index, and can be defined as a *generalized case*, in the sense that it summarizes (i.e. it indexes) a set of cases. In the indexed cases, the feature[1] can be abstracted as in the internal node itself (i.e. resulting in the same string), provided that we work at the same time granularity and symbol taxonomy level of the internal node being considered.

This means that the same case is typically indexed by different nodes in one index (and in the other indexes of the forest). This supports flexible querying, since, depending on the level at which the query is issued, one of the nodes can be more suited for providing a quick answer.

We also advocate a progressive and on-demand definition of the index structures. In particular, in the beginning it makes sense to provide a forest of trees, composed by skeletal indexes, each one rooted at a set of symbols, at the coarsest detail level, in both dimensions. Such indexes develop in the leading dimension (i.e. in time in our current approach), and are as much detailed as the domain knowledge suggests. Further index refinement can then be automatically

---

[1] For the sake of clarity, in our description we will focus on cases with a single feature.

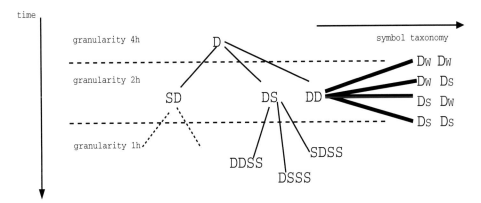

Fig. 6. An example multi-level orthogonal index structure

triggered by the types of queries which have been issued so far. If queries have often involved a time granularity which is not yet represented in the index(es), the corresponding level can be created. A proper frequency threshold for counting the queries has to be set to this end. We proceed analogously by creating an orthogonal index from each node which fits the frequent queries time granularity, but does not match their symbol taxonomy level.

This policy allows to augment the indexes discriminating power only when it is needed, while keeping the memory occupancy of the index structures as limited as possible.

We will now illustrate query answering in our approach, by means of a case study, taken from the haemodialysis domain. In particular, we will focus on a single case feature, for the sake of clarity: namely, haematic volume (HV).

In a good session, HV fits a model where, after an initial period of D_S (strong decrease), which lasts for the first half of the session, a D_W (weak decrease) of the volume follows. An example query summarizing the correct HV behaviour is thus the following: $D_S\ D_W$, where each symbol represents a 2-hours-long episode (globally covering the overall 4 hours duration of the haemodialysis session).

To answer a query, in order to enter the index structure, we first progressively generalize the query itself in the symbol taxonomy direction (see figure 7 - step 1), while keeping time granularity fixed. Then, we generalize the query in the time dimension as well (see figure 7 - step 2).

Then, following the generalization steps backwards, we can enter one of the indexes in the forest from its root, and descend along it, until we reach the node which fits the original query time granularity. If an orthogonal index stems from this node, we can descend along it, always following the query generalization steps backwards. We stop when we reach the same detail level in the symbol taxonomy as in the original query. If the query detail level is not represented in the index, because the index is not complete, we stop at the most detailed possible level. We then return all the cases indexed by the selected node.

In our example, the output of the generalization process allows to identify a single index structure in the forest, namely the one whose root is D (i.e. the

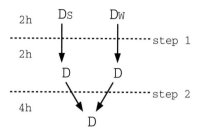

Fig. 7. Generalization steps for the HV query

tree shown in figure 6) as a support for a quick query answering. Matching the steps in the generalization process to the nodes in the index structure (in the time direction), we can descend through the node DD. Now, we can move "horizontally" in the symbol taxonomy direction, to reach the node $D_S\ D_W$, which matches exactly our query. As a result, we can retrieve all the cases indexed by such a node.

We may want to generalize the required behaviour, in order to retrieve a larger number of cases, maybe not perfectly matching the positive HV model. Interactive and progressive query relaxation and refinement are supported in our framework. For instance, we can allow any combination of decreasing episodes in the session. This can be obtained by relaxing the query in the direction of the symbols, using e.g. the sequence DD in a 2 hours granularity. Query relaxation (as well as refinement) can be repeated several times, until the user is satisfied with the obtained results.

Finally, the user may want to retrieve a generalized case, i.e. to stop the search at a proper internal node in the index structure. This node subsumes a set of cases, but the user may just be interested in calculating the distance between the query and the node, which summarizes the retrieval set, without entering the details of all the elements composing it. This functionality is available too in our framework.

The interested reader may find additional technical details about the framework in [31].

4   Conclusions

Time series retrieval is a critical issue in all medical domains in which the observed phenomenon dynamics have to be dealt with.

Case-based Reasoning (CBR), and more specifically case-based retrieval, is recently being recognized as a valuable decision support methodology in these domains, as testified by the growing number of works in the field.

In this chapter, we have analyzed in depth the methodologies used to implement case-based retrieval as a decision support strategy in these applications, dealing with the complexity of case representation and retrieval when most features are in the form of time series.

Classical techniques as well as more innovative ones have been presented.

In particular, we have described a framework in which time series dimensionality is reduced by means of TA. The framework supports multi-level abstractions, both along the time dimension, and along a symbol taxonomy one, thus increasing the flexibility of retrieval. Query answering is interactive and is made faster by the use of orthogonal index structures, which can grow on demand.

In our opinion, flexibility and interactivity represent a relevant advantage of our approach to time series retrieval with respect to more classical techniques, in which end users are typically unable to intervene in the retrieval process, that often operates in a black-box fashion.

In the future, we plan to further test our framework in several different application domains, thus validating its significance, and studying ways of making it more and more efficient and usable.

References

1. Aamodt, A., Plaza, E.: Case-based reasoning: foundational issues, methodological variations and systems approaches. AI Communications 7, 39–59 (1994)
2. Agrawal, R., Faloutsos, C., Swami, A.N.: Efficient similarity search in sequence databases. In: Lomet, D. (ed.) FODO 1993. LNCS, vol. 730, pp. 69–84. Springer, Heidelberg (1993)
3. Allen, J.F.: Towards a general theory of action and time. Artificial Intelligence 23, 123–154 (1984)
4. Belal, S.Y., Taktak, A.F.G., Nevill, A., Spencer, A.: An intelligent ventilation and oxygenation management system in neonatal intensive care using fuzzy trend template fitting. Physiological Measurements 26, 555–570 (2005)
5. Bellazzi, R., Larizza, C., Magni, P., Montani, S., Stefanelli, M.: Intelligent analysis of clinical time series: an application in the diabetes mellitus domain. Artificial Intelligence in Medicine 20, 37–57 (2000)
6. Bellazzi, R., Larizza, C., Riva, A.: Temporal abstractions for interpreting diabetic patients monitoring data. Intelligent Data Analysis 2, 97–122 (1998)
7. Berchtold, S., Keim, D.A., Kriegel, H.P.: The x-tree: an index structure for high-dimensional data. In: Proc. VLDB 1996, pp. 28–39. Morgan Kaufman, San Mateo (1996)
8. Bichindaritz, I., Conlon, E.: Temporal knowledge representation and organization for case-based reasoning. In: Proc. TIME 1996, pp. 152–159. IEEE Computer Society Press, Washington (1996)
9. Branting, L.K., Hastings, J.D.: An empirical evaluation of model-based case matching and adaptation. In: Proc. Workshop on Case-Based Reasoning, AAAI 1994 (1994)
10. Chan, K.P., Fu, A.W.C.: Efficient time series matching by wavelets. In: Proc. ICDE 1999, pp. 126–133. IEEE Computer Society Press, Washington (1999)
11. Daw, C.S., Finney, C.E., Tracy, E.R.: Symbolic analysis of experimental data. Review of Scientific Instruments, 2002-07-22 (2001)
12. Dojat, M., Pachet, F., Guessoum, Z., Touchard, D., Harf, A., Brochard, L.: Neoganesh: a working system for the automated control of assisted ventilation in icus. Artificial Intelligence in Medicine 11, 97–117 (1997)
13. Fuch, B., Mille, A., Chiron, B.: Operator decision aiding by adaptation of supervision strategies. In: Aamodt, A., Veloso, M.M. (eds.) ICCBR 1995. LNCS (LNAI), vol. 1010, pp. 23–32. Springer, Heidelberg (1995)

14. Funk, P., Xiong, N.: Extracting knowledge from sensor signals for case-based reasoning with longitudinal time series data. In: Perner, P. (ed.) Case-Based Reasoning in Signals and Images, pp. 247–284. Springer, Heidelberg (2008)

15. Goldin, D.Q., Kanellakis, P.C.: On similarity queries for time-series data: constraint specification and implementation. In: Montanari, U., Rossi, F. (eds.) CP 1995. LNCS, vol. 976, pp. 137–153. Springer, Heidelberg (1995)

16. Guttman, A.: R-trees: a dynamic index structure for spatial searching. In: Proc. ACM SIGMOD, pp. 47–57. ACM Press, New York (1984)

17. Hetland, M.L.: A survey of recent methods for efficient retrieval of similar time sequences. In: Last, M., Kandel, A., Bunke, H. (eds.) Data Mining in Time Series Databases. World Scientific, London (2003)

18. Jaczynski, M.: A framework for the management of past experiences with time-extended situations. In: Proc. ACM conference on Information and Knowledge Management (CIKM) 1997, pp. 32–38. ACM Press, New York (1997)

19. Jaere, M.D., Aamodt, A., Skalle, P.: Representing temporal knowledge for case-based prediction. In: Craw, S., Preece, A.D. (eds.) ECCBR 2002. LNCS (LNAI), vol. 2416, pp. 174–188. Springer, Heidelberg (2002)

20. Jagadish, H.V., Mendelzon, A.O., Milo, T.: Similarity based queries. In: Proc. 14th ACM Symp. on Principles of Database Systems, San Jose, CA (1995)

21. Kadar, S., Wang, J., Showalter, K.: Noise-supported travelling waves in sub-excitable media. Nature 391, 770–772 (1998)

22. Keogh, E.: Fast similarity search in the presence of longitudinal scaling in time series databases. In: Proc. Int. Conf. on Tools with Artificial Intelligence, pp. 578–584. IEEE Computer Society Press, Washington (1997)

23. Keogh, E., Chakrabarti, K., Pazzani, M., Mehrotra, S.: Dimensionality reduction for fast similarity search in large time series databases. Knowledge and Information Systems 3(3), 263–286 (2000)

24. Keravnou, E.T.: Modeling medical concepts as time objects. In: Wyatt, J.C., Stefanelli, M., Barahona, P. (eds.) AIME 1995. LNCS (LNAI), vol. 934, pp. 67–90. Springer, Heidelberg (1995)

25. Leake, D.B., Smyth, B., Wilson, D.C., Yang, Q. (eds.): Special issue on maintaining case based reasoning systems. Computational Intelligence 17(2), 193–398 (2001)

26. Lin, J., Keogh, E., Lonardi, S., Chiu, B.: A symbolic representation of time series, with implications for streaming algorithms. In: Proc. of ACM-DMKD, San Diego (2003)

27. Ma, J., Knight, B.: A framework for historical case-based reasoning. In: Ashley, K.D., Bridge, D.G. (eds.) ICCBR 2003. LNCS, vol. 2689, pp. 246–260. Springer, Heidelberg (2003)

28. Miksch, S., Horn, W., Popow, C., Paky, F.: Utilizing temporal data abstractions for data validation and therapy planning for artificially ventilated newborn infants. Artificial Intelligence in Medicine 8, 543–576 (1996)

29. Montani, S.: Exploring new roles for case-based reasoning in heterogeneous ai systems for medical decision support. Applied Intelligence 28, 275–285 (2008)

30. Montani, S., Bottrighi, A., Leonardi, G., Portinale, L.: A cbr-based, closed loop architecture for temporal abstractions configuration. Computational Intelligence 25(3), 235–249 (2009)

31. Montani, S., Bottrighi, A., Leonardi, G., Portinale, L., Terenziani, P.: Multi-level abstractions and multi-dimensional retrieval of cases with time series features. In: McGinty, L., Wilson, D. (eds.) Case-Based Reasoning Research and Development. LNCS, vol. 5650, pp. 225–239. Springer, Heidelberg (2009)

32. Montani, S., Portinale, L.: Accounting for the temporal dimension in case-based retrieval: a framework for medical applications. Computational Intelligence 22, 208–223 (2006)
33. Montani, S., Portinale, L., Leonardi, G., Bellazzi, R., Bellazzi, R.: Case-based retrieval to support the treatment of end stage renal failure patients. Artificial Intelligence in Medicine 37, 31–42 (2006)
34. Nakhaeizadeh, G.: Learning prediction from time series: a theoretical and empirical comparison of cbr with some other approaches. In: Wess, S., Richter, M., Althoff, K.-D. (eds.) EWCBR 1993. LNCS (LNAI), vol. 837, pp. 65–76. Springer, Heidelberg (1994)
35. Nilsson, M.: Retrieving short and dynamic biomedical sequences. In: Proc. 18th international florida artificial intelligence research society conference–special track on case-based reasoning. AAAI Press, Menlo Park (2005)
36. Nilsson, M., Funk, P.: A case-based classification of respiratory sinus arrhythmia. In: Funk, P., González Calero, P.A. (eds.) ECCBR 2004. LNCS (LNAI), vol. 3155, pp. 673–685. Springer, Heidelberg (2004)
37. Nilsson, M., Funk, P., Xiong, N.: Clinical decision support by time series classification using wavelets. In: Chen, C.S., Filipe, J., Seruca, I., Cordeiro, J. (eds.) Proc. Seventh International Conference on Enterprise Information Systems (ICEIS 2005), pp. 169–175. INSTICC Press (2005)
38. Oppenheim, A.V., Shafer, R.W.: Digital signal processing. Prentice-Hall, London (1975)
39. Palma, J., Juarez, J.M., Campos, M., Marin, R.: A fuzzy approach to temporal model-based diagnosis for intensive care units. In: Lopez de Mantaras, R., Saitta, L. (eds.) Proc. European Conference on Artificial Intelligence (ECAI) 2004, pp. 868–872. IOS Press, Amsterdam (2004)
40. Portinale, L., Montani, S., Bottrighi, A., Leonardi, G., Juarez, J.: A case-based architecture for temporal abstraction configuration and processing. In: Proc. IEEE International Conference on Tools with Artificial Intelligent (ICTAI), pp. 667–674. IEEE Computer Society, Los Alamitos (2006)
41. Rafiei, D., Mendelzon, A.: Similarity-based queries for time series data. In: Proc. ACM SIGMOD, pp. 13–24. ACM Press, New York (1997)
42. Ram, A., Santamaria, J.C.: Continuous case-based reasoning. In: Proc. AAAI Case-Based Reasoning Workshop, pp. 86–93 (1993)
43. Rougegrez, S.: Similarity evaluation between observed behaviours for the prediction of processes. In: Wess, S., Richter, M., Althoff, K.-D. (eds.) EWCBR 1993. LNCS (LNAI), vol. 837, pp. 155–166. Springer, Heidelberg (1994)
44. Schmidt, R., Gierl, L.: Temporal abstractions and case-based reasoning for medical course data. two prognostic applications. In: Perner, P. (ed.) MLDM 2001. LNCS (LNAI), vol. 2123, pp. 23–34. Springer, Heidelberg (2001)
45. Seyfang, A., Miksch, S., Marcos, M.: Combining diagnosis and treatment using asbru. International Journal of Medical Informatics 68, 49–57 (2002)
46. Shahar, Y.: A framework for knowledge-based temporal abstractions. Artificial Intelligence 90, 79–133 (1997)
47. Shahar, Y., Musen, M.A.: Knowledge-based temporal abstraction in clinical domains. Artificial Intelligence in Medicine 8, 267–298 (1996)
48. Stacey, M.: Knowledge based temporal abstractions within the neonatal intesive care domain. In: Proc. CSTE Innovation Conference, University of Western Sidney (2005)
49. Stephen, G.A.: String searching algorithms. Lecture Notes Series in Computing, vol. 3. World Scientific, Singapore (1994)

50. Subrahmanian, V.S.: Principles of Multimedia Database Systems. Morgan Kaufmann, San Mateo (1998)
51. Terenziani, P., German, E., Shahar, Y.: The temporal aspects of clinical guidelines. In: Ten Teije, A., Miksch, S., Lucas, P. (eds.) Computer-based Medical Guidelines and Protocols: A Primer and Current Trends (2008)
52. Ukkonen, E.: Algorithms for approximate string matching. Information Control 64, 100–118 (1985)
53. Ukkonen, E.: Approximate matching over suffix trees. In: Apostolico, A., Crochemore, M., Galil, Z., Manber, U. (eds.) CPM 1993. LNCS, vol. 684, pp. 228–242. Springer, Heidelberg (1993)
54. Watson, I.: Applying Case-Based Reasoning: techniques for enterprise systems. Morgan Kaufmann, San Francisco (1997)
55. Xia, B.B.: Similarity search in time series data sets. Technical report, School of Computer Science, Simon Fraser University (1997)

Chapter 11
Meta-learning for Image Processing Based on Case-Based Reasoning

Anja Attig and Petra Perner

Institute of Computer Vision and Applied Computer Sciences, IBaI, Leipzig, Germany
pperner@ibai-institut.de
www.ibai-institut.de

Abstract. We propose a framework for model building in image processing by meta-learning based on case-based reasoning. The model-building process is seen as a classification process during which the signal characteristics are mapped to the right image-processing parameters to ensure the best image-processing output. The mapping function is realized by case-based reasoning. Case-based reasoning is especially suitable for this kind of process, since it incrementally allows one to learn the model based on the incoming data stream. To find the right signal/image description of the signal/image characteristics that are in relationship to the signal-processing parameters is one important aspect of this work. In connection with this work intensive studies of the theoretical, structural, and syntactical behavior of the chosen image-processing algorithm have to be done. Based on this analysis we can propose several signal/image descriptions. The selected image description should summarize the cases into groups of similar case and map these to the same processing parameters. Having found groups of similar cases, these should be summarized by prototypes that allow fast retrieval of several groups of cases. This generalization process should permit building up the model over the course of time based on the incrementally obtained data stream. We studied this task for image segmentation based on the Watershed-Transformation. First, we studied the theoretical and the implementation aspects of the Watershed Transformation and drew conclusions for suitable image descriptions. Four different descriptions were chosen - statistical and texture features, marginal distributions of columns, rows, and diagonal similarity between the regional minima of two images, and the shape descriptor based on central moments. Our study showed that the weighted statistical and texture features and the shape descriptor based on central moments have yielded the best image description so far for the Watershed Transformation. It can best separate the cases into groups having the same segmentation parameters and it sorts out rotated and rescaled images. Generalization over cases can also be performed over the groups of case. It helps to speed up the retrieval process and to learn incrementally the general model.

1 Introduction

The aim of image processing is to develop methods for automatically extracting from an image or a video the desired information. The developed system should assist a

I. Bichindaritz et al. (Eds.): Computational Intelligence in Healthcare 4, SCI 309, pp. 229–264.
springerlink.com   © Springer-Verlag Berlin Heidelberg 2010

user in processing or understanding the content of a complex signal, such as an image. Usually, an image consists of thousands of pixels. This information can hardly be quantitatively analyzed by the user. In fact, some problems related to the subjective factor or to the tiredness of the user arise, which may influence reproducibility. Therefore, an automatic procedure for analyzing an image is necessary.

Although in some cases it might make sense to process a single image and to adjust the parameters of the image processing algorithm to this single image manually, mostly the automation of the image analysis makes only sense if the developed methods have to be applied to more than one single image. This is still an open problem in image processing. The parameters involved in the selected processing method have to be adjusted to the specific image. It is often hardly possible to select the parameters for a class of images in such a way that the best result can be ensured for all images of the class. Therefore, methods for parameter learning are required that can assist a system developer in building a model [1] for the image processing task.

While the meta-learning task has been extensively studied for classifier selection, it has not been studied so extensively for parameter learning. Soares et. al [2] studied parameter selection for the identification of the kernel width of a support-vector machine, while Perner [3] studied parameter selection for image segmentation.

The meta-learning problem for parameter selection can be formalized as follows: For a given signal that is characterized by specific signal properties A and domain properties B find the parameters P of the processing algorithm that ensure the best quality of the resulting output signal/information:

$$f : A \cup B \rightarrow P \tag{1}$$

Meta-data for images may consist of image-related meta-data (gray-level statistics) and non-image related meta-data (sensor, object data) [4]. In general, the processing of meta-data from signals and images should not require too heavy processing and should allow characterizing the properties of the signal that influence the signal processing algorithm.

The mapping function f can be realized by any classification algorithm, but the incremental behavior of case-based reasoning (CBR) fits best to many data/signal processing problems, where the signal-class cannot be characterized ad-hoc, since the data appear incrementally. The right similarity metric that allows mapping data to parameter-groups and, as a consequence, allows obtaining good output results, should be studied more extensively. Performance measures that allow to judge the achieved output and to automatically criticize the systems performance are another important problem [5].

Abstraction of cases to learn domain theory would allow better understanding the behavior of many signal processing algorithms that cannot anymore be described by means of the standard system theory [6].

The aim of our research is to develop methods that allow us to learn a model for the desired task from cases without heavy human interaction (see Fig. 1). The specific emphasis of this work is to develop a methodology for finding the right image description for the case that group similar images in terms of parameters within the same group and map the case to the right parameters in question.

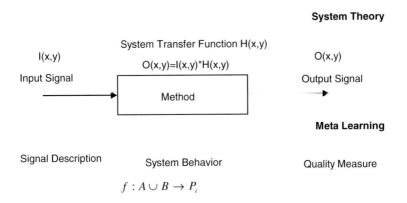

Fig. 1. Problem description in modeling

In section 2, we describe the image segmentation based on case-based reasoning. In section 3, we review the theoretical and behavioral aspects of the Watershed Transformation and how to use case-based reasoning to form the image segmentation model. An overview about some of the test images and the corresponding best segmentation parameters is given in section 4, where also the problems concerning the evaluation of the results are briefly addressed. The derived image descriptions from the theoretical and behavioral study in section 3 are given in section 5. A discussion of the result is done in section 6. The process of generalization is described in section 7. Finally, we give conclusions in section 8.

2 CBR-Based Image Segmentation

2.1 Case-Based Meta-control of Image Segmentation

The segmentation problem can be seen as a classification problem for which we have to learn the best classifier. Depending on the segmentation task, the output of the classifier can be the labels for the image regions, the segmentation algorithm selected as the most adequate, or the parameters for the selected segmentation algorithm. In any case, the final result is a segmented image. The learning of the classifier should be done on a sufficiently large test data set, which should represent the entire domain well enough, in order to be able to build up a general model for the segmentation problem. However, often it is not possible to obtain a sufficiently large data set and, therefore, the segmentation model does not fit the entire data set and needs to be adjusted to process new data. We note that a general model does not guarantee the best segmentation for each image; rather, it guarantees an average best fit over the entire set of images.

Another aspect of the problem is related to the changes in image quality caused by variations in environmental conditions, image devices, etc. Thus, the segmentation performance needs to be adapted to changes in image quality. All this suggests the use of case-based reasoning [7] as a basic methodology for image segmentation, since CBR can be seen as a method for problem solving as well as a method to capture new

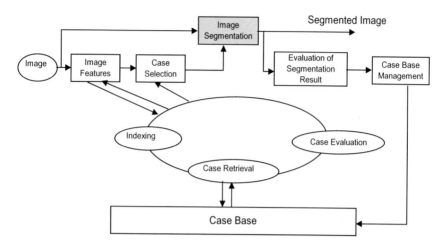

Fig. 2. Scheme of case-based image segmentation

experience. It can be seen as a learning and knowledge discovery approach. The CBR process consists of six phases: extracting the case description, indexing, retrieval, learning, adaptation and application of the solution.

The CBR process for image segmentation is shown in Fig. 2. The actual image characteristics are described by mean features computed on the whole image. These features are used for indexing the case-base and for retrieval of a set of cases close to the current problem, based on a proper similarity measure.

To adjust the segmentation parameters, indexing should find out images sharing the same segmentation parameters. Among the cases close to the current problem, the closest one is selected and its associated solution is given as control input to the image segmentation unit. The image segmentation unit takes the current image and processes it according to the current control state. Finally, the output is the segmented image.

A case consists of a description of the image characteristics and the solution. The description of the image characteristics can take into account non-image and image information. Based on image description, we can reduce our complex solution space to a subspace of relevant cases, where variation in image quality among the cases is limited.

The solution of a case can be one of the outputs of the classifiers described above. Supposing that our aim is to control the parameters of the segmentation unit, the solution is the set of parameters applicable for the segmentation of the current image. The solution is given as an input to the segmentation unit and the current image is processed by the segmentation unit, based on the selected parameters.

If we want to control the selection of the best algorithm in a set of possible algorithms, then the solution given to the image segmentation unit would be the selected algorithm. If we want to label the regions, then the output would be the labeled regions.

After the image has been processed, the segmentation result is evaluated. This means that the segmentation quality is judged either by an expert or automatically. Depending on the obtained evaluation, the knowledge containers (case description, similarity, solution) are modified to ensure a better segmentation result by processing again the same image. This task is done by the case-base maintenance unit.

The case-base maintenance unit is shown in Fig. 3. Different from a conventional segmentation process, CBR also includes the evaluation of the segmentation result and takes it as a feedback to improve the system performance semi-automatically or automatically. Usually this is an open problem in many segmentation applications.

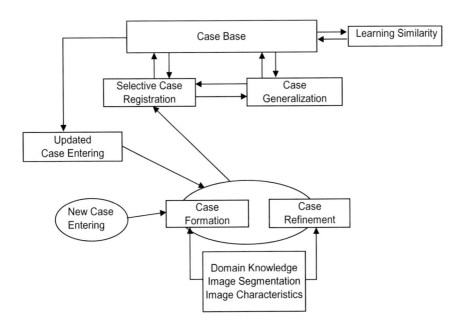

Fig. 3. Case-base maintenance

When the evaluation of the segmentation result is done manually, the expert compares the original image with the labeled image on display. If the expert detects significant differences in the two images, the result is tagged as incorrect and the case-base management will start.

The evaluation procedure can also be done automatically. However, there is no general procedure available and evaluation can be done automatically only in a domain-dependent fashion.

2.2 Case-Based Maintenance and Model Learning

Case-based maintenance is done for several purposes: 1. to enter a new case, when no similar cases are available in the case-base, 2. to update an existing case by case refinement, and 3. to obtain case generalization.

Once an incorrect result is observed for an input image either by the user or by the automatic evaluation procedure, the case is tagged as a bad case. In a successive step, the best segmentation parameters for that image are determined and the attributes, necessary for similarity determination, are computed from the image. Both the segmentation parameters and the attributes calculated from the image are stored into the case-base as a new case. In addition to that, non-image information is extracted from the file header or from any other associated source of information and is stored together with the other information in the case-base. If the case-base is organized hierarchically, the new case has to be stored at the position in the hierarchy suggested by its similarity-relation to the other cases in the case-base.

During storage, case generalization is done to ensure that the case-base does not become too large unnecessarily. Cases that are similar to each other are grouped together in a case class and, for this case-class, a prototype is computed by averaging the values of the attributes. Case generalization ensures that a case is applicable to a wider range of segmentation problems.

It can also happen that several cases are quite similar to each other and, therefore, they get retrieved for a new problem at the same time. Then, learning the similarity by updating the local weights associated to each attribute is advised.

3   The Watershed Algorithm: What Influences the Result of the Segmentation?

An easy way to explain the idea of the Watershed Transform is the interpretation of the image as 3D landscape. Therefore we allocate for every pixel its grey value as z-coordinate. Now we flood the landscape from the regional minima, after having bored the local minima and sunk the landscape into water. Lakes are created (basins, catchment basins) in correspondence with the regional minima. We build dams (watershed lines or simply watersheds), where two lakes meet. Alternatively, instead of sinking the landscape, the latter can be flooded by rainfall and the watershed lines will be the lines of attracting the rain that will fall on the landscape. Whichever of the paradigmas is used – the immersion or rainfall paradigma - to obtain its simulation two approaches are possible: either the basins are identified, then the watershed lines are obtained by taking a set complement, or the complete image partition is computed, then successively the watersheds are found by detecting boundaries between basins.

Many algorithms were developed for computing the Watershed Transform. For a survey see e.g. [8]. In this work we deal mainly with the Watershed Transformation scheme suggested by Vincent and Soille in [9], and use this scheme also for the new implementation that we have done for the segmentation algorithm from Frucci et al. [10], [11].

The first definition of the so called Watershed Transform by immersion was given by Vincent and Soille [9]. Let D be a digital grey value image with h_{min} and h_{max} as the minimal and maximal gray value. MIN_h is the union of all regional minima with grey value h with $h \in [h_{min}, h_{max}]$. Furthermore, let $B \subseteq D$ and suppose that B is partitioned in k connected sets B_i ($i \in [1,\ldots,k]$). Then, the geodesic influence zone of the set B_i within D $iz_D(B_i)$ is computed as:

$$iz_D(B_i) = \{p \in D \mid \forall j \in [1\ldots k]/\{i\}: d_D(p,B_i) < d_D(p,B_j)\}, \tag{2}$$

where $d_D(p,B_i) = \min_{q \in B_i} d_D(p,q)$ with $d_D(p,q)$ as the minimum path among all paths within D between p and q.

The union of the geodesic influence zones of the connected components B_i, $IZ_D(B)$, is computed as follows:

$$IZ_D(B) = \sum_{i=1}^{k} iz_D(B_i) \tag{3}$$

The Watershed Transform by immersion is defined by the following recursion:

$$\begin{aligned} X_{h_{min}} &= \{p \in D \mid f(p) = h_{min}\} = T_{h_{min}} \\ X_{h+1} &= MIN_{h+1} \cup IZ_{T_{h+1}}(X_h), \quad h \in [h_{min}, h_{max}) \end{aligned} \tag{4}$$

where T_h, defined as $T_h = \{p \in D \mid f(p) \le h\}$, is the set of pixels with grey-level smaller than or equal to h, and MIN_h is the union of all the regional minima at level h. The watershed line of D is then the complement of $X_{h_{max}}$ in D.

The Vincent-Soille algorithm, which does not strictly implement equation (4) (for details see below and [8]), consists of two steps:

1. The pixels of the input image are sorted in increasing order of grey values.
2. A Flooding step is done, level after level, starting from level hmin and terminating at level hmax. For every gray value, breadth-first-search is done to determine the label (label of existing basin, new label or watershed label) to be ascribed to the pixel.

The location of regional minima is important for segmentation by Watershed Transform. To extract the objects of interest in the image, the minima should not lie along the border line of the objects (see Fig. 4 and Fig. 5). On the contrary, regional maxima should be located on the border lines. To correctly identify the minima far from the border lines, in practice the gradient image of the original image is used as an input image for the Watershed Transformation (compare Fig. 5 and Fig. 6).

The Watershed Transform is also dependent on the connectivity. For example, the gradient image in Fig. 4 has three regional minima if 4-connectedness is used, but only one minimum if 8-connectedness is used. In the following, we always use 4-connectedness.

An advantage of the Vincent-Soille algorithm is that it runs in linear running time respectively to the number of pixels of the input image (if the used sorting algorithm

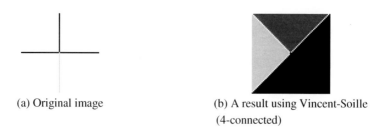

(a) Original image   (b) A result using Vincent-Soille
                                          (4-connected)

Fig. 4. An image and a segmentation result using the Vincent-Soille algorithm (4-connected)

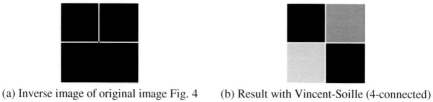

(a) Inverse image of original image Fig. 4   (b) Result with Vincent-Soille (4-connected)

Fig. 5. An image and the segmentation result using the Vincent-Soille algorithm (4-connected)

(a) Gradient image (with Prewitt Edge Detec-   (b) Result with Vincent-Soille (4-connected)
tor) of original image in Fig. 4

Fig. 6. An image and a segmentation result using the Vincent-Soille algorithm (4-connected)

3	3	2	2
3	3	1	2
0	0	1	0
0	0	1	0

(a) Original image

W	B	B	B
A	W	B	B
A	A	W	B
A	A	W	B

(b) Result using theoretical
recursion (4-connected)

A	W	W	B
A	A	W	B
A	A	W	B
A	A	W	B

(c) Result using
Vincent-Soille (4-connected)

Fig. 7. Comparing the results of the theoretical recursion with Vincent-Soille algorithm under condition 1

is linear). To obtain linear computation time, Vincent and Soille modified the theoretical recursion of expression 4, so as to access each pixel only once. To this aim, at iteration t, only pixels labeled h are checked, while expression 4 requires that pixels labeled less than or equal to h are checked. This modification to the recursion

2	0	2
0	1	0
2	1	2

(a) Original image

W	B	W
A	W	C
A	W	C

(b) Result by using theoretical recursion (4-connected)

W	B	W
A	C	C
W	C	C

(c) Result by using Vincent-Soille (4-connected)

Fig. 8. Comparing the results of the theoretical recursion with Vincent-Soille algorithm under condition 2

schemes introduces some drawbacks. Specifically, watershed lines thicker than just one pixel can be created and differently labeled basins (see Fig. 7). A pixel that becomes during an iteration *t* the watershed label and is neighbor of 2, 4, or more odd-numbered pixels with different labels, can get the wrong label during the same iteration after having visited all adjacent basins (see Fig. 8).

Another example of thick watershed lines created by the above modification is shown in Fig. 9.

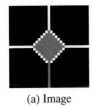

(a) Image

(b) Result (red: Watershed lines)

Fig. 9. A segmentation result using the Vincent-Soille algorithm (4-connected)

Theoretically, the results of the Watershed Transformation do not depend on the order in which the neighbors of a pixel are visited. Because of the constraints introduced by Vincent-Soille into the implementation of the algorithm, the order of visitation heavily influences the result. For example, if for a pixel (x, y) its neighbors are visited, in the order $\{(x-1, y), (x, y+1), (x+1, y), (x, y-1)\}$ (see Fig. 10b), or in the order $\{(x, y+1), (x-1, y), (x, y-1), (x+1, y)\}$ (see Fig. 10c), different results will be obtained.

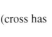

(a) Original image (cross has one pixel width)

(b) Result with pixel visiting order 1

(c) Result with pixel visiting order 2

Fig. 10. Cross image and segmentation results using the Vincent-Soille algorithm (4-connected) when different pixel visiting orders are used

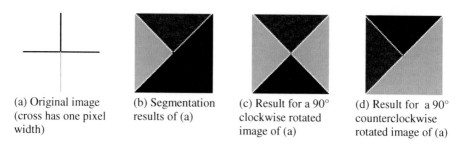

(a) Original image
(cross has one pixel
width)

(b) Segmentation
results of (a)

(c) Result for a 90°
clockwise rotated
image of (a)

(d) Result for a 90°
counterclockwise
rotated image of (a)

Fig. 11. Cross image and segmentation results using the Vincent-Soille algorithm (4-connected) for rotated images

(a) Original image - a two pixels wide cross

(b) Result using Vincent-Soille algorithm
(4-connected)

Fig. 12. A scaled image and the segmentation result using the Vincent-Soille algorithm (4-connected)

This property also explains why the algorithm is not invariant with respect to rotation (see Fig. 11) and scaling (see Fig. 12).

The cross in image Fig. 12 has double the width in comparison with the cross in Fig. 10. The light-colored pixel at the intersection of the light-colored and dark-colored branches of the cross has now only two darker neighbors. In such a condition we obtain the correct result for the Watershed Transformation.

Scaling algorithms generally use interpolations, which can produce more regional minima in the rescaled image than in the original image. As a consequence, a larger number of components can be obtained for the scaled image, which will result in a different segmentation from that of the original image.

The Vincent-Soille algorithm does not generate always connected watershed lines. A reason for that is the constraint demonstrated in Fig. 6. No watershed line separates the two basins A and B, if all the highest grey pixels between the two basins belong to the geodesic influence zone of either A or B. For example, consider Fig. 13 (a), showing an image completely black except for a grey stripe that is four pixels wide. For this image the Vincent-Soille algorithm creates no watershed line between the two basins, because no pixel of the stripe has the same distance to the two basins (compare Fig. 13b and c).

To solve the two above drawbacks, Roerdink and Meijster [8] proposed a slightly modified algorithm, which is, however, remarkably more expensive with regard to

A	1	2	3	4	B
A	1	2	3	4	B
A	1	2	3	4	B
A	1	2	3	4	B

A	4	3	2	1	B
A	4	3	2	1	B
A	4	3	2	1	B
A	4	3	2	1	B

(a) Image   (b) Portion of (a) with the geodesic distance from pixel of the stripe to basin A   (c) Portion of (a) with the geodesic distance from pixel of the stripe to basin B   (d) Result

Fig. 13. An image, the geodesic distances from pixel of the stripe to the different basins and the segmentation result using the Vincent-Soille algorithm

computation, since its cost is $O(N^2)$, where N is the number of pixels in the image. The original version of Roerdink´s and Meijster´s algorithm is not quite correct. Therefore, Andreä and Haufe give a corrected version in [12].

As we already pointed out, watershed segmentation performs better when using the gradient image of the input image. During our study we tested different edge detectors. The Prewitt (with Chessboard Distance) and the Sobel (with Euclidian Distance) (described e.g. in [13]) edge detectors produced the best results coupled with the use of the new implementation of algorithms [10] with the Vincent-Soille Watershed Transformation. But neither of them was clearly better than the other. All of the following tests were performed with the Prewitt detector, because we obtained the best results with it when working with our test images.

Furthermore, independently of the selected approach, Watershed Transformation tends to highly oversegment due to many regional minima that can possibly be interpreted as noisy minima. To solve this problem different approaches exist, like intensive preprocessing (e.g. [14]), marker controlled watershed (e.g. [15]) or region-merging (e.g. [16], [17]). For preprocessing in order to reduce the number of local minima, smoothing algorithms or extended edge detectors eliminating unnecessary edges, sharpen edges or produce edges with less gaps are adopted. Often a combination of different preprocessing methods is used. A problem of the majority of the preprocessings methods is the dependence on the result of the particular kind of images. By the marker-controlled watershed a set of regions called markers are used in place of the set of minima. These regions are often manually determined by the user. Therefore this Watershed Transform approach is often qualified for interactive use and less for automation.

To solve the problem of oversegmentation, Frucci [17] combines an iterative computation of the Watershed Transform with processes called digging and flooding. Flooding merges adjacent basins. This is achieved by letting water increase the level, so that it can overflow from one basin into an adjacent one if the level of water is higher than the lowest height along the watershed line separating the two basins. Also digging merges adjacent regions. In this case, to merge a basin A, regarded as non-significant, with a basin B, a canal is dug in the watershed line separating A and B to allow water to flow from B into A. The effect of merging is that the number of local minima found at each iteration diminishes. Flooding and digging are iterated until only significant basins are left.

The algorithm involves expensive computation, but it has the advantage of producing acceptable segmentation results independently of the kind of image. In fact, the approach followed in [17] rather than identifying the watershed lines during the Watershed Transformation, first builds the complete partition of the image into basins and only after that detects the watershed lines by boundary detection. In this way, both drawbacks affecting the Vincent-Soille approach are overcome at the expense of higher computation costs. Therefore, neither the Frucci algorithm presented in [17], nor the extension of the Frucci algorithm introduced in [10], are suitable for real-time processing.

We have used the new implementation of the algorithm [10], [11] for our case–based reasoning studies, since the computation costs are much lower then, due to the use of the Watershed Transform computed by the Vincent and Soille scheme.

Let X and Y be two adjacent basins in the watershed partition of a grey-level image D and W and Z some other basins. As in [17], we denote LO_{XY}, the *local overflow of X with respect to Y*, as the pixel with the minimal grey value along the border line between X and Y. The value of the pixel with the lowest value is the *overflow of X*, O_X. Furthermore, R_X is the grey value of the regional minimum of X, $SA_{XY} = |R_X - R_Y|$ denotes the *similarity parameter* and $D_{XY} = LO_{XY} - R_X$ defines the relative depth of X at LO_{XY} (see Fig. 14).

In order to determine if a basin X has to be merged with a basin Y, Frucci et al. [10] introduce the notion of *relative significance* of X with respect to Y and perform the following check.:

$$\frac{1}{2}\left(a \cdot \frac{SA_{XY}}{At} + b \cdot \frac{D_{XY}}{Dt} \right) \geq T \text{ , with } a,b,T \geq 0 \qquad (5)$$

where At and Dt are the threshold value (for the automatic computation see [17]) a, b and T constants, and the left side of 5 is the relative significance of X with respect to Y.

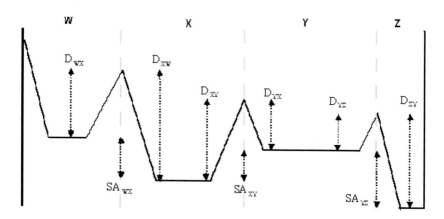

Fig. 14. Similarity parameter and relative depth

If condition 5 is satisfied, the basin X is significant with respect to Y. The relative significance f X is evaluated with respect to all its adjacent basins. Three cases, as shown in Table 1, are possible. When merging is possible, Table 1 also specifies if digging or flooding has to be performed. After flooding or digging have been performed for all basins that are not strongly significant, the Watershed Transformation is executed again with an obviously smaller number of local minima.

Table 1. Cases for the significance of X by taking into account the relative significance with respect to all its adjacent basins

X is denoted	if	type of merging
strongly significant	X is significant with respect to each adjacent region Y.	no merging
non significant	X is non-significant with respect to each adjacent region Y.	flooding
partially significant	all other cases	digging

Flooding: All the pixels of X with a lower grey value than O_X are set to the value O_X. If Watershed Transformation is executed again, the basin X results to be merged with any adjacent basin Y for which the value of LO_{XY} is O_X.

Digging: The basin X is only merged with any adjacent basin Y, being non- significant with respect to X and in such a way that $R_X \geq R_Y$. Therefore, a canal is dug from the regional minimum of X to the regional minimum of Y passing through LO_{XY}. All the pixels of the canal whose grey values are greater than R_X are set to R_X.

We have implemented the segmentation algorithm [10] by computing the Watershed Transform according to the scheme of Vincent and Soille, so as to reduce the overall computation cost. However, using such a watershed model creates some problems due to the fact that watershed lines may be missing or thick, which inhibits in

6	6	6	6	32
6	7	7	32	0
13	13	12	3	0
8	8	8	32	0
8	8	8	8	32

a) Portion of an image

6	6	6	6	32
6	6	7	32	0
13	13	12	3	0
12	12	12	32	0
12	12	12	12	32

(b) Result after flooding

A	A	A	A	W
A	A	A	W	B
W	W	W	B	B
W	W	W	W	B
W	W	W	W	W

(c) Result basin A and B and watershed lines

Fig. 15. Successive results for an image after flooding and Watershed Transformation based on the Vincent-Soille algorithm

some cases the possibility to check adjacent basins and, hence, to apply flooding or digging. For an example of thick watershed lines, see Fig. 15, where LO_{XY} is equal to 12, the basins X and Y are those respectively characterized by the local minima equal to 8, and 6.

If, instead of flooding, Table 1 had suggested to apply digging, we would have obtained mainly the same result for the image in Fig. 15 (b). The only difference would have been that pixels labeled 12 would have been labeled 8. In that case one obtaines the parameters At=Dt=8 if the surrounding image of this cutout shown in Fig. 15 is suitable.

Furthermore, it should be noted that digging over O_X is not always the best way. Other minimal criteria for path digging are explained by Bleau and Leon in [16].

In our study, we are interested in analyzing the image properties in order to detect the proper values for the constants a, b and T. The constants a and b control the influence of the similarity parameter and the depth. T can be regarded as a threshold. If T is 0 and $a, b \geq 0$, then we obviously get the same segmentation like the one produced by the Vincent-Soille algorithm. For $a, b = 2$ and $T = 1$ we often obtain similar results to those achieved by using the algorithm [17].

Since we have used the Vincent-Soille Watershed Transformation, which is not invariant for image rotation and scaling, in our implementation of algorithms [10] and [11], the best value of a, b and T can be different for two images after scaling or rotation.

To decide which watershed-based segmentation algorithm to use, we have also considered the algorithm described in [10] in its original implementation. Making a compromise between computation costs and quality of the obtained segmentation results, we have finally opted for the Vincent-Soille algorithm as a basis for the CBR-based watershed algorithm. In future work, we will carry out further tests on the different behavior of the basic watershed algorithms. The hope is that the choice of the basic algorithm can be included as a parameter into a CBR-based watershed algorithm.

4   Test Images and Parameters for Watershed Segmentation

For our study we used a data base comprised of different types of images, such as e.g. landscape, medical and biological images, and face images. Nine of these images are shown in Fig. 16a-j and are used for demonstration purposes of the results throughout this chapter. The neurone images {neu1;neu2;neu3;neu4;neu4-r180} seem to belong to the same class, except that neu4_r180 is the 180 degree rotated image of neu4 and neu4 seems to be a rescaled cut-out of one of the image neurons.

The parameters for the Watershed segmentation were obtained by running the CBR-based Watershed segmentation and adjusting the parameters until the result had the best segmentation quality. The resulting parameters are shown in Table 2.

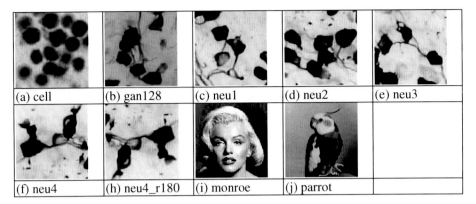

| (a) cell | (b) gan128 | (c) neu1 | (d) neu2 | (e) neu3 |
| (f) neu4 | (h) neu4_r180 | (i) monroe | (j) parrot | |

Fig. 16. Images used for the study

Table 2. Segmentation parameters a, b, and T of the test images shown in Fig. 16

ImageName	a	b	T
monroe	0,5	2	1
gan128	0,75	0,75	1
parrot	0,75	2	1
cellr	1	1	1
neu1	2	1	1
neu2	0,25	1	1
neu3	2	1	1
neu4	0,75	2	1
neu4_r180	1	0,5	1

Table 3 shows the Images having the same segmentation parameters. Based on segmentation parameters the images neu1 and neu3 and neu4 and parrot should be grouped together by the image description.

Table 3. Images having the same segmentation parameters

ImageName	a	b	T
parrot	0,75	2	1
neu4	0,75	2	1
neu1	2	1	1
neu3	2	1	1

Fig. 17 and Table 3 demonstrate the clustering of images grouped according to their parameters. Based on this result we found an image description which grouped the images monroe, parrot and neu4 as well as the images neu1 and neu3.

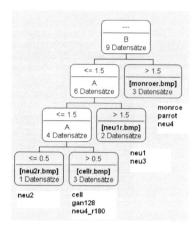

Fig. 17. Clustering of Test Images into Groups based on the Segmentation Parameters

Table 4. Parameters for the image class neurone Fig. 18a) to Fig. 18d)

ImageName	a	b	T
neu1r.bmp	2	1	1
neu2r.bmp	0,25	1	1
neu3r.bmp	2	1	1
neu4r.bmp	0,75	2	1

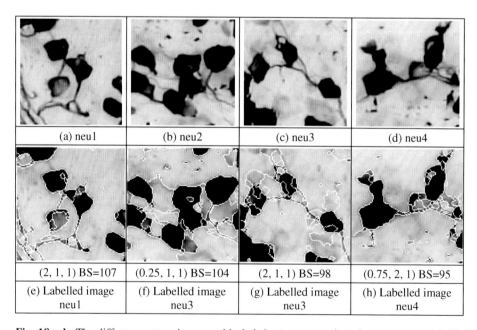

Fig. 18 a-h. The different neuron images with their best segmentation, the parameters (a,b,T), and the number of basins BS

We noted that the image monroe provides also a good result (with only one basin more) with the parameters a=0.75, b=2 and T=1.

Table 4 and Fig. 18 show the four images of the type "neurone", where only two images have the same parameters. One reason is that image "neu4" contains larger objects than the other neurone images. So image neu4 must not get the same parameters, because the Vincent-Soille algorithm is not invariant with respect to scaling. Image neu2 differs from neu1 and neu3 by more connected objects.

We also tested a simple pre-processing method, which reduced well the overseg-mentation of many images.

By our preprocessing method we eliminated some small edges in the gradient image, by setting all pixels having a grey value no greater than a threshold to zero. The threshold must be quite small (compare Fig. 19 and Fig. 20), eliminating only edges caused by background noise and not too many significant edges in the image.

A problem related to the determination of the segmentation parameters for the CBR-based watershed algorithm is how to judge the best segmentation quality. Evaluation done by humans is subjective and can result in different segmented images of the same input image. This is of importance if we only want to separate the parrot (see Fig. 23 a) from the background (Fig. 23 b), or segment parts of the parrot as well

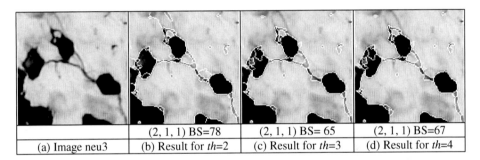

(a) Image neu3	(2, 1, 1) BS=78	(2, 1, 1) BS= 65	(2, 1, 1) BS=67
	(b) Result for *th*=2	(c) Result for *th*=3	(d) Result for *th*=4

Fig. 19. Different segmentation results by elimination of smaller edges in the gradient image with threshold *th*

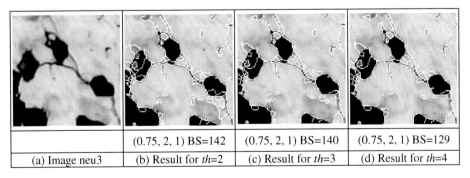

(a) Image neu3	(0.75, 2, 1) BS=142	(0.75, 2, 1) BS=140	(0.75, 2, 1) BS=129
	(b) Result for *th*=2	(c) Result for *th*=3	(d) Result for *th*=4

Fig. 20. Different segmentation results by elimination of smaller edges in the gradient image with threshold *th*

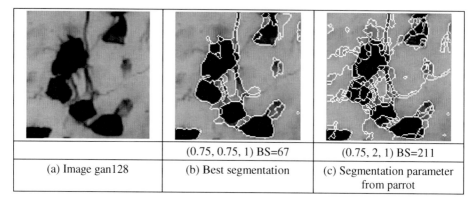

| (a) Image gan128 | (0.75, 0.75, 1) BS=67
 (b) Best segmentation | (0.75, 2, 1) BS=211
 (c) Segmentation parameter from parrot |

Fig. 21. The influence of the selected parameter-set to the segmentation result and the number of basins shown on image gan128

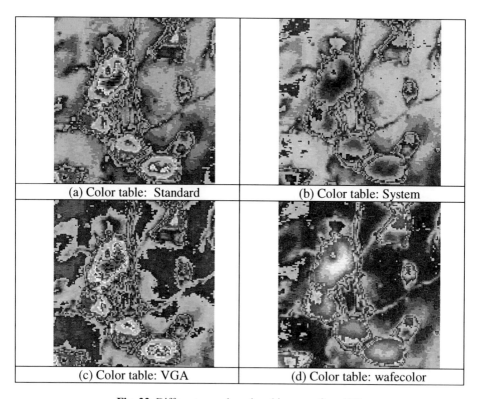

| (a) Color table: Standard | (b) Color table: System |
| (c) Color table: VGA | (d) Color table: wafecolor |

Fig. 22. Different pseudo-colored images of gan128

(see Fig. 23c), for example the check. The result of the automatic evaluation is shown in Fig. 23d.

Another aspect is that interesting textures in the image may not be visible for the human eye (compare Fig. 21 with the Pseudo Color Images from Fig. 22).

Even the automatic evaluation has some weak points. The automatic evaluation proposed in [10] takes the original images, produces an edge image out of it based on the chosen standard edge operation, and labels the edges based on a simple thresholding algorithm (see Fig. 23d, with Otsu´s thresholding algorithm) and then compares this image with the output image of the Watershed Transformation based on case-based reasoning according to Zamperoni´s similarity measure [18]. For each of these processing steps different standard image processing operations can be used, producing different results for the same image.

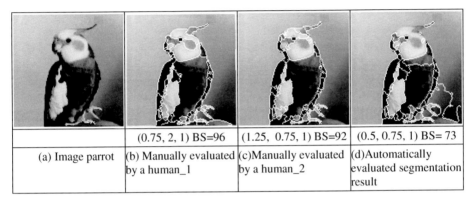

	(0.75, 2, 1) BS=96	(1.25, 0.75, 1) BS=92	(0.5, 0.75, 1) BS= 73
(a) Image parrot	(b) Manually evaluated by a human_1	(c)Manually evaluated by a human_2	(d)Automatically evaluated segmentation result

Fig. 23. Different manually evaluated and automatically evaluated segmentation results of image parrot

5   Elicitation of Image Descriptions and Assessment of Similarity for Watershed Transform

The aim of the image description is to find out from a set of images the group of images that needs the same processing parameters for achieving the best segmentation results. To give an example, the images neu1, neu3, neu4 and parrot should be grouped together based on the best parameters a, b, and T.

We consider different image descriptions in our study that should allow us to group images based on the image parameters and by doing so learn a model for image segmentation from samples.

Cases are normally composed of

- non-image information
- parameters specifying image characteristics, and
- parameters for solution (image segmentation parameters).

Non-image information is different depending on the application. In our study we use images from different domains like landscape, faces or biology. Our aim is to describe image similarity only by general image properties. Hence our cases are composed of

- parameters specifying image characteristics and
- parameters a, b, T for segmentation.

Images, which are classified as being similar based on the image features, should be segmented with the same parameters of the segmentation algorithm, which computes then the best segmentation for any of them.

To understand these properties we use hierarchical clustering. This gives us a graphical representation of the different image groups. Single linkage is used to show outliers, while the distance between two classes is defined as the minimal distance.

The question is: What are the right image properties that allow us to map the images to the right image segmentation parameters for the Watershed Transform?

The image description should reflect the behavioral approach of the Watershed Transformation and the particular image characteristics, respectively. Therefore we studied the theoretical details and the implementation limits of the Watershed Transformation in section 4 to get insights into this question. We came to the conclusion that the distribution of the regional minima is an important criterion for the behavior of the algorithm.

From this work we decided to test four image descriptions described in the following Sections:

- Statistical Feature Image Description,
- Image Description as Marginal Distribution for Column and Lines,
- Image Description by Similarity between the Regional Minima of two Images, and
- Image Description by Central Moments.

5.1 Statistical and Texture Feature Image Description

According to Perner [3], who used this description for meta-learning of the segmentation parameter for a case-based image segmentation model, we applied statistical features like centroid, energy, entropy, kurtosis, mean, skewness, variance and variation coefficient and texture features (energy, correlation, homogeneity, contrast) for case description. The input image is the gradient image of the original image since the Watershed Transformation works on that image. First results on this image description are reported in Frucci et al.[10]. The texture feature has been chosen to describe the particular distribution of the regional minima in an image, while the statistical features describe the signal characteristics.

Like Perner [3], we determined the distance between two images A and B as follows:

$$dist_{AB} = \frac{1}{k}\sum_{i=1}^{k}\omega_i\left|\frac{C_{iA}-C_{iB}}{C_{i\max}-C_{i\min}}\right|, \tag{6}$$

where k is the number of properties in the data base, $C_{i\max}$ and $C_{i\min}$ are the maximum and minimum value of all the images for the ith features in the data base, C_{iA} is the value of the ith feature of image A (analogous for B) and the ω_i are weights with

$$\sum_{i=1}^{k} \omega_i = 1. \tag{7}$$

We use $\omega_i = 1/k \ \forall i \in [1, \ldots, k]$.

Results are reported in Fig. 24.

If we virtually cut the dendrogram by the cophenetic similarity of 0.0043, we obtain the groups G1={neu4; neu4_r_180; neu1; neu3}, G2={neu2}, G=3{parrot}, G4={gan128}, G5={monroe}, and G6={cell}.

The images neu4 and the image neu4_r_180 rotated by 180 degree are grouped into the same group, although they have completely different segmentation parameters. We obtained the best result for neu4 with the parameter-set a=0.75, b= 2 and T=1, while for neu4_r180 the best segmentation was obtained with the parameter-set a=1, b=0.5 and T=1. By using this latter parameter-set for neu4, we would get an undersegmented result (compare Fig. 26(c)). Overall we observed that not all the images having the same image segmentation parameters are grouped into one group such as neu4 and gan128.

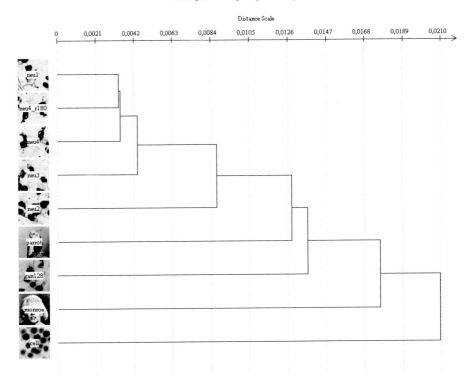

Fig. 24. Dendrogram for image description based on texture and statistical features

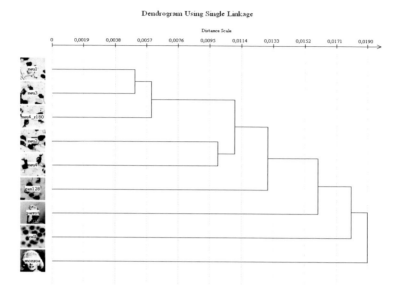

Fig. 25. Dendrogram for image description based on weighted texture, centroid and statistical features

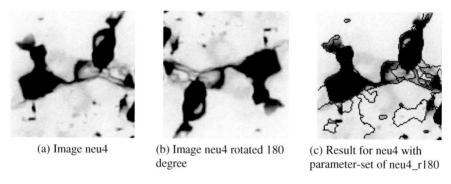

(a) Image neu4

(b) Image neu4 rotated 180 degree

(c) Result for neu4 with parameter-set of neu4_r180

Fig. 26. Orignal image and rotated image and influence of the parameter set

To sort out rotated images from the group including the un-rotated images, we have to give more emphasis to the feature centroid, because this feature is the only one which is not invariant for rotations. Therefore, we divide the image features set into three groups: texture features, centroid, and the remaining statistical features. Each group gets a total weight ω_g of 1/3. The local weights ω_{gi} in each group are computed as follow

$$\omega_g = \sum_{i=1}^{l} \omega_{gi} = \sum_{i=1}^{l} \frac{1}{3 * l} = \frac{1}{3}, \qquad (8)$$

where l is the number of features in the group.

In the resulting dendrogram the images neu4 and neu4_r180 are clustered in different groups (see Fig. 25).

If we virtually cut the dendrogram by a cophenetic similarity value of 0,0057, we obtain the following groups G1={neu1;neu3}, G2={neu4_r180}, G3={neu2}, G4={neu4}, G5={gan128}, G6={parrot}, G7={cell}, and G8={monroe}. Except for the images neu4 and parrot, these groups seem to better reflect the relationship between the image description and the parameter-set. The proper weighting of the features can improve the grouping of the images. For this purpose we need to work out a strategy in a further study.

5.2 Image Description as a Marginal Distribution for Columns and Lines, and Diagonals

As another way to summarize the regional minima into an image description, we chose to calculate the marginal distribution over x- and y-direction of an image as well as over the diagonal. The marginal distribution is calculated by counting the foreground pixels by column for the y-direction and row by row for the x-direction of an image as well as for the diagonal. As a result, we have histograms over the columns, the rows and the diagonal showing the frequency of foreground pixels in the gradient image. The normalized marginal histogram for x- and y-direction for image neu3 is presented in Fig. 27.

In the next step we compare the histograms for the columns, rows and diagonals between two images by different distance functions.

Before we can calculate the marginal distribution for the foreground pixels, we need to binarize the gradient image in order to decide which pixels are foreground or background pixels. We used the thresholding algorithm of Otsu for the automatic binarization. It is clear that this will put another constraint to our approach. However, if it gives us a good image description and an automatic procedure, this is acceptable.

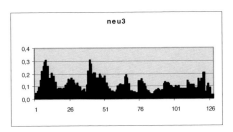
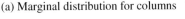
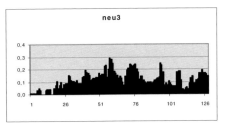

(a) Marginal distribution for columns   (b) Marginal distribution for rows

Fig. 27. Diagram of the Marginal Distribution of image neu3

The Kullback-Leibler divergence is usually the measure of choice when comparing two histograms. The Kullback-Leibler divergence is defined as:

$$Sim_{H_1 H_2} = \sum_{i=1}^{n} (H_2(i) - H_1(i)) \ln \frac{H_2(i)}{H_1(i)} \qquad (9)$$

where H_1 and H_2 are two histograms, n the size of the diagrams and $H_1(i)$ the ith row in the histogram H_1 (analogous for H_2). The problem of this measure is that it cannot handle functional values of zero in the histogram. Then the multiplicand in formula (9) is not defined. A functional value of zero means that for a column or a row no foreground pixel exists, which can always happen in a binarized image. Therefore, although this measure is often cited in the literature as the preferred measure when comparing two histograms, for the purpose proposed in this paper we cannot use this measure.

We used different distance functions, like (squared) Euclidean Distance, city block or Chebyshev Distance to compare two histograms.

The dendrograms of the single-linkage method in Figures Fig. 28 to Fig. 31 show the results of the marginal distribution using the Euclidean Distance, where Fig. 28 (and Fig. 29 and Fig. 31, respectively) shows the results comparing the column histogram (and row and diagonal histograms, respectively) and Fig. 30 shows the results comparing the column and row histograms together.

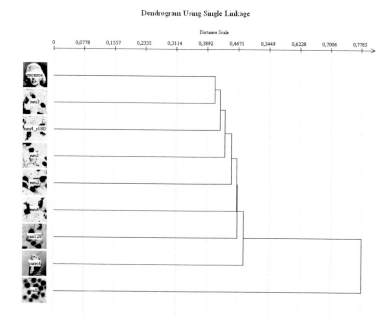

Fig. 28. Dendrogram for image description. Marginal distribution for column using the similarity measure Euclidean Distance

We virtually cut the dendrogram in Fig. 28 by the cophenetic-similarity value equal to 0.455. However, with this cophenetic-similarity value, images for which we got different best segmentation parameters were also clustered in different cases. Therefore the cut-off will be by the cophenetic-similarity value equal to 0.389, because monroe and neu3 have different best segmentation parameters. By this choice

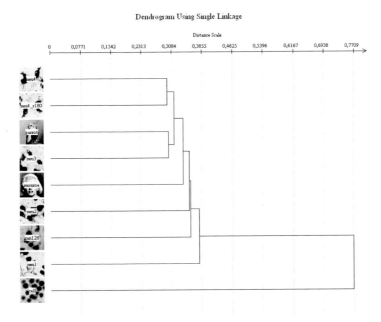

Fig. 29. Dendrogram for image description on marginal distribution for rows using the similarity measure Euclidean

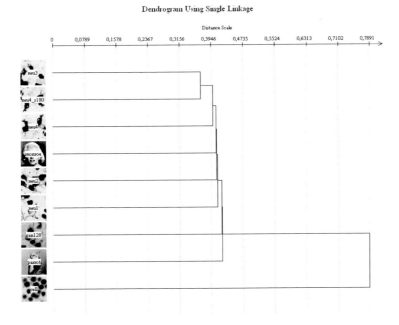

Fig. 30. Dendrogram for image description of marginal distribution of column and row together using the similarity measure of the Euclidean Distance

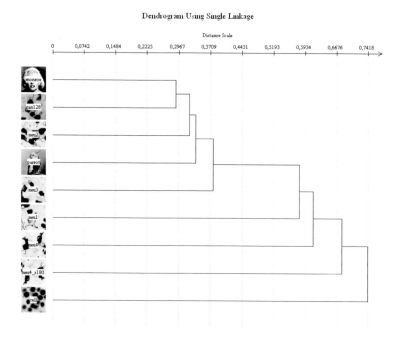

Fig. 31. Dendrogram for image description of marginal distribution of the diagonal use of the similarity measure of the Euclidean Distance

of the cophenetic-similarity value all images are in different clusters, including images with the same best segmentation parameters like neu4 and parrot.

By taking into account the row histograms in Fig. 29, the cut-off should be done by the cophenetic-similarity value equal to 0.25, which is able to separate the images neu4 and neu4_r180. However, with this choice again all the images would be assigned to different clusters.

By comparing column and row histograms together in Fig. 30, we should cut the dendrogram by the cophenetic-similarity value equal to 0.39, in order to separate the rotated images. Then only neu4_r180 and neu3 would be clustered together, but these two images have different best segmentation parameters and hence, should not be assigned to the same case. Thus, the final cut-off should be done by the cophenetic-similarity value equal to 0.34. However, this choice would again, lead to having all images in different clusters.

By considering the diagonal histograms in Fig. 31, we should cut the dendrogram by the cophenetic-similarity equal to 0.66 to separate the images neu4 and neu4_r180. With this choice we would get neu4 and parrot, which have the same best segmentation parameters in the same cluster, as desired. However, also monroe, gan128, neu2, neu3 and neu1 would be assigned to that cluster. Since monroe would result as under-segmented as concerns the hair by the best segmentation parameters of gan128 (compare Fig. 32), we have to cut the dendrogram by the cophenetic-similarity equal to 0.275. Then again all images would be in different clusters.

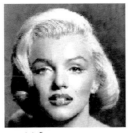

(a) Image monroe

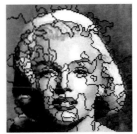

(b) Segmentation with parameters of gan128

Fig. 32. The influence of the selected parameter-set to the segmentation result shown on image Monroe

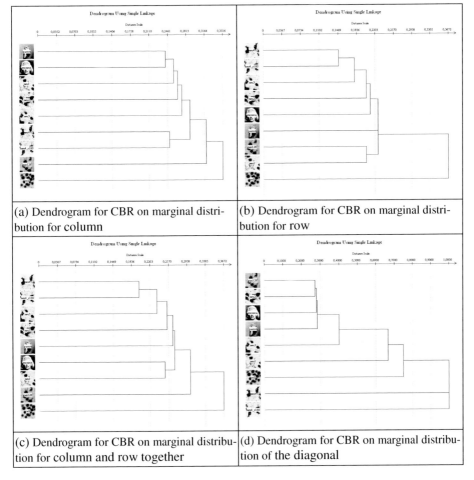

(a) Dendrogram for CBR on marginal distribution for column

(b) Dendrogram for CBR on marginal distribution for row

(c) Dendrogram for CBR on marginal distribution for column and row together

(d) Dendrogram for CBR on marginal distribution of the diagonal

Fig. 33. Dendrogram for image description on marginal distribution using the similarity measure Chebyshev distance

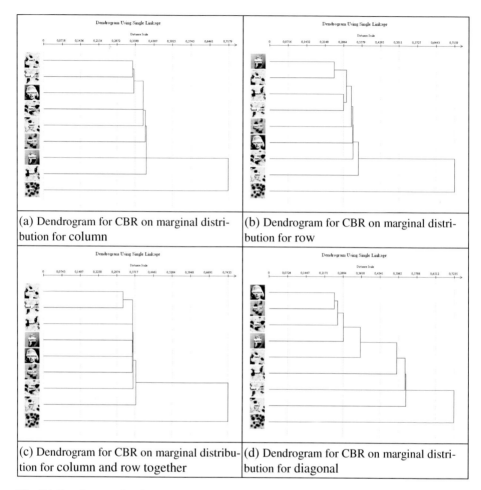

Fig. 34. Dendrogram for CBR on marginal distribution using the similarity measure city block distance

In conclusion, the marginal distribution using the Euclidean Distance enables us to separate rotated images, but we did not get images having the same settings in the same group. We got similar results for the marginal distribution using the Chebyshev Distance (compare with Fig. 33) and the city block Distance (compare with Fig. 34).

In conclusion we have to say, that the marginal distribution is a nice method to summarize the image content in x- and y-direction as well as over the diagonal, but it does not help us in properly grouping images for watershed CBR segmentation.

5.3 Image Description by Similarity between the Regional Minima of Two Images

Obviously the position of the regional minima has an influence on the segmentation result. Thus, we study the starting-points of the Watershed Transform (regional minima). A simple idea is to determine the similarity between two images A and B (having the same size) as follows:

$$SIM = \frac{\text{No Coincidence Points}}{\text{Number Minima Pixel A} + \text{Number Mimima Pixel B}} \tag{10}$$

with $0 \leq Sim \leq 1$. The similarity measure is null zero if the images A and B are equal and one if A and B have no coincidence by the local minima.

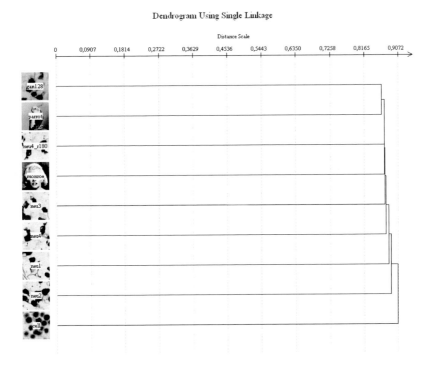

Fig. 35. Dendrogram based on equation 3

The result is shown in Fig. 35. Our test images are all very dissimilar with this measure as the dendrogram in Fig. 35 shows. The lowest cophenetic similarity value is 0.8627 between the gan128 and parrot image. On closer inspection of the regional minima images from the testing images this result is not surprising, because there are not many coincidences (compare Fig. 36).

If we use the similarity measure from [18] for the evaluation of testing the local minima images we are getting from the similarity matrix, all images excluding the parrot are most similar to the cell. That is the image with the smallest number of local minima in our set of test images. Furthermore, we observe that the images are in general all dissimilar as the dendrogram in Fig. 37 shows. Therefore, we consider this measure as unsuitable to distinguish between the groups of images versa their segmentation parameters.

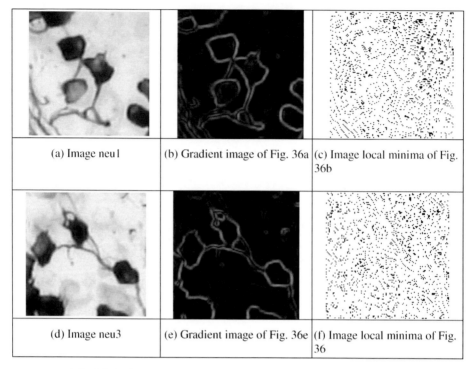

| (a) Image neu1 | (b) Gradient image of Fig. 36a | (c) Image local minima of Fig. 36b |
| (d) Image neu3 | (e) Gradient image of Fig. 36e | (f) Image local minima of Fig. 36 |

Fig. 36. Orginal image and the local minimas from the gradient image

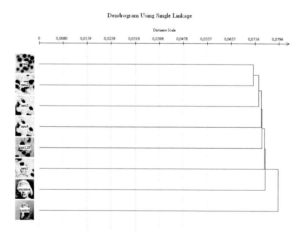

Fig. 37. Dendrogram from similarity measure from [18]

More promising are probably the determination of the distances from one regional minima to all the surrounding minima up to a predefined area and the calculation of the statistical distribution. Then the problem would be to compare the distribution of two images. We will further evaluate this idea in another study.

5.4 Image Description by Central Moments

Next we study central moments for the shape description.

An image can be interpreted as a two-dimensional density function. So we can compute the geometric moments

$$M_{pq} = \int\int x^p y^q g(x,y) \quad p,q = 0,1,2,\ldots \tag{11}$$

with continuous image function $g(x,y)$.

In the case of digital images, we can replace the integrals by sums:

$$m_{pq} = \sum_x \sum_y x^p y^q f(x,y) \quad p,q = 0,1,2,\ldots \tag{12}$$

where $f(x,y)$ is the discrete function of the gray levels.

The seven-moment invariants from Hu [19] have the property of being invariant to translation, rotation and scale. Since our implementation of an algorithm [10] is not invariant with respect to rotation and scale, the invariant moments are unsuitable for our image description.

We can consider the central moments, which are the only ones translation invariant:

$$m_{pq} = \sum_x \sum_y (x - x_c)^p (y - y_c)^q f(x,y) \quad p,q = 0,1,2,\ldots \tag{13}$$

where

$$x_c = \frac{\sum_x \sum_y x f(x,y)}{\sum_x \sum_y f(x,y)} \quad \text{and} \quad y_c = \frac{\sum_x \sum_y y f(x,y)}{\sum_x \sum_y f(x,y)}. \tag{14}$$

For our study we use central moments m_{pq} with p and q between 0 and 3 and as input image the binarized gradient image obtained with the thresholding algorithm of Otsu. To determine the similarity between two images we use the normalized city-block distance in equation 6 its the weights $\omega_i = 1/k \ \forall i \in [1,\ldots,k]$.

Fig. 38 shows the dendrogram of this test. If we virtually cut the dendrogram by the cophenetic similarity measure of 0.0129, we obtain the following groups G1={Monroe, parrot}, G2={neu3, neu4}, G3={gan128}, G4={neu4_r180}, G5={neu2}, G6={neu1}, and G7={cell}. Compared to the statistical and texture features for image description we obtain one more group, but neu4_r180 gets separated from neu4. The resulting groups seem to represent better the relationship between the image characteristic and the image segmentation parameters.

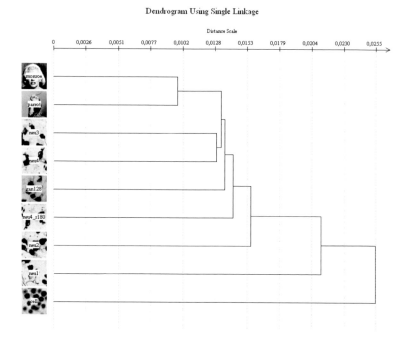

Fig. 38. Dendrogram for CBR based on central moments (on binary gradient image)

Problematic is only neu3, which appears in the same group as neu4. Fig. 39 shows in (b) the best possible segmentation result and in (c) the segmentation result with the parameter (0.75, 2, 1). Fig. 39(c) is more oversegmented than Fig. 39 (b). To get a better result, we can use a threshold for small edges (compare with section 5 and Fig. 20).

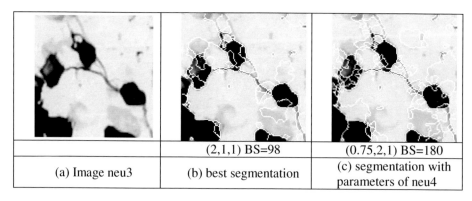

	(2,1,1) BS=98	(0.75,2,1) BS=180
(a) Image neu3	(b) best segmentation	(c) segmentation with parameters of neu4

Fig. 39. The influence of the selected parameter-set on the segmentation result and the number of basins shown in image neu3

6 Discussion

The image descriptions that work well for the Watershed Transformation are the statistical and texture feature description (STDescript) and the image description based on Central Moments (CMDescript). While the STDescript is only rotation and scale invariant, the STDescript weighted and the CMDescript is not. The obtained groups for the two descriptions are:

STDescript
G1={neu4; neu4_r_180; neu1; neu3}, G2={neu2}, G=3{ parrot}, G4={gan128}, G5={monroe}, and G6={cell}

STDescript weighted
G1={neu1;neu3}, G2={neu4_r180}, G3={neu2}, G4={neu4}, G5={gan128}, G6={parrot}, G7={cell}, and G8={monroe}

CMDescript
G1={Monroe, parrot}, G2={neu3, neu4}, G3={gan128}, G4={neu4_r_180}, G5={neu2}, G6={neu1}, and G7={cell}.

The obtained groups of the STDescript weighted seem to reflect better the relationship between the image characteristics and the segmentation parameters than the obtained groups by the CMDescript.

The computation time of both image descriptions is more or less the same.

In conclusion, we can say that the statistical and texture feature description weighted and the central moments are the best image description which we have found so far during our study.

7 Case Generalizations and Incremental Model Learning

For each case group we can compute a case-class representative that will be used during case retrieval as matching candidate. The case representative can be the mean over all cases or the median (see for example table 5). If all cases in a case group share the same segmentation parameters, matching will stop after having found the closest case representative among all case representatives. If not all the cases in a case group share the same segmentation parameters, matching will proceed until the closest case of all the cases in a group of cases is found (see Figure 40 for example of the case base based on the image description of STDescript weighted. Over the course of time new cases can be learnt during the application of the Watershed Transformation based on CBR. The matching procedure is done based on the similarity measure described in Section 5.1.

Table 5. Case group with its case description and prototype

ImageName	Mean	StdDev	Kurtosis	VarCoef	...	Energy	Contrast	LocHomog	xCentroid	yCentroid
neu1r.bmp	16,55	23,58	4,48	1,43	...	0,00748	267,45	268,45	56,98	75,67
neu3r.bmp	15,06	22,43	6,59	1,49	...	0,00558	268,04	269,04	58,55	71,86
Prototype Σ	15,80	23,01	5,54	1,46	...	0,00653	267,75	268,75	57,77	73,76

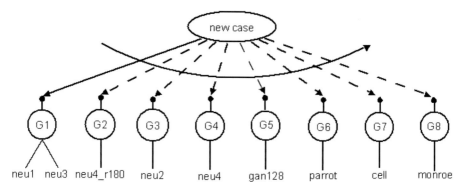

Fig. 40. Retrieval of the case base

8 Conclusion

We have proposed a framework for model building in image processing by meta-learning based on case-based reasoning. The model-building process is seen as a classification process during which the signal characteristics are mapped to the right image-processing parameters to ensure the best image-processing output. The mapping function is realized by case-based reasoning. Case-based reasoning is especially suitable for this kind of process, since it incrementally allows learning the model based on the incoming data stream. To find the right signal/image description of the signal/image characteristics that are in relationship to the signal-processing parameters is one important aspect of this work. In connection with this work one has to do an intensive study of the theoretical, structural, and syntactical behavior [20] of the chosen image processing algorithm. Based on this analysis we can propose several signal/image descriptions. The selected image description should summarize the cases into groups of similar cases and map these similar cases to the same processing parameters. Having found groups of similar cases, these should be summarized by prototypes that allow fast retrieval over several groups of cases. This generalization process should allow building up the model over time based on the incrementally obtained data stream.

Our theoretical study of different algorithms of the Watershed Transformation showed that the WT produces different results if the image is rotated or rescaled. The particular implementation of the algorithm puts constraints on the behavior of the algorithm. As a result of our study we conclude that we need an image description that describes the distribution of the regional minima and that is not invariant against rotation and scaling.

We studied four different image descriptions: statistical and texture feature description, image description as a marginal description between columns, rows, and diagonals, similarity of regional minima in two images, and central moments.

Two image descriptions of the four image descriptions did not lead to any success.

The description based on statistical and texture features is useful but is invariant against rotation and scaling. The best image descriptions are the description based on statistical and texture features weighted and the description based on central moments. These image descriptions seem to well represent the relationship between the image characteristics of the particular image and the segmentation parameters. Cases having the same segmentation parameters could be grouped based on the image descriptions into the same group. This will make possible a generalization on these groups of cases that will lead to a complete image-segmentation model. However, to automatically choose the right weight values for the statistical and texture feature description is up to now an open question.

References

[1] Perner, P.: Why Case-Based Reasoning is Attractive for Image Interpretation. In: Aha, D., Watson, I. (eds.) ICCBR 2001. LNCS (LNAI), vol. 2080, pp. 27–44. Springer, Heidelberg (2001)

[2] Soares, C., Brazdil, P.B., Kuba, P.: A meta-learning method to select the kernel width in support vector regression. Machine Learning 54, 195–209 (2004)

[3] Perner, P.: An Architecture for a CBR Image Segmentation System. Engineering Applications of Artificial Intelligence 12(6), 749–759 (1999)

[4] Perner, P.: Case-Based Reasoning for Image Analysis and Interpretation. In: Chen, C., Wang, P.S.P. (eds.) Handbook on Pattern Recognition and Computer Vision, 3rd edn., pp. 95–114. World Scientific Publisher, Singapore (2005)

[5] Perner, P.: Case-based reasoning and the statistical challenges. Journal Quality and Reliability Engineering International 24(6), 705–720 (2008)

[6] Wunsch, G.: Systemtheorie. Akademische Verlagsgesellschaft, Leipzig (1975)

[7] Perner, P.: Introduction to Case-Based Reasoning for Signals and Images. In: Perner, P. (ed.) Case-Based Reasoning on Images and Signals. SCI, vol. 73, pp. 319–353. Springer, Berlin (2008)

[8] Roerdink, J.B.T.M., Meijster, A.: The watershed transform: definitions, algorithms and parallelization strategies. Fundamenta Informaticae 41, 187–228 (2001)

[9] Vincent, L., Soille, P.: Watersheds in digital spaces: an efficient algorithm based on immersion simulations. IEEE Trans. Patt. Anal. Mach. Intell 13(6), 583–598 (1991)

[10] Frucci, M., Perner, P., di Baja, G.S.: Case-based Reasoning for Image Segmentation by Watershed Transformation. In: Perner, P. (ed.) Case-Based Reasoning on Images and Signals. SCI, vol. 73, pp. 319–353. Springer, Berlin (2008)

[11] Frucci, M., Perner, P., di Baja, G.S.: Case-based Reasoning for Image Segmentation. International Journal of Pattern Recognition and Artificial Intelligence 22(5), 1–14 (2008)

[12] Andreä, S., Haufe, S.: Analyse, Implementierung und Visualisierung der watershed transform. Projektarbeit im Fach Informatik, Martin-Luther-Universität Halle-Wittenberg (2005),
http://users.informatik.uni-halle.de/~andreae/aivwshed.pdf
(Last retrieved: 16.4.2008)

[13] Zamperoni, P.: Methoden der digitalen Bildsignalverarbeitung. Vieweg, Braunschweig (2001)

[14] Wang, D.: A multiscale gradient algorithm for image segmentation using watersheds. Pattern Recognition 30(12), 2043–2052 (1997)

[15] Soille, P.: Morphological Image Analysis, Principles and Applications. Springer, Berlin (2004)

[16] Bleau, A., Leon, L.J.: Watershed-Based Segmentation and Region Merging. Computer Vision and Image Understanding 77(3), 317–370 (2000)

[17] Frucci, M.: Oversegmentation Reduction by Flooding Regions and Digging Watershed Lines. International Journal of Pattern Recognition and Artificial Intelligence 20(1), 15–38 (2006)

[18] Zamperoni, P., Starovotov, V.: How dissimilar are two gray-scale images. In: Proc. 17th DAGM Symposium, pp. 448–454. Springer, Berlin (1995)

[19] Hu, M.K.: Visual pattern recognition by moment invariants. IEEE Trans. Information Theory 8, 179–187 (1962)

[20] Vogt, R.: Die Systemwissenschaften – Grundlagen und wissenschaftstheoretische Einordnung. Haag – Herchen Verlag, Frankfurt am Main (1983)

Chapter 12
Explaining Medical Model Exceptions

Rainer Schmidt and Olga Vorobieva

Institute for Medical Informatics and Biometry, University of Rostock, Germany
rainer.schmidt@medizin.uni-rostock.de

Abstract. In this chapter, a system named ISOR is presented, that supports research doctors to investigate and to explain cases that do not fit a theoretical
hypothesis. The system is designed for situations where neither a well-
developed theory nor reliable knowledge nor, at the beginning, a case base is
available. Instead of theoretical knowledge and intelligent experience, just a
theoretical hypothesis and a set of measurements are given. ISOR is a Case-
Based Reasoning system. That means, when attempting to find an explanation
for an exceptional case, solutions of already explained similar exceptional cases
are considered. However, ISOR uses further knowledge sources, especially a
dialog where the user (a research doctor) can make suggestions for an explanation. ISOR is domain independent and can be applied to various research problems. However, in this chapter, it is focused on the hypothesis that a specific
exercise program improves the physical condition of dialysis patients. Since
many data are missing for this research problem, a method to impute missing
data was developed and is also presented here. This method combines general
domain independent techniques with domain knowledge provided by a medical
expert. For the latter technique Case-based Reasoning is applied again.

1 Introduction

Case-based Reasoning (CBR) uses previous experience represented as cases to understand and solve new problems. A case-based reasoner remembers former cases similar
to the current problem and attempts to modify solutions of former cases to fit the current problem.

The fundamental ideas of CBR originated in the late eighties [1]. In the early nine-
ties CBR emerged as a method that was firstly described by Kolodner [2]. Later on
Aamodt and Plaza presented a more formal characterisation of the CBR method [3],
which consists of four steps: retrieving former similar cases, adapting their solutions
to the current problem, revising a proposed solution, and retaining new learned cases.
However, there are two main subtasks in Case-based Reasoning [2, 3]: The retrieval,
the search for a similar case, and the adaptation, the modification of solutions of retrieved cases. For retrieval a lot similarity measures and sophisticated retrieval algorithms, have been developed within the CBR community. The most common ones are
indexing methods [2] like tree-hash retrieval [4], which are useful for nominal

I. Bichindaritz et al. (Eds.): Computational Intelligence in Healthcare 4, SCI 309, pp. 265–287.
springerlink.com

parameter values, retrieval nets [5], which are useful for ordered nominal values, and Nearest Neighbour Search [6], which is useful for metric parameter values.

The second task, the adaptation is a modification of solutions of former similar cases to fit for a query case. If there are no important differences between a query case and a similar case, a simple solution transfer is sufficient. Sometimes only few substitutions are required, but sometimes the adaptation is a very complicated process. So far, for adaptation still only very few domain independent methods like compositional adaptation [7] exist.

1.1 Case-Based Reasoning for Medical Applications

Especially in medicine, the knowledge of experts does not only consist of rules, but of a mixture of textbook knowledge and experience. The latter consists of cases, typical and exceptional ones, and the reasoning of physicians takes them into account [8]. In medical knowledge based systems there are two sorts of knowledge, objective knowledge, which can be found in textbooks, and subjective knowledge, which is limited in space and time, and which frequently changes.

The problem of updating the changeable subjective knowledge can partly be solved by incrementally incorporating new up-to-date cases [8]. Both sorts of knowledge can be clearly separated: Objective textbook knowledge can be represented in form of rules or functions, whereas subjective knowledge is contained in cases.

So, the arguments for case-oriented methods are as follows:

1. Reasoning with cases corresponds with the decision making process of physicians.
2. Incorporating new cases means automatically updating parts of the changeable knowledge.
3. Objective and subjective knowledge can be clearly separated.
4. Since cases are routinely stored, integration into clinic communication systems should be easy.

Since differences between two cases are sometimes very complex, especially in medical domains, many case-based systems are so called retrieval-only systems. They just perform the retrieval task, visualise query cases in comparison with retrieved similar cases, and sometimes additionally point out the important differences between them.

However, a string of medical CBR systems have already been developed (for overviews see [9, 10, 11]).

1.2 The ISOR Approach

In our previous work on knowledge-based systems [12], it is demonstrated how a dialogue-oriented Case-Based Reasoning system can help in situations where a theoretically approved medical therapy does not produce the desired and usually expected results. In medical studies and in research, exceptions need to be explained. We have developed ISOR, a conversational case-based system that helps doctors to explain exceptional cases. Conversational CBR systems have begun to become popular in recent years [13]. However, so far no common conversational methodology exists but just the common idea to incorporate the user into a conversational solution search.

ISOR deals with situations where neither a well-developed theory nor reliable knowledge nor a proper case base is available. So, instead of theoretical knowledge and intelligent experience, just a theoretical hypothesis and a set of measurements are given. In such situations the usual question is, "how do measured data fit to a theoretical hypothesis?" To statistically confirm a hypothesis it is necessary that the majority of cases fit the hypothesis. Mathematical statistics determines the exact quantity of necessary confirmation [14]. However, usually a few cases do not satisfy the hypothesis. These cases need to be examined to find out why they do not fit the hypothesis. ISOR offers a dialogue to guide the search for possible reasons in all components of the data system. The exceptional cases belong to the case base. This approach is justified by a certain mistrust of statistical models by doctors, because modelling results are usually non-specific and "average oriented" [15], which reflects a lack of attention to individual "imperceptible" features of specific patients.

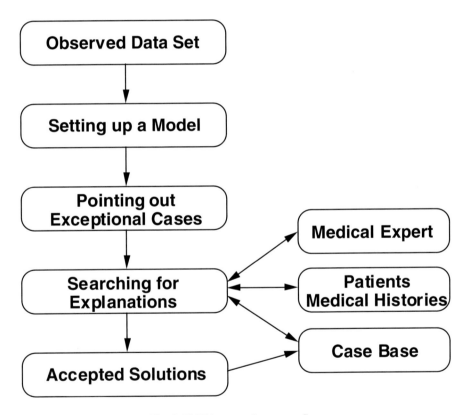

Fig. 1. ISOR's general program flow

The usual Case-Based Reasoning assumption is that a case base with complete solutions is available [2, 3, 16]. Our approach starts in a situation where such a case base is not available but has to be set up incrementally. The general program flow is shown in figure 1. The main steps are:

1. Construct a model,
2. Point out the exceptions,
3. Find causes why the exceptional cases do not fit the model, and
4. Set up a case base.

So, Case-Based Reasoning is combined with a model, in this specific situation with a statistical one. The idea to combine CBR with other methods is not new. Care-Partner, for example, resorts to a multi-modal reasoning framework for the co-operation of CBR and rule-based reasoning (RBR) [17]. Montani et al. [18] rather use CBR to provide evidences for a hybrid system in the domain of diabetes. Another way of combining hybrid rule bases with CBR is discussed by Prentzas and Hat-zilgeroudis [19]. The combination of CBR and model-based reasoning is discussed in [20]. However, statistical methods are used within CBR mainly for retrieval and re-tention [21,22]. Arshadi and Jurisica [23] propose a method that combines CBR with statistical methods like clustering and logistic regression.

The first application of ISOR is on hemodialysis and fitness. Unfortunately, the data set contains many missing data, which makes the process of finding explanations for exceptional cases difficult. So, we decided to attempt to first solve the missing data problem. This is done by partly applying CBR again.

2   Incremental Development of an Explanation Model for Exceptional Dialysis Patients

Hemodialysis means stress for a patient's organism and has significant adverse ef-fects. Fitness is the most available and a relative cheap way of support. It is meant to improve a physiological condition of a patient and to compensate negative dialysis effects. One of the intended goals of this research is to convince patients of the posi-tive effects of fitness and to encourage them to make efforts and to actively partici-pate in the fitness program. This is important because dialysis patients usually feel sick, they are physically weak, and they do not want any additional physical load [24].

At the University clinic in St. Petersburg, a specially developed complex of physio-therapy exercises including simulators, walking, swimming, and so on is offered to all dialysis patients but only some of them actively participate, whereas some others par-ticipate but are not really active. The purpose of this fitness offer is to improve the physical conditions of the patients and to increase the quality of their lives. The hy-pothesis is that actively participating in the fitness program improves the physical condition of dialysis patients.

For each patient a set of physiological parameters is measured. These parameters contain information about burned calories, maximal power achieved by the patient, oxygen uptake, oxygen pulse (volume of oxygen consumption per heart beat), lung ventilation, and others. There are also biochemical parameters like haemoglobin and other laboratory measurements. More than 100 parameters were planned for every patient. But not all of them were actually measured.

Parameters are supposed to be measured four times during the first year of partici-pating in the fitness program. There is an initial measurement followed by one after three months, then after six months and finally after a year. Unfortunately, since some measurements did not happen, many data are missing. Therefore the patient records often contain different sets of measured parameters.

It is necessary to note that parameter values of dialysis patients essentially differ from those of non-dialysis patients, especially of healthy people, because dialysis interferes with the natural, physiological processes in an organism. In fact, for dialysis patients, all physiological processes behave abnormally. Therefore, the correlation between parameters differs too.

For statistics, this means difficulties in applying statistical methods based on correlation and it limits the usage of a knowledge base developed for normal people. Non-homogeneity of observed data, many missing data, many parameters for a relatively small sample size, all this makes the data set practically impossible for usual statistical analysis.

Since the data set is incomplete, additional or substitutional information has to be found in other available data sources. These are databases, namely the already existent individual base and the sequentially created case base, and the medical expert as a special source of information.

2.1 Setting up a Model

Usually, a medical problem needs to be solved based on given data. In this example it is:

"Does a specific fitness programs improve the physiological condition of dialysis patients?"

So, the physical conditions of active and non-active patients need to be compared. Patients are divided into two groups, depending on their activity, active and non-active patients.

According to the assumption, active patients should feel better after some months of participating in the fitness program, whereas non-active ones should feel rather worse. The meaning of "feeling better" and "feeling worse" has to be defined in this context. Therefore, a medical expert selects appropriate factors from ISOR's menu, which contains the parameter names from the observed database. The expert selects the following main factors

- F1: O2PT - Oxygen pulse by training
- F2: MUO2T - Maximal Uptake of Oxygen by training
- F3: WorkJ – performed Work (Joules) during control training

Subsequently the "research time period" has to be determined. Initially, this period was planned to be twelve months, but after a while the patients tend to give up the fitness program. This means, the longer the time period, the more data are missing. Therefore, a compromise between time period and sample size had to be made; a period of six months was chosen.

The next question is whether the model should be quantitative or qualitative? The observed data are mostly quantitative measurements. The selected factors are also quantitative in nature. On the other side, the goal of this research is to find out whether physical training improves or worsens the physical condition of dialysis patients.

One patient does not have to be compared with another patient. Instead, each patient has to be compared with his/her own situation some months ago, namely just before the start of the fitness program. The success should not be measured in absolute values, because the health statuses of patients are very different. Thus, even a modest improvement for one patient may be as important as the great improvement of another. Therefore, we simply classify the development into two categories: "better" and "worse". Since the usual tendency for dialysis patients is to worsen over time, those very few patients where no changes could be observed are added to the category "better".

The three main factors are supposed to describe the changes of the physical conditions of the patients. The changes are assessed depending on the number of improved factors:

- Weak version of the model: at least one factor has improved
- Medium version of the model: at least two factors have improved
- Strong version of the model: all three factors have improved

Finally, the type of model has to be defined. Popular statistical programs offer a large variety of statistical models. Some of them deal with categorical data. The easiest model is a 2x2-frequency table. The "better/ worse" concept fits this simple model very well. So the 2x2-frequency table is used. The results are presented in table 1. Unfortunately, the most popular Pearson Chi-square test is not applicable here because of the small values "2" and "3" in table 1. But Fisher's exact test [14] can be used. In the three versions shown in table 1 a very strong significance between the patients activity and improvement of their physical condition can be observed. The smaller the value of p is, the more significant the dependency.

Table 1. Results of Fisher's exact test, performed via an interactive web-program: http://www.matforsk.noIola.fisher.htm. The cases in bold have to be explained

Improvement mode	Patient's physical condition	Active	Non-active	Fisher Exact p
Strong	Better	28	1	< 0.0001
	Worse	**22**	21	
Medium	Better	40	10	< 0.005
	Worse	**10**	12	
Weak	Better	47	16	< 0.02
	Worse	**3**	6	

Exceptional cases. The performed Fisher test confirms the hypothesis that patients doing active fitness achieve better physical conditions than non-active ones. However, there are exceptions, namely active patients whose health conditions did not improve. Exceptional cases need to be explained. Explained exceptions build the case base. According to table 1, the stronger the model, the more exceptions can be observed and have to be explained. Every exception is associated with at least two problems. The first one is "Why did the patient's condition get worse?" Of course, "worse" is meant in terms of the chosen model. Since there may be some factors that are not included in the model but have changed positively, the second problem is "What has improved in the patient's condition?" To solve this problem significant factors where the values improved have to be searched.

In the following section the set-up of a case base on the strongest model version is explained.

2.2 Setting up a Case Base

We intend to solve both problems (mentioned above) by means of CBR. So we begin to set up the case base up sequentially. That means, as soon as an exception is explained, it is incorporated into the case base and can be used to help explaining further exceptional cases. Alphabetical order for the exceptional cases was chosen.

Since the case base is rather small, sophisticated retrieval algorithms are not required. So, the retrieval of already explained cases is performed by keywords. The main keywords are "problem code", "diagnosis", and "therapy". In the situation of explaining exceptions for dialysis patients the instantiations of these keywords are "adverse effects of dialysis" (diagnosis), "fitness" (therapy), and two specific problem codes. Besides the main keywords, additional problem specific ones are used. Here the additional keyword is the number of worsened factors. Further keywords are optional. They are just used when the case base becomes bigger and retrieval is no longer simple.

However, ISOR not only uses the case base as a knowledge source but further sources are involved, namely the patient's individual base (his medical history) and observed data (partly gained by dialogue with medical experts). Since in the domain of kidney disease and dialysis the medical knowledge is very detailed and much investigated but still incomplete, it is unreasonable to attempt to create an adequate knowledge base. Therefore, a medical expert, observed data, and just a few rules serve as medical knowledge sources.

2.2.1 Expert Knowledge and Artificial Cases

In ISOR, an expert's knowledge can be used in many different ways. Firstly, it is used to acquire rules, and secondly, it can be used to select appropriate items from the list of retrieved solutions, to propose new solutions, and last but not least, to create artificial cases.

Initially, an expert creates artificial cases; afterwards they can be used in the same way as real cases. They are created in the following situation. An expert points out a factor F as a possible solution for a query patient. Since many data are missing, it may happen that just for the query patient values of factor F are missing. In such a situation the doctor's knowledge can not be applied, but it is sensible to save it anyway. In essence, there are two different ways to do this. The first one is to generate a correspondent rule and to insert it into ISOR's algorithms. Unfortunately, this is very complicated, especially to find an appropriate way for inserting such a rule. The better alternative is to create an artificial case. Instead of the name of a patient an artificial case number is generated. The other attributes are either inherited from the query case or declared as missing. The retrieval attributes are inherited. This can be done by a short dialogue (figure 3) and ISOR's algorithms remain intact. Artificial cases can be treated in the same way as real cases: they can be revised, deleted, generalised, and so on.

2.2.2 Solving the Problem "Why Did Some Patients Conditions Became Worse?"

A set of explanations of different origin and different nature is obtained. There are three categories of explanations: additional factor, model failure, and wrong data.

Additional factor. The most important and most frequent solution is the influence of an additional factor. However three main factors are obviously not enough to describe all medical cases. Unfortunately, for different patients different additional factors are important. When ISOR has discovered an additional factor as explanation for an exceptional case, the factor has to be confirmed by the medical expert before it can be accepted as a solution. One of these factors is Parathyroid Hormone (PTH). An increased PTH level sometimes can explain a worsened condition of a patient [24]. PTH is a significant factor, but unfortunately it was measured for only some patients.

Another additional factor as a solution is phosphorus blood level. The principle of artificial cases was used to introduce the factor phosphorus as a new solution. One patient's record contained many missing data. The retrieved solution meant high PTH, but PTH data in the current patient's record was missing too. The expert proposed an increased phosphorus level as a possible solution. Since data about phosphorus data was also missing, an artificial case was created, that inherited all retrieval attributes of the query case, whereas the other attributes were recorded as missing. According to the expert, high phosphorus can provide an explanation. Therefore it is accepted as an artificial solution or a solution of an artificial case.

Some exceptions can be explained by indirect indications, which can be considered as another sort of additional factor. One of them is a very long time of dialysis (more than 60 months) before a patient began with the fitness program.

Model failure. We regard two types of model failures. One of them is deliberately neglected data. As a compromise we just considered data of six months, whereas further data of a patient might be important. In fact, three patients did not show an improvement in the considered six months but in the following six months. So, they were wrongly classified and should really belong to the "better" category. The second type of model failure is based on the fact that the two-category model was not precise enough. Some exceptions could be explained by a tiny and not really significant change in one of the main factors.

Wrong data are usually due to a technical mistake or to data not really proved. One patient, for example, was reported as actively participating in the fitness program but really was not.

2.2.3 Solving the Problem "What in the Patient's Condition Improved?"

There are at least two criteria to select factors for the model. First, a factor has to be significant, and second there must be enough patients for which this factor was measured at least for six months. So, some principally important factors were initially not taken into account because of missing data. The list of solutions includes these factors (figure 3): haemoglobin and maximal power (watt) achieved during control training. Oxygen pulse and oxygen uptake were measured in two different situations, namely during the training and before training in a state of rest. Therefore we have two pairs of factors: oxygen pulse in state of rest (O2PR) and during training (O2PT), maximal oxygen uptake in state of rest (MUO2R) and during training (MUO2T). Measurements made in a state of rest are more indicative and significant than those made during training. Unfortunately, most measurements were made during training. Only for some patients did corresponding measurements in a state of rest exist. Therefore O2PT and MUO2T were accepted as main factors and were incorporated into the model. On the other side, O2PR and MUO2R are solutions for the current problem "What in the patient's condition improved?"

In the case base every patient is represented by a set of cases, and every case represents a specific problem. This means that a patient is described from different points of view, and accordingly different keywords are used for retrieval.

2.3 Another Problem

Just one of many problems that can arise based on the observed data set and that can be solved and analysed by the dialogue (figure 3) is described above. Another interesting research question is "Does it make sense to begin with the fitness program during the first year of dialysis?" The question arises, because the conditions of the patients are considered to be unstable during their first year of dialysis. So, the question is expressed in this way "When should patients begin with the fitness program, earlier or later?" The term "earlier" is defined as "during the first year of dialysis". The term "later" means after at least one year of dialysis. To answer this question two groups of active patients are considered, namely those who began their training within the first year of dialysis and those who began it later (table 2).

According to Fisher's exact test dependence can be observed, with $p < 0.05$. However, the result is not as it was initially expected. Since patients are considered as unstable during their first year of dialysis, the assumption was that an earlier beginning might worsen the conditions of the patients. But the test revealed that the conditions of active patients who began with their fitness program within the first year of dialysis improved even more than the conditions of patients starting later.

Table 2. Changed conditions for active patients

	Earlier	Later
Better	18	10
Worse	6	16

However, there are six exceptional cases, namely active patients starting early and their conditions worsened. These exceptions belong to the case base; the explanations of them are high PTH or high phosphorus level.

2.4 Example

The following example demonstrates how ISOR attempts to find explanations for exceptional cases. Because of data protection no real patient can be used. It is an artificial case but nevertheless is a typical situation.

Query patient: a 34-year old woman started with fitness after five months of dialysis. Two factors worsened, namely Oxygen pulse and Oxygen uptake, and consequently the condition of the patient was assessed as worsened too.

Problem: Why the patient's condition deteriorated after six months of physical training?

Retrieval: The number of worsened factors is used as an additional keyword in order to retrieve all cases with at least two worsened factors.

Case base: It does not only contain cases but more importantly a list of general solutions. For each of the general solutions there exists a list that contains specific solutions based on the cases in the case base. The list of general solutions contains these five items (figure 2):

1) Concentration of Parathyroid Hormone (PTH),
2) Period of dialysis is too long,
3) An additional disease,
4) A patient was not very active during the fitness program, and
5) A patient is very old.

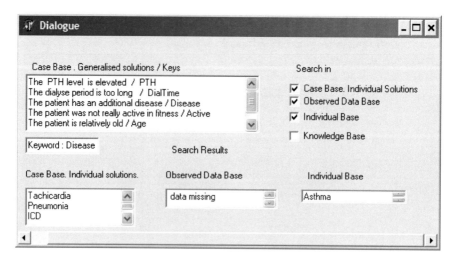

Fig. 2. Dialog menu to search for general solutions

Individual base. The patient suffers from a chronic disease, namely from asthma.

Adaptation. Since the patient started with a fitness program already after five months of dialysis, the second general solution can be excluded. The first general solution might be possible, though the individual base does not contain any information about PTH. Further lab tests showed PTH = 870, which means that PTH is a solution.

Since an additional disease, bronchial asthma, is found in the individual base, this solution is checked. Asthma is not contained as a solution in the case base, but the expert concludes that asthma can be considered as a solution. Concerning the remaining general solutions, the patient is not too old and proclaims that she was active at fitness.

Adapted case. The solution consists of a combination of two factors, namely a high PTH concentration and an additional disease, asthma.

3 Illustration of ISOR's Program Flow

ISOR's main dialogue menu is shown in figure 3. At first, the user sets up a model (steps 1 to 4), subsequently he/she gets the result and an analysis of the model (steps 5 to 8), and then he/she attempts to find explanations for the exceptional cases (steps 9 and 10). Finally, the case base is updated (steps eleven and twelve). For illustration purposes the steps are numbered (in figure 3) and in the following they are explained in detail.

At first the user has to set up a model. To do this he/she has to select a grouping variable. In this example CODACT was chosen. It stands for "activity code" and means that active and non-active patients are to be compared. Provided alternatives are the sex and the beginning of the fitness program (within the first year of dialysis or later). In another menu the user can define further alternatives. Furthermore, the user has to select a model type (alternatives are "strong", "medium", and "weak"), the length of the time period that should be considered (3, 6 or 12 months), and the main factors have to be selected. The list contains the factors from the observed database. In the example, three factors are chosen: O2PT (oxygen pulse by training), MUO2T (maximal oxygen uptake by training), and WorkJ (work in joules during the test training). In the menu list, the first two factors have alternatives: "R" and "T", where "R" stands for state of rest and "T" for state of training.

When the user has selected these items, ISOR calculates the table. "Better" and "worse" are meant in the sense of the chosen model, in the example of the strong model. ISOR does not only calculate the table but additionally extracts the exceptional cases from the observed database. In the menu, the list of exceptions shows the code names of the patients. In the example, patient "D5" is selected and all further data belong to this patient.

The goal is to find an explanation for the exceptional case "D5". In step 7 of the menu it is shown that all selected factors worsened (-1), and in step 8 the factor values according to different time intervals are depicted. All data for twelve months are missing (-9999).

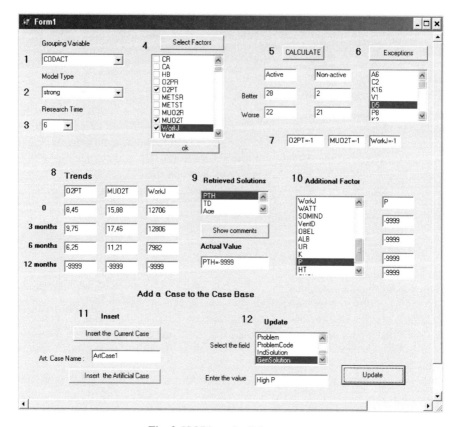

Fig. 3. ISOR's main dialogue menu

The next step means creating an explanation for the selected patient "D5". From the case base ISOR retrieves general solutions. The first retrieved solution in this example, the PTH factor, denotes that the increased parathyroid hormone blood level may explain the failure. Further theoretical information (e.g. normal values) about a selected item can be received by pressing the button "show comments". The PTH value of patient "D5" is missing (-9999). In step 10 the expert user can select further probable solutions. In the example, an increased phosphorus level (P) is suggested. Unfortunately, phosphorus data are missing too. However, the idea of an increased phosphorus level as a possible solution should not be lost. So, an artificial case should be generated.

The final step means inserting new cases into the case base. There are two sorts of cases, query cases and artificial cases. Query cases are stored records of real patients from the observed database. Artificial cases inherit the key attributes from the query cases (step 7 in the menu). Other data may be declared as missing. By the update function the missing data can be inserted later on. In the example of figure 3, the generalised solution "High P" is inherited; it may be retrieved as a possible solution (step 9 of the menu) for future cases.

4 Missing Data

Databases with many variables have specific problems. Since it is very difficult to overview their content, usually a priory a user does not know how complete is a data set. Is there any data missing? How many of them and where are they located?

In the dialysis data set, many data are missing randomly and without any known regularity. The main cause is that many measurements did not happen.

It can be assumed that the data set contains groups of interdependent variables but a priory it is not known how many such groups there are, what kind of variables are dependent, and in which way they are dependent. However, we intend to make use of all possible forms of dependency to impute missing data, because the more complete the observed data base is, the easier it should be to find explanations for exceptional cases and furthermore the better the explanations should be. Even for setting up the model the expert user should select those parameters as main factors with only few missing data. So, the more data are imputed, the better the choice for setting up the model can be.

A data analysis method is often assessed according to its tolerance to missing data (e.g. in [25]). In principle, there are two main approaches to the missing data problem. The first approach is a statistical imputation of missing data. Usually it is based on non-missing data from other records.

The second approach suggests methods that accept the absence of some data. The methods of this approach can be differently advanced, from simply excluding cases with missing values up to rather sophisticated statistical models [26, 27].

Gediga and Düntsch [28] propose the use of CBR to impute missing data. Since their approach does not require any external information, they call it a "non-invasive imputation method". Missing data are supposed to be replaced by their correspondent values of the most similar retrieved cases. However, the dialysis data set contains rather few patients, which means that the "most similar" case for a query case might not be very similar in fact.

So, why don't we just apply statistical methods? Statistical methods require homogeneity of the sample. However, there are no reasons to expect the set of dialysis patients to be a homogenous sample. Since the data consists of many parameters, sometimes missing values can be calculated or estimated from other parameter values. Furthermore, the number of cases in the data set is rather small, whereas usually statistical methods are more appropriate the bigger the number of cases.

4.1 The Data Set

For each patient a set of physiological parameters is measured. These parameters contain information about burned calories, maximal power, oxygen pulse (volume of oxygen consumption per heartbeat), lung ventilation, and many others. Furthermore, there are biochemical parameters like haemoglobin and other laboratory measurements. All these parameters are supposed to be measured four times during the first year of participating in the fitness program. There is an initial measurement followed by a next one after three months, then after six months, and finally after a year. Since some parameters, e.g. the height of a patient, are supposed to remain constant within a year, they were measured just once. The other ones are regarded as factors with four grades, they are denoted as F0 – the initial measurement of factor F, and F3, F6, and F12 – the measurements of factor F after 3, 6, and 12 months.

All performed measurements are stored in the observed database, which contains 150 records (one patient – one record) with 460 variables per record. 12 variables are constants; the other 448 variables represent 112 different parameters.

The factors can not be considered as completely independent from each other, but there are different types of dependency among specific factors. Even a strict mathematical dependency can occur, for example the triple: "time of controlled training, work performed during this time, and average achieved power", can be expressed as Power = Work/Time. Less strict are relations between factors of biochemical nature. An increase of parathyroid hormone, for example, implies an increase of blood phosphorus. Such relations between factors enable us to fill some missing data in the data set.

4.2 Imputation of Missing Data

In ISOR, again CBR is applied, now to impute missing data; the calculated values are filled in the observed database. The knowledge is contained in the case base, namely in form of solutions of former cases.

4.2.1 Types of Solutions

There are three types of numerical solutions: exact, estimated, and binary. Some examples and imputation formulas are shown in table 3. All types of solutions are demonstrated by examples in the next section.

When a missing value can be completely imputed, it is called an exact solution. Exact solutions are based on other parameters. A medical expert has defined them as specific relations between parameters, using ISOR. As soon as they have been used once, they are stored in the case base of ISOR and can be retrieved for further cases.

Table 3. Some examples of solutions and imputation formulas. Abbreviations: BC = Breath consumption, BF = Breath frequency, BV = Breath volume, HAT = Hematocrit, P = Phosphorus, PTH = Parathyroid hormone, PV = plasma volume

Missing parameter	Type of solution	Numeric solution (examples)	Description	Parameters	Time points
PTH	Binary	1	If P(T) >= P(t) then PTH(T) >= PTH(t) Else PTH(T) < PTH(t)	P, PTH	0 and 6
HT	Exact	36,2	HT = 100 * (1–PV/0.065 * Weight)	PV, Weight	6
HT	Estimated	29,1	Y(6) = Y(3)*0.66 + Y(12) * 0.33	HT	3 and 12
WorkJ	Exact	30447,1	WorkJ = MaxPower * Time * 0.5	Time, MaxPower	12
BC	Exact	15,6	BC = BF * BV	BF, BV	12
Oxygen pulse	Estimated	10,29	Linear regression	O2plus	0 and 3 and 12

Since estimated solutions are usually based on domain independent interpolation, extrapolation, or regression methods, a medical expert is not involved. An estimated solution is not considered as full reconstruction but just as estimation.

A binary solution is a partial reconstruction of a missing value. Sometimes ISOR is not able to construct either an exact or an estimated solution, but the expert may draw a conclusion about an increase or a decrease of a missing value. So, a binary solution expresses just the assumed trend. "1" means that the missing value should have increased since the last measurement, whereas "0" means that it should have decreased. Binary solutions are used in the qualitative models of ISOR.

4.2.2 Examples

The following three typical examples demonstrate how missing data are imputed.

First example: Exact solution

The value of hematocrit (HT) after six months is missing. Hematocrit is the proportion of the blood volume that consists of red blood cells. So, the hematocrit measurements are expressed in percentage.

The retrieved solution (fourth column of table 3) requires two additional parameters, namely plasma volume (PV) and the weight of the patient. For the query patient these values (measured after six months) are weight = 74 kg and PV = 3,367. These values are inserted in the formula and the result is a hematocrit value of 30%.

This imputation is domain dependent, it combines three parameters in such a specific way that it can not be applied to any other parameters. However, the formula can of course be transformed in two other ways and so it can be applied to impute values of PV and the weight of the patient. The formula contains specific medical knowledge that was once given as a case solution by an expert.

Second example: Estimated solution

This is the same situation as in the first example. The value of hematocrit that should have been measured after six months is missing. Unlike the first example, now the PV value that is required to apply the domain dependent formula is also missing. Since no other solution for exact calculation can be retrieved, ISOR attempts to generate an estimated solution. Of course, estimated solutions are not as good as exact ones but are acceptable. ISOR retrieves a domain independent formula (fourth column of table 3) that states that a missing value after six months should be calculated as the sum of two-thirds of the value measured after three months and one-third of the value measured after twelve months. This general calculation can be used for many parameters.

Third example: Binary solution

The value of parathyroid hormone (PTH) after six months is missing and needs to be imputed. The retrieved solution involves the initial PTH measurement and the additional parameter phosphorus (P), namely the measurement after six months, P(6), and the initial measurement, P(0). Informally, the solution states that with an increase of phosphorus goes along an increase of PTH too. More formally, the retrieved solution states:

If $P(6) >= P(0)$
  then $PTH(6) >= PTH(0)$
  else $PTH(6) < (PTH(0)$

So, here a complete imputation of the missing PTH value is not possible but just a binary solution that indicates the trend, where "1" stands for an increase and "0" for a decrease.

4.2.3 Case-Based Reasoning

In ISOR, cases are mainly used to explain further exceptional cases that do not fit the initial model. A secondary application is the imputation of missing data. The solutions given by the medical expert are stored in form of cases so that they can be retrieved for solving further missing data cases. Such a case stored in the case base has the following structure:

1. Name of the patient
2. Diagnosis
3. Therapy
4. Problem: missing value
5. Name of the parameter of the missing value
6. Measurement time point of the missing value
7. Formula of the solution (the description column of table 3)
8. Reference to the internal implementation of the formula
9. Parameters used in the formula
10. Solution: Imputed value
11. Type of solution (exact, estimated, or binary)

Since the number of stored cases is rather small (at most 150), retrieval is not crucial. In fact, the retrieval is simply performed by keywords. The four main keywords are: Problem code (here: "missing value"), diagnosis, therapy, and time period. As an additional keyword the parameter where the value is missing can be used. Solutions that are retrieved by using the additional keyword are domain dependent. They contain medical knowledge that has been provided by the medical expert. The domain independent solutions are retrieved by using just the four main keywords.

What happens when the retrieval provides more than one solution? Though only very few solutions are expected to be retrieved at the same time, only one solution should be selected. At first ISOR checks whether the required parameter values of the retrieved solutions are available. A solution is accepted if all required values are available. If more than one solution is accepted, the expert selects one of them. If no solution is accepted, ISOR attempts to apply the one with the fewest required parameter values.

Each sort of solution has its specific adaptation. A numerical solution is just a result of a calculation according to a formula. This kind of adaptation is performed automatically. If all required parameter values are available, the calculation is carried out and the query case receives its numerical solution.

The second kind of adaptation modifies an imputation formula. This kind of adaptation can not be done entirely automatically but the expert has to be involved. When a (usually short) list of solutions is retrieved, ISOR at first checks whether all required values of the exact calculation formulae are available. If required parameter values are not available, there are three alternatives to proceed. First, to find an exact solution formula where all required parameter values are available, second to find an estimation formula, and third to attempt to impute the required values too. Since for the third alternative there is the danger that this might lead to an endless loop, this process can be manually stopped by pressing a button in the dialogue menu. When for an estimated solution required values are missing, ISOR asks the expert.

The expert can suggest an exact or an estimated solution. Of course, such an expert solution also has to be checked for the availability of the required data. However, the expert can even provide just a numerical solution, a value to replace the missing data – with or without an explanation of this suggested value.

Furthermore, adaptation can be differentiated according to its domain dependency. Domain dependent adaptation rules have to be provided by the expert and they are only applicable to specific parameters. Domain independent adaptation uses general mathematical formulae that can be applied to many parameters. Two or more adaptation methods can be combined.

In ISOR a revision occurs. However, it is a rather simple one. It is not as sophisticated as, for example, the theoretically one described by Lieber [29]. Here, it is just an attempt to find better solutions. An exact solution is obviously better than an estimated one. So, if a value has been imputed by estimation and later on (for a later case) the expert has provided an appropriate exact formula, this formula should be applied to the former case too. Some estimation rules are better than others. So it may happen that later on a more appropriate rule is incorporated in ISOR. In principle, the more new solution methods are included in ISOR, the more former already imputed values can be revised.

Artificial cases. Since every piece of knowledge provided by a medical expert is supposed to be valuable, ISOR saves it for future use. If an expert solution cannot be used for adaptation for the query case (required values for this solution might be missing too), the expert user can generate an artificial case. In ISOR exists a special dialogue menu to do this. Artificial cases have the same structure as real ones, and they are also stored in the case base.

5   Results

At first, we undertook some experiments to assess the quality of our imputation method, subsequently we attempted to impute the real missing data and finally we set up a new model for the original hypothesis that actively participating in the fitness program improves the conditions of the patients.

5.1 Experimental Results

Since ISOR is a dialogue system and the solutions are generated within a conversation process with the expert user, the quality of the solutions not only depends on ISOR but also on the expert user.

To test the method a random set of parameter values was deleted from the observed data set. Subsequently, the method was applied and it was attempted to impute the deleted values - but not the ones actually missing!

Table summarises how many deleted values could be imputed. Since for those 12 parameters that were only measured once and remain constant no values were deleted (and none of them are really missing), they are not considered in table 4. More than half of the deleted values could be at least partly imputed, nearly a third of the deleted values could be completely imputed, about 58% of imputation occurred automatically. However, 39% of the deleted values could not be imputed at all. The main reasons are that for some parameters no proper method is available and that specific additional parameter values are required that are sometimes also missing.

Another question concerns the quality of the imputation. That means how close are the imputed values to the real values? It has to be differentiated between exact, estimated and binary imputed values. Just one of the 13 binary imputed values was wrong. However, this mainly shows the "quality" of the expert user, who probably was rather cautious and made binary assessments only when he/she felt very sure.

Table 4. Summary of randomly deleted and imputed values. Only the deleted values were attempted to impute, but not the really missing ones.

Number of Parameters	112
Number of values	448
Number of really missing values	104
Number of randomly deleted values	97
Number of completely imputed values	29
Number of estimated values	17
Number of partly imputed values (binary)	13
Number of automatically imputed values	34
Number of expert assistance	25
Number of values that could not be imputed	38

Table 5. Closeness of the imputed values. The numbers in brackets show the deviations on average in percentage.

Deviation	Number of exactly imputed values	Number of estimated values
< 3 %	14 (2.2)	9 (1.8)
< 5 %	13 (5.7)	5 (6.1)
< 10 %	2 (8.5)	2 (7.4)
> 10 %	0	1 (12.3)

The deviation (percentage) between the imputed values and the real ones is shown in table 5. Concerning the two exactly imputed values with more than 5% deviation, we consulted the expert user, who consequently altered one formula, which had been applied for both values. For the estimated values, it is conspicuous that for few values the deviation is rather big. The probable reason is that general estimation methods have problems with varying parameter courses.

5.2   Imputation of Real Missing Data and Setting up a New Model

As a consequence of the experimental results, we assumed that our method is not perfect but at least practical. So, it was attempted to impute real missing data. The result is shown in table 6.

It is no surprise that more missing values could be imputed (table 6) than randomly deleted ones (see table 2), because all imputation methods rely on other parameter values and in general holds that with an increased number of given values the chance of imputing missing values increases too. In the experiment (table 4) not just the randomly deleted values were missing but also the real missing ones.

Table 6. Summary of missing and imputed values.

Number of Parameters	112
Number of values	448
Number of missing values	104
Number of completely imputed values	37
Number of estimated values	24
Number of partly imputed values (binary)	19
Number of automatically imputed values	49
Number of expert assistance	31
Number of values that could not be imputed	24

After this imputation we return to the original problem, namely to set up a model for the hypothesis that actively participating in the fitness program improves the conditions of the patients (see section 2.1). Since many missing values have been imputed, the expert user can chose other main factors to set up the model, namely also those ones where many data had been missing before. In fact, the expert user now chose a different third factor than before, namely PTH instead of WorkJ. The resulting strongest model is shown in table 7.

Table 7. Results of Fisher's exact test, for p < 0.0001.

Patient's physical condition	Active	Non-active	Fisher Exact p
Better	39	1	< 0.0001
Worse	11	21	

The result is obviously much better than the model before (see table 1 in section 2.1). Since the missing data problem is not responsible for all exceptional cases, also for this model some (eleven) exceptional cases still have to be explained.

6 Discussion

Though statistics is the traditional method for data analysis, other intelligent data analysis methods have become popular, especially for large quantities of data, e.g. for online analytic processing [30]. Such "data mining" methods include artificial neural networks, Bayesian networks, decision trees, genetic algorithms, and statistical pattern recognition [31]. However, ISOR is designed for medical studies. Usually, there are just a few cases involved in such studies and the data sets are rather small.

Outlier detection and outlier management are interesting research topics, especially in medicine, because often measuring errors occur due to nurses and doctors being under stress. A strange data value that stands out because it is not like the rest of the data in some sense is commonly called an outlier [32]. However, in the strongest model version in the presented application of dialyse and fitness 22 out of 72 cases (this means about 30 %) contradict the hypothesis (table 1). Since the threshold of most statistical tests is 5%, in the presented application the contradicting cases should not be treated as outliers.

Furthermore, the idea of ISOR is to support research doctors in their search for reasons why cases are deviating from a research hypothesis. Usually, the doctors are not interested in this question when there are just few outlier cases. They are becoming curious when the number of such cases is rather big.

How about the ethical point of view? Patients without health insurance or with serious co-morbidities can become fiscal disasters to those who care for them. Papadimos and Marco [33] presented a philosophical discourse, with emphasis on the writings of Immanuel Kant and G.F.W. Hegel, as to why physicians have the moral imperative to give such "outliers" considerate and thoughtful care. However, the seriously ill dialyse patients should not be blamed if they do not go in for sports actively, because they might feel too week due to their physical condition.

Furthermore, ISOR is a general program applicable on medical studies. In the dialyse and fitness application the patients had the choice to actively participate in the fitness program or to do so rather passively. Usually, in medical studies patients have just the choice between different treatments (often a rather new one and an established one). Beforehand it often cannot be said which choice will lead to an outlier group.

7 Conclusion

In this chapter, it has been proposed to use CBR to explain cases that do not fit a statistical model. Here one of the simplest models was presented. However, it is relatively effective, because it demonstrates statistically significant dependencies. In the example of fitness activity and health improvement of dialysis patients the model covers about two thirds of the patients, whereas the other third can be explained by applying CBR.

The presented method makes use of different sources of knowledge and information, including medical experts. This approach seems to be a very promising method to deal with a poorly structured database, with many missing data, and with situations where cases contain different sets of attributes.

Additionally a method to impute missing values was developed. This method combines general domain independent techniques with expert knowledge, which is delivered as formulae for specific situations (treated as cases) and can be used for later similar situations too. The expert knowledge is gained within a conversational process between the medical expert, ISOR, and the system developer. Since the time of the expert is valuable, he/she is only consulted when absolutely necessary.

In ISOR, all main CBR steps are performed: retrieval, adaptation, and revision. Retrieval (of usually a list of solutions) occurs by the help of keywords. Adaptation (just like part of the imputation process of missing data) is an interactive process between ISOR, a medical expert, and the system developer. In contrast to many CBR systems, in ISOR revision plays an important role.

In principle, the active incorporation of a medical expert into the decision making process seems to be a promising idea. Already in our previous work [12], a successful Case-Based Reasoning system was developed that performed a dialog with a medical expert user to investigate therapy inefficacy.

Since CBR seems to be appropriate for medical applications (see section 2.1) and many medical CBR systems have already been developed, it stands to reason to combine both ideas, namely to build systems that are both, case-oriented and dialog-oriented.

Acknowledgements

We thank Professor Alexander Rumyantsev from the Pavlov State Medical University for his close co-operation. Furthermore we thank Professor Aleksey Smirnov, director of the Institute for Nephrology of St-Petersburg Medical University and Natalia Korosteleva, researcher at the same Institute, for collecting and managing the data.

References

1. Schank, R.C., Leake, D.B.: Creativity and learning in a case-based explainer. Artificial Intelligence 40, 353–385 (1989)
2. Kolodner, J.: Case-Based Reasoning. Morgan Kaufmann Publishers, San Mateo (1989)
3. Aamodt, A., Plaza, E.: Case-Based Reasoning: foundation issues. Methodological variation and system approaches. AI Commun. 7(1), 39–59 (1994)
4. Stottler, R.H., Henke, A.L., King, J.A.: Rapid retrieval algorithms for case-based reasoning. In: Proc of 11th Int Joint Conference on Artificial Intelligence, pp. 233–237. Morgan Kaufmann, San Mateo (1989)
5. Lenz, M., Auriol, E., Manago, M.: Diagnosis and decision support. In: Lenz, M., et al. (eds.) Case-Based Reasoning Technology. LNCS (LNAI), vol. 1400, pp. 51–90. Springer, Heidelberg (1998)
6. Broder, A.: Strategies for efficient incremental nearest neighbor search. Pattern Recognition 23, 171–178 (1990)
7. Wilke, W., Smyth, B., Cunningham, P.: Using Configuration Techniques for Adaptation. In: Lenz, M., Bartsch-Spörl, B., Burkhard, H.-D., Wess, S. (eds.) Case-Based Reasoning Technology, From Foundations to Applications, pp. 139–168. Springer, Heidelberg (1998)

8. Gierl, L.: Klassifikationsverfahren in Expertensystemen für die Medizin. Mellen Univ. Press, Lewiston (1992)
9. Gierl, L., Bull, M., Schmidt, R.: CBR in Medicine. In: Lenz, M., Bartsch-Spörl, B., Burkhard, H.-D., Wess, S. (eds.) Case-Based Reasoning Technology. LNCS (LNAI), vol. 1400, pp. 273–297. Springer, Heidelberg (1998)
10. Schmidt, R., Montani, S., Bellazzi, R., Portinale, L., Gierl, L.: Case-Based Reasoning for Medical Knowledge-based Systems. International Journal of Medical Informatics 64(2-3), 355–367 (2001)
11. Nilsson, M., Sollenborn, N.: Advancements and trends in medical case-based reasoning: An overview of systems and system developments. In: Proceedings Seventeenth International Florida Artificial Intelligence Research Society Conference, pp. 178–183. AAAI Press, Menlo Park (2004)
12. Schmidt, R., Vorobieva, O.: Case-Based Reasoning Investigation of Therapy Inefficacy. Knowledge-Based Systems 19(5), 333–340 (2006)
13. Aha, D.W., McSherry, D., Yang, Q.: Advances in conversational Case-Based Reasoning. Knowledge Engineering Review 20, 247–254 (2005)
14. Kendall, M.G., Stuart, A.: The advanced theory of statistics. Macmillan publishing, New York (1979)
15. Hai, G.A.: Logic of diagnostic and decision making in clinical medicine. Politheknica publishing, St. Petersburg (2002)
16. Perner, P. (ed.): Case-Based Reasoning on Images and Signals. Springer, Heidelberg (2007)
17. Bichindaritz, I., Kansu, E., Sullivan, K.M.: Case-based Reasoning in Care-Partner. In: Smyth, B., Cunningham, P. (eds.) EWCBR 1998. LNCS (LNAI), vol. 1488, pp. 334–345. Springer, Heidelberg (1998)
18. Montai, S., Magni, P., Bellazzi, R., Larizza, C., Roudsari, C., Carsson, E.R.: Integration model-based decision support in multi-modal reasoning system for managing type 1 diabetic patients. Artificial Intelligence in Medicine 29(1-2), 131–151 (2003)
19. Prentzas, J., Hatzilgeroudis, I.: Integrating Hybrid Rule-Based with Case-Based Reasoning. In: Craw, S., Preeece, A. (eds.) ECCBR 2002. LNCS (LNAI), vol. 2416, pp. 336–349. Springer, Heidelberg (2002)
20. Shuguang, L., Qing, J., George, C.: Combining case-based and model-based reasoning: a formal specification. In: Proc APSEC 2000, p. 416 (2000)
21. Corchado, J.M., Corchado, E.S., Aiken, J., Fyfe, C., Fernandez, F., Gonzalez, M.: Maximum likelihood Hebbian learning based retrieval method for CBR systems. In: Ashley, K.D., Bridge, D.G. (eds.) ICCBR 2003. LNCS, vol. 2689, pp. 107–121. Springer, Heidelberg (2003)
22. Rezvani, S., Prasad, G.: A hybrid system with multivariate data validation and Case-based Reasoning for an efficient and realistic product formulation. In: Ashley, K.D., Bridge, D.G. (eds.) ICCBR 2003. LNCS, vol. 2689, pp. 465–478. Springer, Heidelberg (2003)
23. Arshadi, N., Jurisica, I.: Data Mining for Case-based Reasoning in high-dimensional biological domains. IEEE Transactions on Knowledge and Data Engineering 17(8), 1127–1137 (2005)
24. Davidson, A.M., Cameron, J.S., Grünfeld, J.-P. (eds.): Oxford Textbook of Nephrology, vol. 3. Oxford University Press, Oxford (2005)
25. McSherry, D.: Interactive Case-Based Reasoning in sequential diagnosis. Applied Intelligence 14(1), 65–76 (2001)
26. Little, R., Rubin, D.: Statistical analysis with missing data. John Wiley & Sons, Chichester (1987)

27. Fleiss, J.: The design and analysis of clinical experiments. John Wiley & Sons, Chichester (1986)
28. Gediga, G., Düntsch, I.: Maximum Consistency of Incomplete Data via Non-Invasive Imputation. Artificial Intelligence Review 19(1), 93–107 (2003)
29. Lieber, J.: Application of the revision theory to adaptation in Case-Based Reasoning: The conservative adaptation. In: Weber, R.O., Richter, M.M. (eds.) ICCBR 2007. LNCS (LNAI), vol. 4626, pp. 239–253. Springer, Heidelberg (2007)
30. Codd, E.F.: Providing OLAP (On-Line Analytic Processing) to User-Analysts: Am IT Mandate. E.F. Codd and Associates (1994)
31. Piatetsky-Shapiro, G., Frawley, W.J.: Knowledge Discovery in Databases. AAAI Press/The MIT Press (1991)
32. Cheng, J.G.: Outlier Management in Intelligent Data Analysis. PhD Thesis (2000), http://www.dcs.bbk.ac.uk/research/recentphds/gcheng.pdf (last visited May 2008)
33. Papadimos, T.J., Marco, A.P.: The obligation of phyicians to medical outliers: a Kantian and Hegelian synthesis. BMC Medical Ethics 5(3) (2004)

Chapter 13
Computational Intelligence Techniques for Classification in Microarray Analysis

Juan F. De Paz[1], Javier Bajo[2], Sara Rodríguez[1], and Juan M. Corchado[1]

[1] Departamento de Informática y Automática, Universidad de Salamanca
Plaza de la Merced s/n, 37008, Salamanca, España
[2] Universidad Pontificia de Salamanca
Compañía 5, 37002, Salamanca, España
{fcofds,srg,corchado}@usal.es, jbajope@upsa.es

Abstract. During the last few years there has been a growing need for using computational intelligence techniques to analyze microarray data. The aim of the system presented in this study is to provide innovative decision support techniques for classifying data from microarrays and for extracting knowledge about the classification process. The computational intelligence techniques used in this chapter follow the case-based reasoning paradigm to emulate the steps followed in expression analysis. This work presents a novel filtering technique based on statistical methods, a new clustering technique that uses ESOINN (Enhanced Self-Organizing Incremental Neuronal Network), and a knowledge extraction technique based on the RIPPER algorithm. The system presented within this chapter has been applied to classify CLL patients and extract knowledge about the classification process. The results obtained permit us to conclude that the system provides a notable reduction of the dimensionality of the data obtained from microarrays. Moreover, the classification process takes the detection of relevant and irrelevant probes into account, which is fundamental for subsequent classification and an extraction of knowledge tool with a graphical interface to explain the classification process, and has been much appreciated by the human experts. Finally, the philosophy of the CBR systems facilitates the resolution of new problems using past experiences, which is very appropriate regarding the classification of leukemia.

Keywords: Case-based Reasoning, HG U133, ESOINN, CLL leukemia classification, decision rules.

1 Introduction

The use of computational intelligence techniques has become fundamental in medicine, since there is a growing need of decision support tool that facilitate the monitoring of patients and the automatic processing of patient's data [1] [2] [3]. One of the fields in medicine requiring computational intelligence is the analysis of microarrays, and more specifically expression arrays, for the analysis of different sequences of

I. Bichindaritz et al. (Eds.): Computational Intelligence in Healthcare 4, SCI 309, pp. 289–312.
springerlink.com   © Springer-Verlag Berlin Heidelberg 2010

oligonucleotides [1] [4]. The data obtained from microarrays are an important source of knowledge to prevent and detect cancer. The analysis of this information allows the detection of patterns that characterize certain diseases and, most importantly, the genes associated with these different diseases. Since the amount of data obtained from microarrays is huge and the time required to analyze the data is very high, it is necessary to obtained novel computational techniques that can provide automatic processing and artificial intelligence techniques that provide behaviours similar to the human ones.

An expression analysis basically consists of three stages: normalization and filtering; clustering and classification; and extraction of knowledge. These stages are carried out from the luminescence values found in the probes. Presently, the number of probes containing expression arrays has increased considerably to the extent that it has become necessary to use new methods and techniques to analyze the information more efficiently [5]. It is necessary to develop new techniques to analyze large volumes of data, extract the relevant information, and delete the information which has no relevance to the classification process. Moreover, the knowledge obtained during the classification process is of great importance for subsequent classifications. There are various artificial intelligence techniques such as artificial neural networks [6] [7], bayesian networks [8], and fuzzy logic [9] which have been applied to microarray analysis. While these techniques can be applied at various stages of expression analysis, the knowledge obtained cannot be incorporated into successive tests and included in subsequent analyses.

The system proposed in the context of this work focuses on the detection of carcinogenic patterns in the data from microarrays for patients, and is constructed from a CBR system that provides a classification technique based on previous experiences [11]. The system is an evolution of our previous work in the classification of leukemia patients [12], where a mixture of experts was used. The incorporation of the CBR paradigm to health care [13] [14] provides additional learning and adaptation capabilities. Moreover. The filtering and extraction of knowledge models have been improved and new techniques have been incorporated. The purpose of case-based reasoning (CBR) is to solve new problems by adapting solutions that have been used to solve similar problems in the past [10]. A CBR manages cases (past experiences) to solve new problems. The way cases are managed is known as the CBR cycle, and consists of four sequential steps which are recalled every time that a problem needs to be solved: retrieve, reuse, revise and retain. Each of the steps of the CBR life cycle requires a model or method in order to perform its mission.

The approach presented in this work focuses on the classification of subtypes of leukemia, specifically, to detect patterns and extract subgroups within the CLL type of leukemia, and incorporates various techniques of computational intelligence at different stages of the reasoning cycle of a CBR system. In the retrieve phase, new pre-processing and filtering techniques are incorporated in order to select the probes with relevant information for classifying patients. This innovative method notably reduces the dimensionality of the data, which makes it possible to use techniques with greater computational complexity in later stages of the CBR cycle, which would otherwise be unviable. The reuse stage incorporates a classification technique based on ESOINN [15] neural networks, that proposes a novel method for generating clusters, and for identifying the nearest cluster for the final classification. An additional grouping technique known as PAM [16] (Partition around medoids), is also used, resulting in a more accurate classification, since the results suggested by the ESOINN network are compared to those obtained using the PAM technique. The revise phase initiates a RIPPER [43] algorithm for extracting knowledge about the classification process. Moreover, the revise stage includes a MDS (Multidimensional Scaling) technique [18] [19] [20] for presenting information in low dimensionality. Additionally, a human expert analyzes this information and evaluates the proposed classification as well as the validity of the rules generated. Finally, in the retain stage, if the human expert considers the proposed solution valid, the system stores the case information and the rules that have been obtained.

The chapter is structured as follows: the next section briefly introduces the problem that motivates this research. Section 3 presents the approach presented in this work and describes the novel strategies incorporated in the stages of the CBR cycle. Section 4 details the innovative computational intelligence techniques presented in this work. Section 5 describes a case study specifically developed to evaluate the CBR system presented within this study, consisting of a classification of CLL leukemia patients. Finally, Section 6 presents the results and conclusions obtained after testing the model.

2 Related Work

Microarray has become an essential tool in genomic research, making it possible to investigate global gene expression in all aspects of human disease [21]. Microarray technology is based on a database of gene fragments called ESTs (Expressed Sequence Tags), which are used to measure target abundance using the scanned fluorescence intensities from tagged molecules hybridized to ESTs [22]. Specifically, the HG U133 plus 2.0 [5] are chips used for expression analysis. These chips analyze the expression level of over 47.000 transcripts and variants, including 38.500 well-characterized human genes. It is comprised of more than 54.000 probe sets and 1.300.000 distinct oligonucleotide features. The HG U133 plus 2.0 provides multiple, independent measurements for each transcript. The use of Multiple probes provides a complete data set with accurate, reliable, reproducible results from every experiment. Microarray technology is a critical element for genomic analysis and allows an in-depth study of molecular characterization of RNA expression, genomic changes, epigenetic modifications or protein/DNA unions.

Expression arrays [5] are a type of microarrays that have been used in different approaches to identify the genes that characterize certain diseases [23] [24] [25]. In all cases, the data analysis process is essentially composed of three stages: normalization and filtering; clustering; and classification. The first step is critical to achieve both a good normalization of data and an initial filtering to reduce the dimensionality of the data set with which to work [26]. Since the problem at hand is working with high-dimensional arrays, it is important to have a good pre-processing technique that can facilitate automatic decision-making about the variables that will be vital for the classification process. In light of these decisions it will be possible to reduce the original dataset. Moreover, the choice of a clustering technique allows data to be grouped according to certain variables that dominate the behaviour of the group. After organizing into groups it is possible to extract knowledge and classify patients within the group which presents the most similarities.

Case-based reasoning [11] is particularly applicable to this problem domain because it (i) supports a rich and evolvable representation of experiences, problems, solutions and feedback; (ii) provides efficient and flexible ways to retrieve these experiences; and (iii) applies analogical reasoning to solve new problems [27]. CBR systems can be used to propose new solutions or evaluate solutions to avoid potential problems. The chapter of CBR in health care is discussed in [13] [14], where the advantages of this paradigm are remarked. The research in [28] suggests that analogical reasoning is particularly applicable to the biological domain, in part because biological systems are often homologous (rooted in evolution). Moreover, biologists often use a form of reasoning similar to CBR, where experiments are designed and performed based on the similarity between features of a new system and those of known systems. In [29] a mixture of experts for case-based reasoning (MOE4CBR) is proposed. It is a method that combines an ensemble of CBR classifiers with spectral clustering and logistic regression, but does not incorporates extraction of knowledge techniques and does not focus on dimensionality reduction. Some approaches such as [11] provide CBR solutions and knowledge extraction techniques, facilitating the comprehension of the classification process. This chapter presents a CBR solution which also incorporates new knowledge extraction techniques, but additionally focuses on the definition of innovative strategies for dimensionality reduction and clustering. The following section presents a detailed account of the CBR system proposed in this work.

3   CBR System as Paradigm for Classifying Microarray Data

This section presents the CBR system proposed in the context of this research and provides a classification technique based on previous experiences for data from microarrays. The CBR developed system imitates the behaviour of human experts in the laboratory and incorporates innovative knowledge discovery techniques. The system receives data from the analysis of chips and is responsible for classifying individuals based on evidence and existing data.

The purpose of CBR is to solve new problems by taking into account similar problems that were previously resolved in the past [10]. The primary concept when working with CBRs is the concept of case. A case can be defined as a past experience, and is composed of three elements: a problem description which describes the initial problem; a solution which provides the sequence of actions carried out in order to solve the problem; and the final stage which describes the state achieved once the solution was applied. A CBR manages cases (past experiences) to solve new problems. The way cases are managed is known as the CBR cycle, and consists of four sequential steps which are recalled every time a problem needs to be solved: retrieve, reuse, revise and retain. Each step of the CBR life cycle requires a model or method in order to perform its mission.

In the CBR system proposed within this study, the retrieve phase filters variables, and recovers important variables from the cases to determine the most influential for the classification. Once the most important variables have been retrieved, the reuse phase begins adapting the solutions for the retrieved cases to obtain the clustering. Once this grouping is accomplished, the next step is knowledge extraction. The revise phase consists of an expert revision for the proposed solution, and finally, the retain phase allows the system to learn from the experiences obtained in the three previous phases, consequently updating the cases memory.

A key element in a CBR system is a case, which can be defined as a past experience [10] and is composed of three elements: problem description, problem solution, and the final state obtained after applying the solution. A case in the system presented in this work contains information related to the patient, the rules, the proposed classification, and the probes marked as irrelevant or important. The case is defined by the following expression:

$$i_j = (id, S = (A_1, ..., A_n), C^p, C^r)$$

where $i_j \in I$ and $I = \{i_1, ..., i_s\}$ is the set of individuals/cases, A is the set of all the probes, A_i represents the probe i, C^p is the predicted class and C^r the actual class.

In addition to the cases memory, our system incorporates a memory of rules that contains the information extracted through the knowledge extraction techniques. The memory of rules is structured as follows:

$$R = \{r_1, ..., r_l\}, \qquad \text{with} \qquad r_i = (l_1 \wedge ... \wedge l_m) \rightarrow c_j \text{ where}$$

$$l_s = (d_{ts}, o_s, \Re) / d_{ts} \in D_t, o_s \in O, S_{Irr} \subseteq A$$

where R is the set of rules from the decision rules, l_s contains a set of discretized probes, an operator and a real value, D_t is the discretization value for the probe A_t, $O = \{=, \neq, >, <, \leq, \geq\}$ operator, and S_{Irr} is the set of probes marked as irrelevant, $c_j \in C^p$.

When a new case is classified, a new decision rules are generated in the revise stage. A set of rules are extracted which provide knowledge about the relevance of the probes in the clustering and classification process. Figure 1 shows a scheme of the techniques applied in the different stages of the CBR cycle. As seen in Figure 1, the important probes that allow the classification of patients are recovered in the Retrieve phase. The Retrieve phase is divided into 6 sub-phases: pre-processing through RMA, removal of irrelevant variables, uniform distribution, probes without meaningful cut-off points, and correlated variables. In the Reuse phase the patients are grouped by means of an ESOINN neural network. Then, the patients with no prior classification are assigned to a group using the nearest cluster. In the Revise phase the RIPPER [43] algorithm is applied for extracting knowledge about the most important probes for the classification, and the MDS technique [18] [19] [20] is used to make a representation in low dimensionality. Finally, in the Retain phase, the knowledge is updated. This knowledge includes the case classification, the decision rules obtained, and the information associated with the importance or irrelevance of certain probes extracted from the rules. Figure 1 shows the scheme of the CBR system proposed within this study.

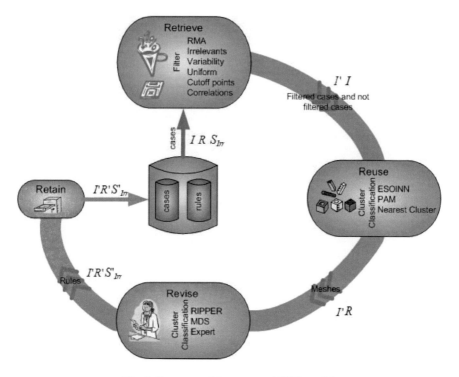

Fig. 1. Structure of the proposed CBR model

3.1 Retrieve

Traditionally, only the cases similar to the current problem are recovered, often because of performance, and then adapted. With regards to expression array, the number of cases is not a critical factor, rather the number of variables. For this reason, we have incorporated an innovative filtering strategy where variables are retrieved at this stage and then, depending on the identified variables, the rest of the stages of the CBR are carried out. The new strategy allows a notable reduction in the dimensionality of the data.

3.2 Reuse

In this phase the clustering of individuals is carried out, along with the classification of new individuals to one of the clusters. This chapter proposes a hybrid solution that takes into account a ESOINN neural network and the PAM method.

3.3 Revise

As shown in Figure 1, the revision is carried out by a human expert who determines if the group assigned by the system is correct. To facilitate the human expert task, the equivalence index and the error rate were calculated in the reuse stage. It is important for the medical human expert to understand the classification process performed in the two previous stages. In this sense, the system presented in this work provides a knowledge extraction method in the Revise phase. This method analyses the steps followed in the retrieve and reuse stages, and extracts knowledge which is then formalized in rules. In this way, the human expert can easily evaluate the classification and extract conclusions concerning the efficiency of the classification process. A RIPPER algorithm is used.

3.4 Retain

If the human expert identifies relevant information at the revise stage, the knowledge is acquired and the information obtained is stored. The information that is stored corresponds to the classifications considered correct, the decision rules generated that are considered relevant, and the probes marked as irrelevant. The information stored is divided into the cases memory I and the memory of rules R and S_{Irr}. Figure 1 shows the structure of the retain stage. Taking the revision of the expert into account, the system learns from the new experience and stores the information that the expert established as relevant. The stored information can include probes, classifications and rules.

4   Innovative Computational Intelligence Techniques for Dimensionality Reduction and Classification Improvement

This chapter details the innovative computational techniques included in the CBR phases of the system. The innovations consist of dimensionality reduction, classification improvements and extraction of knowledge technique. As the computational intelligence algorithms are included in the different phases of a CBR cycle, in this section we are going to present each of the novel algorithms as a part of the phases of the CBR cycle. Figure 1 details the steps followed in each of the stages of the CBR cycle. The structure of the CBR system proposed will now be explained in detail, presenting innovative techniques modelled in each of the stages of the CBR.

4.1 Filtering

This computational intelligence technique is carried out in the retrieve phase of the CBR cycle. The filtering phase is carried out on I together with the new case i_s. The filtering is only applied to those probes not associated with any of the rules. First, a pre-processing of the data is conducted using RMA. Then, the 5 filtering sub-phases are executed: removal of control probes, removal of erroneous probes, removal of low variability probes, removal of probes with a uniform distribution, and removal of correlated probes. These five sub-phases are outlined in the following paragraphs.

4.1.1   RMA

This phase begins once the laboratory experiment with microarrays has been completed. The researcher obtains various files that contain gross intensity values. Prior to analyzing the data, it is important to complete the pre-processing phase, which eliminates defective samples and standardizes the data. This phase is normally divided into 3 sub-phases: background correction, standardization, and summarization. There is currently a limited group of algorithms that investigators use for performing these steps. The most common are MAS5.0 [30] (Microarray Affymetrix Suite 5.0), PLIER [31] (Probe Logarithmic Intensity Error), and RMA) [32] (Robust Multi-array Average).

The RMA [32] algorithm is method for normalizing and summarizing probe-level intensity measurements. It analyzes the values for the PM (Perfect-Match): in the first step, a Background Correction is carried out to remove the noise from the averages of the PM; in the second step, the data is quantile normalized in order to compare data from different microarrays; finally, a summarization is made and the values for each probe-set are generated.

4.1.2 Irrelevant Probes
Once the control and the erroneous probes have been eliminated, the filtering process begins. The first step consists of eliminating the probes marked as irrelevant in previous executions of the CBR cycle. This way, all probes that can pass the filtering phase, but are prone to cause erroneous results during the reuse phase, are removed.

4.1.3 Variability
The second stage is to remove the probes that have low variability. This work is carried out according to the following steps:

1. Calculate the standard deviation for each of the probes j

$$\sigma_{.j} = +\sqrt{\frac{1}{n}\sum_{j=1}^{n}\left(\overline{\mu}_{.j} - x_{ij}\right)^2} \tag{1}$$

Where n is the total number of cases, $\overline{\mu}_{.j}$ is the average population for the variable j, and x_{ij} is the value of the probe j for the individual i.

2. Standardize the above values

$$z_i = \frac{\sigma_{.j} - \mu}{\sigma} \tag{2}$$

Where $\mu = \dfrac{1}{n}\sum_{j=1}^{n}\sigma_{.j}$ and $\sigma_{.j} = +\sqrt{\dfrac{1}{n}\sum_{j=1}^{n}\left(\overline{\mu}_{.j} - x_{ij}\right)^2}$ where $z_i \equiv N(0,1)$

3. Discard probes for which the value of z meets the following condition: $z < -1.0$. This will achieve the removal of about 16% of the probes if the variable follows a normal distribution.

4.1.4 Uniform Distribution
Finally, all remaining variables that follow a uniform distribution are eliminated. The variables that follow a uniform distribution will not allow the separation of individuals. Therefore, the variables that do not follow this distribution will be really useful

variables in the classification of the cases. The contrast of assumptions is explained below, using the Kolmogorov-Smirnov [33] test as an example. H0: the data follow a uniform distribution; H1: the analyzed data do not follow a uniform distribution. Statistical contrast:

$$D = \max\{D^+, D^-\} \tag{3}$$

where $D^+ = \max\limits_{1 \le i \le n}\left\{\dfrac{i}{n} - F_0(x_i)\right\}$ $D^- = \max\limits_{1 \le i \le n}\left\{F_0(x_i) - \dfrac{i-1}{n}\right\}$ with i as the pattern

of entry, n the number of items and $F_0(x_i)$ the probability of observing values less than i with H_0 being true. The value of statistical contrast is compared to the next value:

$$D_\alpha = \frac{C_\alpha}{k(n)} \tag{4}$$

in the special case of uniform distribution $k(n) = \sqrt{n} + 0.12 + \dfrac{0.11}{\sqrt{n}}$ and a level of

significance $\alpha = 0.05$ $C_\alpha = 1.358$.

4.1.5 Cut-Off Points

This step removes the probes that, despite not following a uniform distribution, have no separation between elements, and do not allow the elements to be partitioned. The way to remove the probes is to detect changes in the densities of the data, and to se-lect the final probes. The probes in which cut-offs or high densities are not detected are eliminated, as they do not provide useful information to the classification process. This will keep the probes that allow the separation of individuals. The detection of the separation intervals is performed by calculating the distance between adjacent indi-viduals. Once the distance is calculated, it is possible to determine the potentially relevant values. The selection is carried out by applying confidence intervals for the values of these differences if the values follow a uniform distribution, or by selecting the values above a certain percentile if the values do not follow a normal distribution. This process is formalized as follows:

1. Let I' be the set of individuals with filtered probes together with the new in-dividual, where $x_{.j}$ represents the probe j for all the individuals, and x_{ij} the individual i for the probe j

2. Select the probe $j = 1$, $x_{.j}$

3. Sort in increasing order values $x_{.j}$

4. Calculate the value for $x'_{ij} = x_{i+1j} - x_{ij}$

5. Determine if the variable x'_{ij} follows a uniform distribution by means of the Shapiro-Wilk test [34], otherwise go to step 10.

6. Calculate the value for $\overline{x}'_{\cdot j}$

7. Establish the confidence interval for the variance, which is established as

$$\sigma'^2_{\cdot j} \in \left[\frac{(n-1) \cdot S^2}{\chi^2_{n-1,1-\alpha/2}}, \frac{(n-1) \cdot S^2}{\chi^2_{n-1,\alpha/2}} \right] \text{ with } \alpha = 0.05 \text{ and } n =\# x'_{\cdot j} \text{ and the}$$

number of elements for $x'_{\cdot j}$, S is the sampling variance.

8. Establish the set of elements form x'_{ij} not belonging to the set

$$Q_j = \left\{ x'_{ij} \, / \, x'_{ij} \notin I_{\sigma_j} \right\}$$

9. Go to step 11.

10. Select those values up to the percentile P_α from every $x'_{\cdot j}$ and establish the

set $Q_j = \left\{ x'_{ij} \, / \, x'_{ij} > P_\alpha \right\}$

11. Select the probe $j+1$ in the case of more probes needing revision and go to step 2.

12. Create the new set of probes

$$I' = \bigcup x'_{\cdot j} \, / \, \exists x'_{ij} \in Q_j \, / \, i >\# x' \cdot u \wedge i <\# x' - \# x' \cdot u$$

13. Finalize and return the new set of individuals with the filtered probes I'

4.1.6 Correlations

At the last stage of the filtering process, correlated variables are eliminated so that only the independent variables remain. To this end, the linear correlation index of Pearson is calculated and the probes meeting the following condition are eliminated.

$$r_{x_i y_{\cdot j}} > \alpha \tag{5}$$

given: $\alpha = 0.95$ $\quad r_{x_i y_{\cdot j}} = \dfrac{\sigma_{x_i x_j}}{\sigma_{x_i} \sigma_{x_j}}, \quad \sigma_{x_i x_j} = \dfrac{1}{N} \displaystyle\sum_{s=1}^{n} \left(\overline{\mu}_{\cdot i} - x_{si} \right)\left(\overline{\mu}_{\cdot j} - x_{sj} \right)$ where

$\sigma_{x_i x_j}$ is the covariance between probes i and j.

4.2 Classification

There are several algorithms for clustering, but the most common are the hierarchical algorithms [35] and those based on partitioning [16]. Within the hierarchical algorithms the most common is the dendrogram [35]. The dendrograms are hierarchical methods that initially define conglomerates for each available case. At each stage the method joins the conglomerates with a smaller distance, and calculates the distance of the conglomerate with respect to the others. The new distances are updated in the distance matrix. The process finishes when there is only one conglomerate (agglomerative method) remaining.

Among the partition-based methods it is possible to find alternatives based on RNAs such as SOM [36] (Self-Organizing Map), GNG [37] (Growing Neural Gas) or

SOINN [38] (Self-Organizing Incremental Neuronal Network). Other alternatives are the methods based on heuristics, such as k-means [39] or PAM [16]. These two methods define a series of initial clusters which correspond to a new individual or to existing individuals, and are marked as the cluster representatives, while the remaining individuals are allocated to the nearest cluster. The problem with each of these methods is that they do not consider changes in the distribution of densities of individuals, and usually do not detect clusters with atypical forms, such as elongated clusters.

4.2.1 ESOINN Neural Network

Neural Networks based on GNG, allow detecting clusters with atypical forms, adjusting iteratively to the distribution of the individuals, and detecting low density zones. There are variants of the GNG, such as the GCS [40] (Growing Cell Structure) or SOINN [38] (Self-Organizing Incremental Neuronal Network). Unlike self-organizing maps based on meshes, Growing Grid or GCS do not set the number of neurons, or the degree of connectivity, but they do establish the dimensionality of each mesh. This complicates the separation phase between groups once the neurons are distributed evenly across the surface. The ESOINN neural network [15] (Enhanced Self-Organizing Incremental Neuronal Network) is a variation of the SOINN neural network [38], which allows the creation of a single layer, while ESOINN is able to incorporate both the distribution process along the surface and the separation between low density groups. The learning process of the network is distributed into two stages: the first stage of competition CHL [40] (Competitive Hebbian Learning) where the closest node to the input pattern is selected; and the second adaptation/growing stage similar to a GNG. The training phase and the various algorithms applied at every modified stage are outlined below:

1. Update the weights of neurons by following a process similar to the SOINN, but introducing a new definition for the learning rate in order to provide greater stability for the model. This learning rate has produced good results in other networks such as SOM [42].

$$\Delta W_{a_1} = n_1(M_{a_1})(\xi - W_{a_1})$$
$$\Delta W_{a_i} = n_2(M_{a_1})(\xi - W_{a_i}) \text{ with } a_i \in N_{a_1} \tag{6}$$

Where $n_1(x) = \dfrac{1}{\sqrt{x}}$, $n_2(x) = \dfrac{1}{\sqrt{2 + x^2}}$, a_i is neuron i, ξ is the input pattern,

M_{a_1} is the number of winnings of neuron a_i, N_{a_1} is the set of neighbours of a_i.

2. Delete the connections with higher age. The ages are standardized and those whose values are in the region of rejection with k>0 are removed. The assigned value of α is 0.05, therefore

$$z_i = \frac{e_i - \mu}{\sigma} \text{ , } z \equiv N(0,1) \text{ then } f(z) = \frac{1}{\sqrt{2\pi}} Exp\left[\frac{-z^2}{2}\right] \tag{7}$$

Where $P(z < k) = \alpha / 2 \;\rightarrow\; P(z < k) = 0.975 \;\rightarrow\; \Theta(z) = 0.975$ k=1.96

Therefore all z values that are greater than 1.96 are deleted

3. Once all input patterns have been introduced then a KS-Test [33] is carried out in order to determine if the density distribution for the neurons in each group follows a normal distribution. If so, the learning procedure is finished; otherwise the next pattern is processed. The value of α chosen is 0.05.

Once the cases have been distributed in the meshes, it is necessary to assign each of the meshes to a class according to the following procedure: Let I' be the set of individuals once the probes have been filtered and G^E the set of clusters created by means of the ESOINN neural network, defined as $G^E = \{g^E / g^E \subseteq I'\}$, where $g_i^E \cap g_j^E = \phi, \forall i \neq j$ with $g_i^E, g_j^E \in G^E$. Let C be the set of existing classes for the individuals where $c_j \in C$ is the class j in the set. We can say that the mesh i, g_i^E belongs to a class j, $g_i^E \in c_j$ and is represented as $g_{i_{c_j}}^E$ when

$$\max_{c_j \in C} \frac{\# I_{c_j} / g_i^E}{\# I_{c_j}} \cdot \frac{\# I'_{c_j}}{\# I'} \tag{8}$$

where $I'_{c_j} = \{s \in I / s \in c_j\}$ and I'_{c_j} / g_i^E is the set of individuals from c_j restricted to the group g_i^E.

The set of meshes belonging to the class is denoted as $G_{c_j}^E$ and is defined by the expression (9).

$$G_{c_j}^E = \bigcup_{g_{i_{c_j}}^E \in G^E} g_{i_{c_j}}^E \tag{9}$$

4.2.2 PAM
The PAM algorithm [16] is executed parallel to the clustering in order to facilitate a comparison of the results obtained. The classification made by both methods, PAM and ESOINN, generates an equivalence index between the two methods that determines the consistency of the reuse phase. The algorithm used for PAM is as follows:

1. Select the number of clusters depending on $\# C$.
2. The metric used for the distance is the same as the one used in the ESOINN network
3. Classify the patients taking all of the variables into account, without any filtering $G^P = \{g^P / g^P \subseteq I\}$ with $g_i^P \cap g_j^P = \phi, \forall i \neq j$

4. Once the groups G^P are created, an assignation is made following the procedure indicated in (8).

4.2.3 Equivalence Index
Once the individuals have been classified using both the PAM and the ESOINN neural networks, the equivalence index for both methods eq is calculated, and the error

rate for the ESOINN network is determined as a function of the pre-classified cases. The equivalence index is defined as indicated in (10):

$$eq = \frac{\#\left\{ i \in I' / i \in c_j^E \wedge i \in c_j^P \right\}}{\# I'} \tag{10}$$

Where c_j^E represents the set of meshes belonging to class j through the ESOINN network and c_j^P represents the set of individuals belonging to class j through the PAM algorithm.

4.2.4 Classification
Once the meshes are generated by the clustering process, previously unclassified individuals are now classified by selecting the nearest mesh. When the mesh has been selected, the case is assigned to the class of the mesh selected. The assignment is defined as (11).

$$i_s \in G_{k_{c_j}}^E \rightarrow i_u \in C_j \tag{11}$$

where i_u is the unclassified individual, i_s is the individual closest to the individual i_u calculated using the Euclidean distance.

As shown in Figure 1, the reuse stage receives the filtered and not-filtered data resulting from the retriever stage as inputs. The input is used for both the ESOINN neural network and the PAM technique. The ESOINN neural network generates a set of groups assigned to different classes. These groups are composed of meshes containing different elements together with the information of the previous classification. The PAM technique repeats the same project concurrently and generates the groups for each of the classes. The groups generated by PAM contain the individuals and their previous classification, but do not consider sub-groups. Finally, the equivalence index is calculated and the new patient is classified. The error rate for the ESOINN network is made through (8) to determine the class for each of the groups.

4.3 Knowledge Extraction

The knowledge extraction phase detects anomalous classifications, since it accounts for the existence of probes with irrelevant information, or those that were decisive for the misclassification. Sometimes, the existence of certain probes causes a classification of patients based on erroneous criteria, such as the distinction between men and women. Such a classification, without being wrong, is irrelevant to the problem, which is why the probes that can cause these classifications are analyzed at this stage. If the human expert notes that the probes contain irrelevant information, they are marked as irrelevant and not taken into account in the next iteration of the CBR cycle.

The extraction of knowledge that is presented to the human expert is carried out using the RIPPER [43]. There are other alternatives for the generation of decision rules which operate similar to the decision trees, including J48 [17] and PART [44]. These methods extract similar information to classify individuals according to decision rules. The results are similar for the different methods.

The general objective of extraction of knowledge techniques is to provide a human expert with information about the system-generated classification by means of a set of rules that support the decision-making process. It should be noted that knowledge extraction techniques are not intended to substitute the rationale and experience of a human expert during a diagnosis, rather to complement the process and serve as an additional methodology or guideline for common procedures in analysis.

The process is described in the following steps. Let I' be the set of individuals and s the number of probes once the filtering process has finished:

$$f_r : A_1 \times ... \times A_s \rightarrow A_1' \times ... \times A_s'$$

$$(a_1,...,a_s) \rightarrow f_r(a_1,...,a_s) = (a_1',...,a_s')$$

where $A_i' \in [0,1]$ is the value of the term i using the function f_r and is obtained in the following way:

$$a_i' = \frac{a_i - \min(A_i)}{\max(A_i) - \min(A_i)}$$

Finally the values are discretized by means of f_u in a series of predefined levels t.

$$f_u : A_1' \times ... \times A_s' \rightarrow \overbrace{D \times ... \times D}^{s}$$

$$(a_1',...,a_s') \rightarrow f_u(a_1',...,a_s') = (d_1',...,d_s')$$

where $D = \bigcup_{i \in \{0,...,t-1\}} i \cdot \frac{1}{t-1}$, we can say that $d_i' = d_j$ if applying the function f_u,

with $d_j \in D$ if $d_i' \in [d_j - 1/(2t), \ d_j + 1/(2t)]$.

Once the transformation is finished, the set of individuals is determined by the sub-set $I' \subseteq \overbrace{D \times ... \times D}^{s}$ of the data, and RIPPER is used to generate the rules that classify the individuals. The use of RIPPER, allows rules to be obtained for classifying an individual $i_k \in I'$ to the class c_j by means of rules similar to:

$$r_i = (l_1 \wedge ... \wedge l_m) \rightarrow c_j$$

where d_p is the value for the attribute p for the individual i_k. In this way the set is defined for rules R' that classify the individuals for each of the classes.

The input corresponds to the discretization of the values (if the reuse phase has been successful). Subsequently, knowledge extraction is applied through the RIPPER. Finally, the relevant information extracted is stored (probes inconsequential, important and results of the classification). At this stage a 3D representation with the information retrieved is displayed. The dimensionality is reduced by using MDS [18] [19] [20].

5 Case Study: Computational Intelligence Techniques for Classification of CLL Leukemia

Microarray analysis has made it possible to characterize the molecular mechanisms that cause several cancers. Regarding leukemia, microarray analysis has facilitated the identification of certain characteristic genes in the different variants of leukemia [24] [41] [45]. Cancer experts remark on the importance of the identification of the genes associated to each type of cancer in order to establish the most efficient treatments for the patients [46] [47]. The Cancer Institute in the city of Salamanca was interested in novel tools for decision support in the process of CLL (Chronic Lymphocytic Leukemia) patient classification. In this way, we focus on a concrete leukemia subtype, while our previous works were aimed at classifying patients into leukemia subtypes [12].

The Institute provided us with 91 samples of patient data and asked for a tool to provide decision support in the expression array analysis process and to incorporate innovative techniques to reduce the dimensionality of the data and identify the variables with a higher influence in the patient's classification. The samples corresponded to patients affected by chronic lymphocytic leukemia. CLL is a disease of lymphocytes that appear to be mature but are biologically immature. These B lymphocytes arise from a subset of CD5-B cells that appear to have a role in autoimmunity. The pathogenesis of chronic lymphocytic leukemia is likely a multistep process, initially involving a polyclonal expansion of CD5-B cells followed by the transformation of a single cell [48]. CLL is one of four main types of leukemia. About 15.110 new cases of CLL will be diagnosed in 2008. Approximately 90.179 people are currently living with CLL, more than the number of people living with any other type of leukemia. Most people with CLL are at least 50 years old [49]. CLL starts with a change to a single cell called a lymphocyte. Over time, the CLL cells multiply and replace normal lymphocytes in the marrow and lymph nodes. The high number of CLL cells in the marrow may crowd out normal blood-forming cells, and CLL cells are not able to fight off infection like normal lymphocytes do [49]. The aim of the tests performed in this study is to determine whether our system is able to classify new patients based on previously analyzed and stored cases.

6 Results and Conclusions

This chapter has presented a case-based reasoning system, that evolved from a previous work in leukemia patients classification [12], specifically designed to analyze data from microarrays, facilitating the grouping and classification of individuals. Moreover, the system provides an innovative method for exploring the classification process and extracting knowledge in the form of rules which help the human experts to understand the classification process and obtain conclusions about the relevance of the probes. The human experts in the laboratory have remarked on the advantages of using the system as a decision support system for CLL classification, and have especially noted the facility in acquiring knowledge and explanations.

Section 5 presented the case study considered in this report, which classified 91 CLL leukemia patients into groups. The aim of the case study was to identify the probes that allow classifying the CLL leukemia patients into subgroups. In an initial test, data from 91 patients, where previous classification was not taken into account, were used in the system. The pre-processing phase began with 54.675 probes and the RMA was applied to obtain the luminescence values for each of the probes and to homogenize the values from different chips. After the pre-processing phase, the filtering process was applied, notably reducing the probes to 541, without increasing the error rate.

Once the filtering was executed, it was still difficult to extract knowledge from the data. Figure 2 shows the 91 individuals in a bar graph, where the bars are divided in 541 probes with amplitude proportional to their value. The upper part of Figure 2 shows the classification obtained for each of the individuals, and the bottom of Figure 2 shows the parallel coordinates that represent 561 coordinates and 91 lines for each of the individuals.

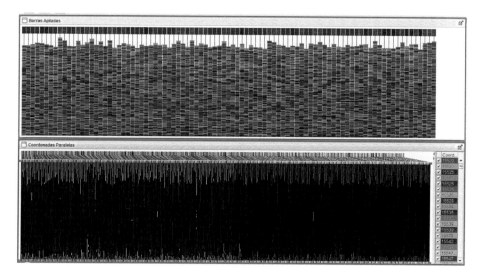

Fig. 2. Values for the probes obtained from the individuals.

The reuse phase begins when the probes have been filtered, and generates the meshes for the groups as well as the distribution of the individuals along the space. The mesh closest to the new case was then selected and the classification was made. To evaluate the proposed model, the system classified 90 individuals together with a new individual, and the results obtained were compared to the previous existing classifications. This process was repeated for each of the 91 individuals considered for the experiment and the results obtained demonstrate that 82 of the 91 individuals were successfully classified.

In the revise phase, the CBR system extracted the knowledge obtained during the classification process, as shown in Figure 3. Figure 3 presents the decision rules obtained in the revision phase that are applied to extract knowledge from the classification carried out in the previous phase.

(209083_at <= 0.25) and (1552280_at <= 0) => Class =C2 (10.0/1.0)
(231592_at >= 1) => Class=C2 (4.0/1.0)
(203213_at >= 0.75) => Class =C3 (29.0/0.0)
(1552619_a_at >= 0.5) => Class =C3 (2.0/0.0)
=> Class =C1 (46.0/1.0)

Fig. 3. Decision Rules obtained in the revision phase.

Figure 4 represents some graphics where the values of the retrieved probes are compared, and the information obtained from the retrieved probes is presented as decision rules. The values of the probes shown in Figure 4 are not the discretized ones used for the decision rules. At the top of Figure 4, both the real classification and the classification predicted by the system are presented by means of decision rules. If the colour matches, then there is a coincidence in the classification. As can be seen, there is an individual misclassified in the first of the classes identified in Figure 4, zero in the second class and two in the third class. At the bottom of Figure 4, it is possible to observe the parallel coordinates and the colours represent the class associated to the individual. As can be seen, it is possible to distinguish the probes associated to each of the classes. In this way, in the first of the coordinates can be seen how a group of individuals is separated from the rest.

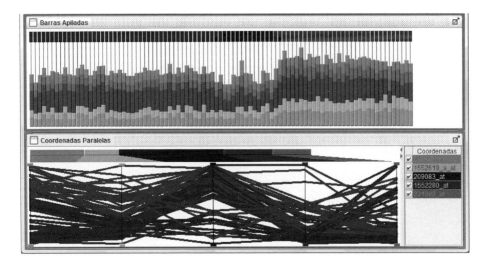

Fig. 4. Representation of the retrieved probes in terms of decision rules for the 91 individuals.

Figure 5 shows the classification of the individuals for the last class. Figure 5a shows the individuals classified to the class C3. In the classification of the individuals, the parallel coordinates establish the top and bottom margins for each of the probes, facilitating a graphical representation of the information contained by the rules. Once the margins are established, the individuals out of the ranks are shown as dimmed in the bars and the parallel coordinates. As can be seen in Figure 5a, when the individuals marked in red colour were selected, some individuals marked in blue (class C1) and marked in violet (class C2) were activated. Looking at the first of the coordinates, it is possible to observe a red line that corresponds to an individual with a low value and that is the responsible of the activation of the individuals of the C1 and C2 classes. Figure 5b shows a selection of the individuals estimated as members of the class C3. As can be seen in Figure 5b, the rest of the individuals remain dimmed, which allows a separation of the rest of the individuals. This is possible because of the information provided by the decision rules.

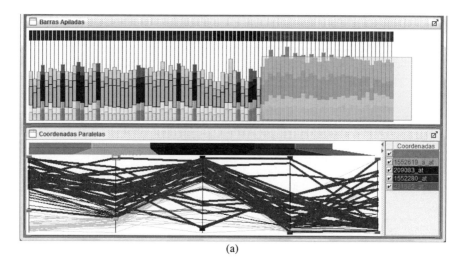

(a)

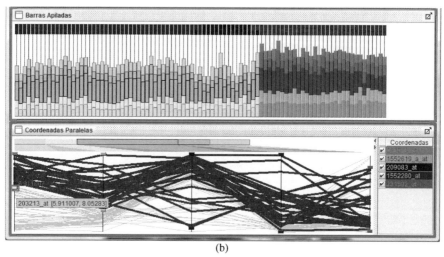

(b)

Fig. 5. Representation of the retrieved probes using the decision rules. (a) represents those individuals that are situated in the same rank of values than the individuals of the class C3. (b) shows the individuals situated in the same rank of values than the individuals estimated as members of the class C3.

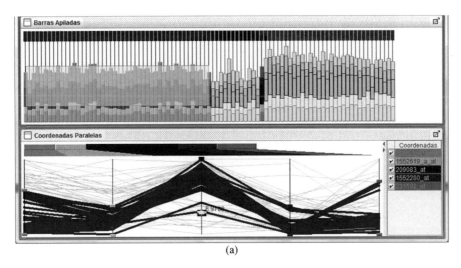

(a)

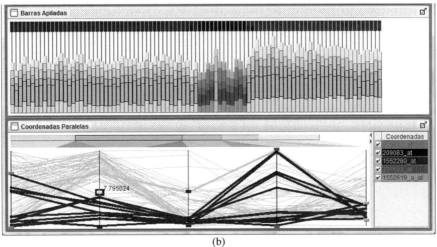

(b)

Fig. 6. Representation of the probes for the individuals of the classes C1 y C2.

Figure 6 represents the classification of individuals for the first class. As can be seen in Figure 6a, when the individuals of the class C1 were selected, only one of the individuals of the rest of the classes was activated. Figure 6b shows the results obtained when the margin of parallel coordinates was configured in order to avoid the activation of individuals of the other classes. As can be seen, only one individual of the class C2 was deactivated, which indicated that it was out of the margins, with a high value for the probe 15552280_at.

To obtain a visual representation of the patient's classification, we use the MDS [18] [19] [20], and the dimensionality of the data is reduced to three. Figures 7a and 8b represent the information once MDS has been applied and, as shown, the individuals of the different clusters are separated in the space. Figure 7 shows a representation

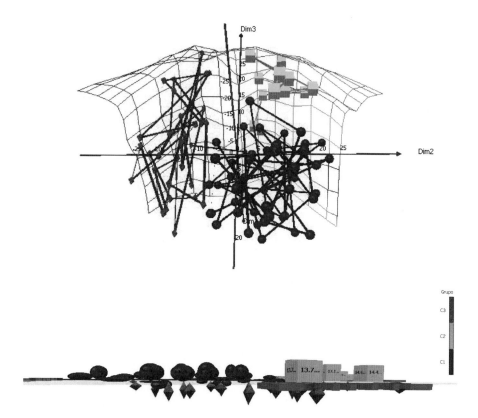

Fig. 7. Representation of low dimentionality probes with MDS

of the classification obtained for the individuals. Figure 7a represents the information obtained in a 3D format and, as can be seen, it is possible to identify three different classes clearly separated. Figure 7b shows a heatmap for the classification. As can be seen, class C1 contains negative values, while the classes C2 and C3 contain positive values.

In order to evaluate the global functioning of the system, we included an additional test. In this test the system contains 45 previously classified individuals, and aims to classify the remaining 46 cases using previous knowledge. Figure 8 presents the error rate identified for each of the interactions of the CBR system. As can be seen in Figure 8, the error rate is reduced after the initial iterations. The user of the CBR paradigm provides the ability for learning from previous experiences, which improves the performance of the classification process. In this sense, the classification provided by the system presented within this chapter improves the classification provided in our previous works 12 and provides a more detailed knowledge about the classification process.

The approach presented in this chapter is a specialized and novel system that integrates the steps of an expression analysis within the stages of a CBR cycle. The system is able to incorporate the knowledge acquired in previous classifications and use

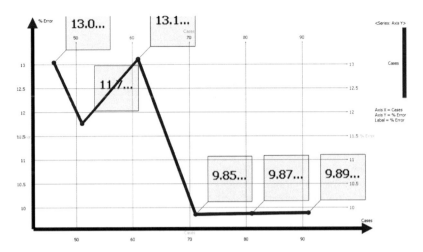

Fig. 8. Error rate for the classification process related to the iterations.

it to perform new classifications, providing a much appreciated decision support tool for doctors. As demonstrated, the proposed system reduces the dimensionality based on the filtering of genes with little variability and those that do not allow a separation of individuals due to the distribution of data. It also presents a clustering technique based on the neuronal network ESOINN, which is validated with a PAM technique. Finally, the system incorporates a technique for knowledge extraction and presents it to the human experts in a very intuitive format.

With the results obtained from empirical studies we can conclude that the CBR system presented in this study provides a tool that detects genes and probes, which are the most important factor for the detection of pathology, and facilitates a classification and reliable diagnosis, as shown by the results presented in this chapter. The system has been applied to classify CLL leukemia patients and allows the human expert to obtain information about the classification process and to identify the probes considered as important or irrelevant for further classifications. Taking into account these results, we can conclude that the incorporation of computational intelligence techniques in the expression analysis can facilitate the working day of the care personnel and provide a robust and reliable decision support tool for the prevention and detection of cancerous patterns.

Acknowledgments. Special thanks to the Institute of Cancer of Salamanca for the information and technology provided.

References

1. Tu, Y.J., Zhou, W., Piramuthu, S.: Identifying RFID-embedded objects in pervasive healthcare applications. Decision Support Systems 46(2), 586–593 (2008)
2. Chakraborty, D., Takahashi, H., Suganuma, T., Takeda, A., Kitagata, G., Hashimoto, K., Shiratori, N.: Context-aware remote healthcare support system based on overlay network. WSEAS Transactions on Computers 7(9), 1505–1514 (2008)

3. Lina, S., Chien, F.: Cluster analysis of genome-wide expression data for feature extraction. Expert Systems with Applications 36(2-2), 3327–3335 (2009)
4. Stadlera, Z.K., Come, S.E.: Review of gene-expression profiling and its clinical use in breast cancer. Critical Reviews in Oncology/Hematology 69(1), 1–11 (2009)
5. Affymetrix. GeneChip® Human Genome U133 Arrays,
   `http://www.affymetrix.com/support/technical/datasheets/`
   `hgu133arrays_datasheet.pdf`
6. Sawa, T., Ohno-Machado, L.: A neural network based similarity index for clustering DNA microarray data. Computers in Biology and Medicine 33(1), 1–15 (2003)
7. Bianchia, D., Calogero, R., Tirozzi, B.: Kohonen neural networks and genetic classification. Mathematical and Computer Modelling 45(1-2), 34–60 (2007)
8. Baladandayuthapani, V., Ray, S., Mallick, B.K.: Bayesian Methods for DNA Microarray Data Analysis. Handbook of Statistics 25(1), 713–742 (2005)
9. Avogadri, R., Valentini, G.: Fuzzy ensemble clustering based on random projections for DNA microarray data analysis. Artificial Intelligence in Medicine 45(2-3), 173–183 (2009)
10. Kolodner, J.: Case-Based Reasoning. Morgan Kaufmann, San Francisco (1993)
11. Riverola, F., Díaz, F., Corchado, J.M.: Gene-CBR: a case-based reasoning tool for cancer diagnosis using microarray datasets. Computational Intelligence 22(3-4), 254–268 (2006)
12. Corchado, J.M., De Paz, J.F., Rodríguez, S., Bajo, J.: Model of Experts for decision support in the diagnosis of leukemia patients. Artificial Intelligence in Medicine 46, 179–200 (2009)
13. Bichindaritz, I.: Role and Significance of Case-based Reasoning in the Health Sciences. KI 23(1), 12–17 (2009)
14. Bichindaritz, I., Marling, C.: Case-based reasoning in the health sciences: What's next? Artificial Intelligence in Medicine 36(2), 127–135 (2006)
15. Furao, S., Ogura, T., Hasegawa, O.: An enhanced self-organizing incremental neural network for online unsupervised learning. Neural Networks 20(8), 893–903 (2007)
16. Kaufman, L., Rousseeuw, P.J.: Finding Groups in Data: An Introduction to Cluster Analysis. Wiley, New York (1990)
17. Saravanan, N., Cholairajana, S., Ramachandran, K.I.: Vibration-based fault diagnosis of spur bevel gear box using fuzzy technique. Expert Systems with Applications 36(2-2), 3119–3135 (2009)
18. Borg, I., Groenen, P.: Modern multidimensional scaling theory and applications. Springer, Heidelberg (1997)
19. Kruskal, J.B.: Multidimensional scaling by optimizing goodness of fit to nonmetric hypothesis. Psychometrika 29(1), 1–27 (1964)
20. Ture, M., Tokatli, F., Kurt, I.: Using Kaplan–Meier analysis together with decision tree methods (C&RT, CHAID, QUEST, C4.5 and ID3) in determining recurrence-free survival of breast cancer patients. Expert Systems with Applications 36(2), 2017–2026 (2009)
21. Quackenbush, J.: Computational analysis of microarray data. Nature Review Genetics 2(6), 418–427 (2001)
22. Lipshutz, R.J., Fodor, S.P.A., Gingeras, T.R., Lockhart, D.H.: High density synthetic oligonucleotide arrays. Nature Genetics 21(1), 20–24 (1999)
23. Taniguchi, M., Guan, L.L., Basarab, J.A., Dodson, M.V., Moore, S.S.: Comparative analysis on gene expression profiles in cattle subcutaneous fat tissues. Comparative Biochemistry and Physiology Part D: Genomics and Proteomics 3(4), 251–256
24. Avogadri, R., Valentini, G.: Fuzzy ensemble clustering based on random projections for DNA microarray data analysis. Artificial Intelligence in Medicine 45(2-3), 173–183 (2009)

25. Margalit, O., Somech, R., Amariglio, N., Rechav, G.: Microarray based gene expression profiling of hematologic malignancies: basic concepts and clinical applications. Blood Reviews 4(4), 223–234

26. Armstrong, N.J., Van de Wiel, M.A.: Microarray data analysis: From hypotheses to conclusions using gene expression data. Cellular Oncology 26(5-6), 279–290 (2004)

27. Jurisica, I., Glasgow, J.: Applications of case-based reasoning in molecular biology. Artificial Intelligence Magazine, Special issue on Bioinformatics 25(1), 85–95 (2004)

28. Aaronson, J.S., Juergen, H., Overton, G.C.: Knowledge Discovery in GENBANK. In: Proceedings of the First International Conference on Intelligent Systems for Molecular Biology, pp. 3–11 (1993)

29. Arshadi, N., Jurisica, I.: Data Mining for Case-Based Reasoning in High-Dimensional Biological Domains. IEEE Transactions on Knowledge and Data Engineering 17(8), 1127–1137 (2005)

30. Affymetrix. Statistical Algorithms Description Document,
    `http://www.affymetrix.com/support/technical/whitepapers/`
    `sadd_whitepaper.pdf`

31. Affymetrix. Guide to Probe Logarithmic Intensity Error (PLIER) Estimation,
    `http://www.affymetrix.com/support/technical/technotes/`
    `plier_technote.pdf`

32. Irizarry, R.A., Hobbs, B., Collin, F., Beazer-Barclay, Y.D., Antonellis, K.J.: Exploration, Normalization, and Summaries of High density Oligonucleotide Array Probe Level Data. Biostatistics 4, 249–264 (2003)

33. Brunelli, R.: Histogram Analysis for Image Retrieval. Pattern Recognition 34, 1625–1637 (2001)

34. Jurečkováa, J., Picek, J.: Shapiro–Wilk type test of normality under nuisance regression and scale. Computational Statistics & Data Analysis 51(10), 5184–5191 (2007)

35. Saitou, N., Nie, M.: The neighbor-joining method: A new method for reconstructing phylogenetic trees. Molecular Biology and Evolution 4, 406–425 (1987)

36. Kohonen, T.: Self-organized formation of topologically correct feature maps. Biological Cybernetics, 59–69 (1982)

37. Fritzke, B.: A growing neural gas network learns topologies. In: Advances in Neural Information Processing Systems, vol. 7, pp. 625–632 (1995)

38. Shen, F.: An algorithm for incremental unsupervised learning and topology representation, Tokyo: Ph.D. thesis. Tokyo Institute of Technology (2006)

39. Redmond, S.J., Heneghan, C.: A method for initialising the K-means clustering algorithm using kd-trees. Pattern Recognition Letters 28(8), 965–973 (2007)

40. Martinetz, T.: Competitive Hebbian learning rule forms perfectly topology preserving maps. In: ICANN 1993: International Conference on Artificial Neural Networks, pp. 427–434 (1993)

41. Guinn, B., Gilkes, A.F., Woodward, E., Westwood, N.B., Muftia, G.J., Linchc, D., Burnett, A.K., Mills, K.I.: Microarray analysis of tumour antigen expression in presentation acute myeloid leukaemia. Biochemical and Biophysical Research Communication 333(5), 703–713 (2005)

42. Corchado, J.M., Bajo, J., De Paz, Y., De Paz, J.F.: Integrating Case Planning and RPTW Neuronal Networks to Construct an Intelligent Environment for Health Care. Expert Systems with Applications 36(3), 5844–5858 (2009)

43. Holte, R.C.: Very simple classification rules perform well on most commonly used datasets, Machine Learning (1993)

44. Frank, E., Witten, I.H.: Generating accurate rule sets without global optimization, pp. 144–151. Morgan Kaufmann, San Francisco (1998)
45. Vogiatzis, D., Tsapatsoulis, N.: Active learning for microarray data. International Journal of Approximate Reasoning 47(1), 85–96 (2008)
46. Yang, T.Y.: Efficient multi-class cancer diagnosis algorithm, using a global similarity pattern. Computational Statistics & Data Analysis 53(3), 756–765 (2009)
47. Leng, C.: Sparse optimal scoring for multiclass cancer diagnosis and biomarker detection using microarray data. Computational Biology and Chemisty 32(6), 417–425 (2008)
48. Foon, K.A., Rai, K.L., Gale, R.P.: Chronic lymphocytic leukemia: new insights into biology and therapy. Annals of Internal Medicine 113(7), 525–539 (1990)
49. Chronic Lymphocytic Leukemia (2008), The leukemia and lymphoma society, http://www.leukemia-lymphoma.org/all_page.adp?item_id=7059

Part IV
Sample Applications and Case Studies

Chapter 14
The Evolution of Healthcare Applications in the Web 2.0 Era

Iraklis Varlamis[1] and Ioannis Apostolakis[2]

[1] Harokopio University of Athens, Dept. of Informatics and Telematics, Greece
[2] Technical University of Crete, Dept. of Sciences, Greece

Abstract. Healthcare refers to the diagnosis, treatment and management of illness, as well as to the preservation of health through specialized services. Healthcare services are offered by medical practitioners and organizations and directed to individuals or to populations. The advent of the Web increased the pervasiveness of healthcare services and attracted the interest of both practitioners and patients. In its turn, Web 2.0 brought people together in a more dynamic and interactive space. With new services, applications and devices, it promises to enrich our web experience, and to establish an environment where virtual medical communities may flourish away from private interests and financial expectations. This article performs a bird's eye view of Web 2.0 novelties, portrays the structure of a community for healthcare and describes how medical information can be exploited in favor of the community. It discusses the merits and necessities of various approaches and tools and sheds light on pitfalls that should be avoided.

1 Introduction

Medical informatics and Healthcare applications have been devoted to the study and implementation of structures to improve communication, understanding and management of medical information and promote public health. Their main objective is the extraction, storage and manipulation of data and information and the development of tools and platforms that apply knowledge in the decision-making process, at the time and place that a decision needs to be made.

The advent of internet introduced the idea of tele-application of medical practices. Tele-medicine, tele-education of practitioners and nurses, tele-healthcare and tele-consultation are rapidly developing applications of clinical medicine, where medical information is transferred via telephone, the Internet or other networks for the purpose of consulting, and sometimes remote medical procedures or examinations.

Internet has broaden the scope of medical information systems and led to the development of distributed and interoperable information sources and services. In the same time, the need for standards became crucial. Federated medical libraries, biomedical knowledge bases and global healthcare systems, offer a rich information sink and facilitate mobility of patients and practitioners.

I. Bichindaritz et al. (Eds.): Computational Intelligence in Healthcare 4, SCI 309, pp. 315–328.
springerlink.com   © Springer-Verlag Berlin Heidelberg 2010

The Web attracted more patients and increased the popularity of freely available medical advice and knowledge. The abundance of web sites that offer medical content affected the way patients face their doctors, gave them a second opinion and increased their awareness.

Its' successor, Web 2.0, was built on the same technologies and concepts but added a layer of *semantic abstraction*, offered a *network as a platform sensation* and gave a *social networking aspect* to medical information systems.

Patients, instead of seeking medical information and requesting medical advice on their issues, are supplied with useful news, when medical advances take place. Patients are able to discuss their issues with other patients and collectively develop a medical knowledge base with easy to use tools. The plethora of tools and platforms available enhances the inventory of medical practitioners and can be of value to them and their patients if properly exploited. This paper gives an overview of these tools, discusses the merits of their use and the potential hazards that should be avoided.

In the following section we enlist the major technological novelties of Web 2.0 under the prism of certain applications and explain how they led to Heath 2.0. In section 3 we examine a community based approach, which combines the aforementioned novelties, under the prism of intelligent information management and in section 4 we discuss the potential merits of this approach and the issues that should be considered.

2   From Web to Web 2.0, Health 2.0 and Medicine 2.0

Internet and its services had a major impact on health care and medical information. First, it opened public access to medical information, which was previously restricted to health care providers. Of all searches on the Internet, 4.5% have been calculated to be health-related [7]. The patients feel empowered before reaching their doctors [1], since they find or ask for information on the web. They get an idea about their diagnosis and treatment options and want to actively participate in therapeutic decisions. As a result, the way of interaction between the patient and the doctor, has changed. Similarly the way people perceive medical information has changed.

2.1 Medical Information and Web-Based Applications

The seek for direct medical consultation gained place from searching and browsing of medical information and this is another fact of change in the way of communication between doctors and patients. "Ask the doctor services" [25], initially deployed through e-mail, kept record of questions and replies by expert physicians and published results to the web for further reference [26]. Web sites have been also created in order to alert or support patients [12] and offer informative content, provide directions for prevention, cure and symptoms' handling and of course sample questions and feedback from physicians.

Electronic assessment is another healthcare application which gained great attention. Online questionnaires, symptom checklists etc. were used in order to increase the interactivity of web based medical applications. Short screening tests [13], [21], helped people to detect and overcome their addictions, alerted them and reminded

Table 1. Web based medical services

Web applications	Purpose	Services
Ask the doctor	Offer medical consultation on demand	E-mail
Medical chats	Offer medical consultation on demand, group therapy	Chat
Medical forum	Offer medical consultation on demand, retain archive	Forum
Ask the doctor website	Archive medical consultation	Dynamic Web site
Patient support websites and mailing lists for alerts	Provide informative content, support and prevention guidelines	Email, Static Web site
Online assessment	Prevent maladies, detect additions	Active Web Site
Tele-healthcare, medicine, homecare etc.	Remotely provide clinical care, diagnosis, medical education	Tele-conference, Voice and Video over IP

them to visit their doctor. Mailing lists were another solution for supporting patients in a constant manner.

Table 1 summarizes medical applications and services delivered over the web.

Tele-healthcare, tele-medicine [14], tele-homecare and other applications make use of Web and the whole Internet infrastructure in order to offer clinical and non-clinical services (medical education, information and administrative services).The main aim of these application is the transfer of medical information and advices between the hospital and the remote patient, or the remote care provider, thus removing geographical and time zone barriers. In the same direction, interoperable medical information systems have been developed to support exchange and utilization of medical information across different hospitals, different healthcare providers or even across different countries [4], [3]. Web is mainly employed to achieve better coordination of all the participants in the medical process.

All the above applications created a critical mass of people, practitioners, patients, care providers and care givers that requests medical information and advice in health related issues in an everyday basis. People gathered in virtual communities and started seeking for more flexible and collaborative solutions on their issues. The interest for ubiquitous medical information and pervasive solutions [5], created new web applications that facilitate people in sending, processing and receiving medical information. At the same time a lot of Web 2.0 applications and standards emerged.

The original definition of Web 2.0 by O'Reilly [18] summarizes the characteristics of Web 2.0 applications as: (1) data sources that get richer as more people use them, (2) collective intelligence, and (3) lightweight components and APIs that can be easily assembled, (4) rich user experiences. Other researchers view Web 2.0 in its widest sense, incorporating all existing web tools, user produced content (blogs, podcasts and vidcasts), protocols and semantics that allow harnessing collective intelligence [11].

Although the definition of term Health 2.0 is still under development, it is certain that it will stand in the common ground of social-networking and health care. Emerging internet technologies and applications aim to transform health care into a collective social service. Health 2.0 mainly focuses on actors such as patients, care-givers and, care-providers and their roles in the collective approach [22].

The term Medicine 2.0 [8] has been introduced by the Journal of Medical Internet Research (JMIR) (http://www.jmir.org) and the International Medical Informatics Association (http://www.imia.org) as name for a conference series (http://www.medicine20congress.com). Medicine 2.0 has a broader scope than Health 2.0 and its applications, services and tools are Web-based services for health care consumers, caregivers, patients, health professionals, and biomedical researchers, who use Web 2.0 technologies as well as semantic web and virtual reality tools, to enable and facilitate specifically social networking, participation, collaboration, and openness within and between these user groups.

A survey of collaborative services and their applications in Healthcare and Medical communities is presented in the following section.

3   Collaborative Services in Medical and Healthcare Communities

Despite the achievements of web and its services, it was necessary that patients seek for medical information and that patients contact their doctors for consultation, diagnosis or treatment. The advent of Web 2.0 changed this uni-directional flow of information. Now, all community members, even patients are able to feed the community with news, advices and personal experiences. Moreover, the request-serve model has changed towards a push-pull model where information is accumulated by community members and is made available to all community members through intelligent services. Patients receive useful alerts and doctors get notifications on medical advances, new medicines and therapies.

In [18], the term Web 2.0, is perceived to encompass a set of services, which extend Web 1.0 capabilities and emphasize on the community and collaboration aspects. In [22] and [23] authors present how medical communities can be used in favor of patients and how communication and collaboration between members of the healthcare community can be hosted in a community platform. The utter aim of any medical and healthcare community is to assist patients, either directly by providing medical care or indirectly by improving medical knowledge. Depending on the specific targets of the community (e.g. practitioners' education, patients' support, etc.) the members, the roles and the use of web 2.0 services differentiate.

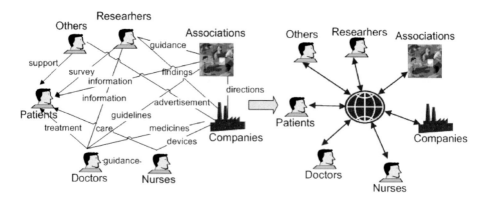

Fig. 1. How the medical mesh transforms into a community

In the following, we provide an overview of the most popular Web 2.0 services, present their main features and give reference to several online implementations in medical applications.

3.1 Web 2.0 Services

There is already an important amount of Web 2.0 applications [6], [7], [15], [16], which are related to medical issues. Blogs, wikis, folksonomies, podcasts and vidcasts are among them. In the following we give details on these applications, on the way information is published, annotated and consumed and on their potential use in favour of the medical community.

The main characteristics of all Web 2.0 services, which are presented in Table 2 are: a) contribution is communal, b) publishing has been replaced by participation and c) access is public or at least is granted to the members of the medical community. Anonymity and identity issues are solved with the use of virtual identities. They are mainly asynchronous since it is infeasible for all community members to be concurrently online.

Blogs
Blogs (Weblogs) are Web sites that function as online journals. They present published content in reverse publication date blogs. One or more persons may contribute with articles (posts), comments, links to other Web sites and multimedia content. Blog participants form virtual groups based on their common interests.

Table 2. Web 2.0 applications. Examples and open source solutions

Web 2.0 apps	Purpose	Online examples/tools
Blogs, photo blogs	Provide medical consultation, news, announcements, photos, allow comments	www.docnotes.net http://casesblog.blogspot.com
		www.wordpress.com www.flickr.com
RSS feeds and news syndication	Instantly receive medical information right after it is published	http://www.doctorslounge.com/rss http://www.rss4medics.com www.medicalnewstoday.com
		http://www.feedforall.com
Podcast and Vidcast	Provide consults, courses and information in audio and video stream format	http://conversations.acc.org/ http://www.annals.org/podcast/index.shtml http://www.clevelandclinic.org
		http://video.google.com/ http://www.archive.org/details/movies
Wiki	Collaboratively construct an archive of medical knowledge	http://askdrwiki.com/mediawiki/ http://www.radiopaedia.org
		http://www.mediawiki.org/ http://www.splitbrain.org/go/dokuwiki
Collaborative Tagging and Social bookmarking	Link to informative content, evaluate sources and organize knowledge	http://www.bibsonomy.org/ http://www.citeulike.org/
		http://www.flickr.com/ http://www.connotea.org/
Cyberspaces	Provide a virtual and interactive learning environment	http://www.secondlife.com http://opensimulator.org/

The easy and immediate publishing made them very popular. The posting of a clinical photo from a digital camera or a mobile phone directly to a blog after optimisation and commenting can be made at the touch of a button. Medical blog examples include Clinical Cases and Images, Family Medicine Notes etc.

RSS

RSS stands for "Really Simple Syndication." It is a standard format used to share content on the Internet. Many websites provide RSS "feeds" that describe their latest news and updates. They play the role of newsletters but offer information in pieces, at the moment it is created (feeds) and can be accessed by various devices and systems grace to the standard format. The doctors' lounge, RSS for medics and Medical News Today are a few medical RSS news syndication services. Most blogging services offer the ability to create RSS feeds and an RSS reader is the only tool needed to process this feed.

Audio and video podcasts

They can be employed similar to RSS for providing medical information on emerging issues. Moreover, the power of image and the ease of listening instead of reading make them ideal for the dissemination of medical information and for online courses. In a project developed at St George's, University of London, UK, named Clinical Skills Online (CSO) [8], online videos demonstrate core Clinical Skills common to a wide range of medical and health-based courses in Higher Education. The video courses are categorized by topic, by user's expertise and occupation and are available to the public. The option of user feedback is available through a questionnaire and a free text comments form. Other interesting examples include: the Annals of Internal Medicine, the podcasts of the American College of Cardiology (Conversations with Experts) and the vidcasts of Cleveland Clinic.

Wikis

Wikis are considered to replace content management applications by allowing users to easily publish articles, images and video. They can start to cover the lack of free online medical information and function as a repository of medical information that could be readily accessed for reference. They are built and populated collaboratively by domain experts and are accessible to patients, doctors or trainees and the public. In a medical wiki, the group of editors creates and contributes with article reviews, disease definitions (symptoms, cure etc), clinical notes, medical images or video. Editors have the ability to alter content published by other editors and have their articles edited by others hoping that the wiki will finally converge into a widely accepted final version.

Social bookmarking

Medical bookmarking is aimed to promote the sharing of medical references mainly amongst practitioners and researchers. Scientists can share information on academic papers, are able to collaboratively catalog medical images with specific tools developed for that purpose. Article readers can organize their libraries, which can comprise Medline articles, with freely chosen tags. The result is a multi-faceted taxonomy, called folksonomy of tags (topics) and associated sources. Many medical information sources support tagging by users (i.e. JSTOR, PLoS, PubMed, and ScienceDirect). Human knowledge, captured in the categorization and characterization of articles, or web sources in general, can be exploited by intelligent agents in order to provide recommendations about related sources or tags.

Cyberspaces

Although the term **cyberspace** dates back into 80's, it is becoming more and more realistic nowadays. The improvement of 3-D visualization technologies and the need to refurbish the link-based Web surfing allowed the development of new platforms and virtual environments, which allow users to replace accounts with avatars, hypertext with interactive 3-D objects and browsing with walking, flying and teleporting. The educational possibilities of these virtual environments are many [2] and the projects and workgroups that have been created are numerous [20] (e.g. the IBM 3D Virtual Healthcare Island in Second Life, the OpenSim project that can be deployed individually).

It is obvious, that all the services presented above, differ from typical web services, in the multitude and nature of information sources they cover and the way of enhancing and exploiting this information.

3.2 The Structure of Medical Community

A medical community that will encompass all the people interested in medical issues should be open to new members. Trustfulness is critical in medical issues and specifically in medical consultation, so the identity of consultants has to be valid and accessible to the community members. In the same time, the anonymity is necessary (or at least helpful) for patients that seek for consultation.

Information/content providers and information consumers are the two main types of users. The former should necessarily use their real identities, whereas the latter can remain anonymous or behind use virtual personas. Information consumers (i.e. patients, people asking about medical issues etc) can potentially become providers, since their questions, remarks and bookmarks are made available to the community. However, the quality of this content is questionable. Moderators, administrators and facilitators stand in-between the two types of users and are responsible for the smooth operation of the community. They control the registration process and guarantee the validity of expert members' identities.

The community members are able to form groups inside the community based on common needs and interests. The needs of each group are different and sometimes contradictory. It is necessary for the community to allow members to communicate their similarities and join their forces, whilst protecting their individuality. A healthcare community can attract scientists and researchers, doctors and nurses, patients and people with personal interests in medicine and healthcare, companies. More specifically:

- Scientists and researchers join the community in order to exchange knowledge and promote their science. They communicate with patients, analyze surveys' results and population statistics and get useful feedback on patient needs, on medical issues that arise etc. They co-operate with other scientists for their experiments and disseminate their findings to companies and individuals. They also give useful directions to medical associations concerning public health.

- Medical associations provide the professionals with guidelines on patient treatment and inform patients on topics such as prevention, self protection etc. They issue specifications for companies that produce medical devices and medications.
- Healthcare companies advertise their products (devices, therapies, medical applications) to doctors, nurses and patients.
- Healthcare practitioners get informed on new findings, emerging therapies and medical approaches and sometimes get online training. In parallel, they guide nurses and patients' families on patient-care and provide researchers and associations with useful feedback on emerging patient needs.
- Patients are *receivers* of support, treatment, care, information and advertisement from all other participants. They contribute to the community, as end users of the community outcomes and as specimens of surveys.

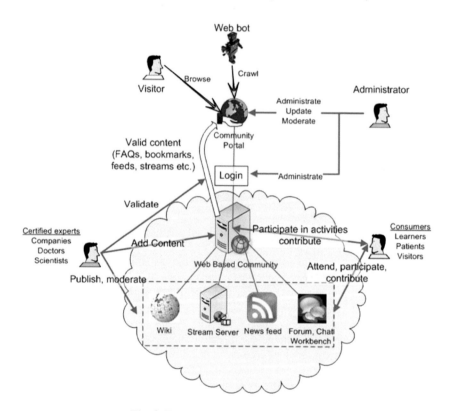

Fig. 2. The medical community structure

As it is depicted in Figure 2, the medical community should provide different level of accessibility to visitors, registered members and special members such as doctors or scientists. The nucleus of the virtual community should be equally accessible to members and visitors. More specifically, the community portal must be accessible to every web visitor or web service (bot) that wishes to browse or process the published content. Community members, should register once and login every time they want to join the community. The registration of new members should be controlled by the administrators. The identity of expert members (doctors, company officials, scientists etc) should be checked and certified by the administrators, where as simple members can join by giving a contact e-mail address.

Once inside the community, registered users are able to participate in the various activities (i.e. chat with doctors or other members, perform public discussions, attend a video podcast or register to news feeds). The community experts create and publish new content and are charged with the moderation of group discussions, and the filtering of content uploaded by non experts. They use the wiki and tagging services to accumulate and organize the knowledge base of the community and inform on new findings using the news feeds.

3.3 The Assembly of Web and Web 2.0 Tools

A **web site** is necessary to welcome web visitors and guide potential members into joining the community. The site should provide informative content on the community aim and structure and can be created as a joint effort of the universities or educational institutes that support the community. The web site will advertise the educational programs and will provide information concerning every day activities of each course, news and announcements of interest to the students.

The web site administration should be performed by technical staff from the educational partners of the community (i.e. the university). Coordination tasks will be held by the registrar office, who will be responsible for the members' accounts, their participation in virtual classes etc.

A smart and cost free solution for the web site is presented in [24]. There, the web site was a blog, created by the university. The blog was visible to anyone, but practically only registered community members were allowed to update content or comment. In an effort to delegate administration tasks, a "weblog umbrella" can replace the community portal (see Figure 3). Another solution, which requires access to a web server, is to deploy the web site in an open source Content Management System.

Blogs (or web logs) are easily updatable websites where administrators can post messages by filling a few forms and without special knowledge on web design technologies. Separate blogs for each field of interest allow **experts** to distribute news and knowledge in an organized manner, to add or drop material, to add short notices or announcements and manage the comments or posts of the community members. The **registered members** are permitted to comment on the blog posts thus providing the community with useful feedback. The **visitors** are able only to read announcement or comments.

Educational activities of the community can be ideally supported by a **web based course management system** (i.e. Moodle, Mahara, WebCT, Blackboard etc). Such systems are specialized in managing and delivering on line courses, and assemble various community tools such as forums, wikis etc. In the majority of courses tutors use the community application solely for provided reading material to students. However, in several cases, students and professors need the forum, chat and other services in order to coordinate their actions. When an integrated course management system is not available, the community can be still operational by combining various open source tools.

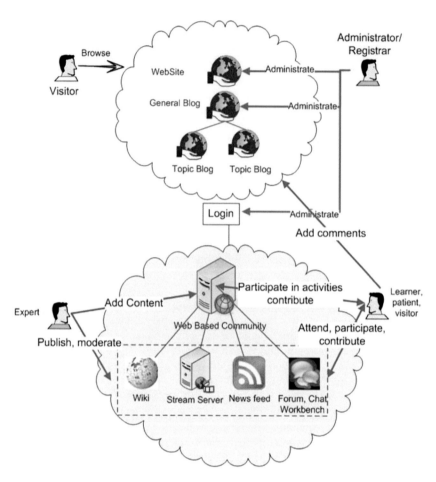

Fig. 3. The 'blog umbrella' alternative to the community portal

Computer-mediated *chat*, *discussion forums* and *newsgroups* can be formed and supported by the community administrators. Such forums will host discussions focused on the healthcare issues [2] and will be used from doctors to provide guidelines. *Mailing lists* and *web feeds* can be in assistance of doctors and patients. For example the doctor will be able to inform patients for an upcoming medical examination.

When there is need for building collaborative knowledge and making it available to medical researchers and practitioners, wikis are a cost-free, open-source solution. A *wiki* is the collaborative coverage of a topic from the members of a community. Any member can contribute or modify the content under conditions (proper reason, provide references etc.). The vast number of medical wikis currently available [17] is an indication of their popularity and their importance for medical matters. A wiki can be created and moderated by the domain experts in order to quickly build a terminology source for students.

Other collaboration services comprise, *virtual workbenches, virtual blackboard* etc. The results and history of collaboration services are usually stored and used as a reference by other community members. Such applications usually require specialized software and dedicated sources and thus are not widely used for medical education. The educational potential of *virtual worlds* has attracted the interest of medical communities, and created new opportunities for medical education in the cyberspace [2], [19].

When a teleconference room is available, distant courses can be performed from the joint institutes. Tutors and students communicate using real-time video over a streamed media server. Educational *multimedia content* (i.e. medical videos from surgeries, recorder sessions or courses etc.) can be stored in media repositories, and made available to community members. Free video hosting servers can be used for this task, however, bandwidth and storage limitations, restricted access and other issues should be considered.

The applications presented in the bottom section of figure 2, can be accessible both to students and tutors, however the degree of participation increases for students as moving from left to the right. All these services (i.e. wikis, streaming media, news feed, forum, chat, workbench etc.) can be offered through separate tools and platforms or ideally through the same Web Based CMS.

The next section illustrates the gains from the use of Web 2.0 tools for individuals, companies, organizations and healthcare and medicine in general.

4 Discussion

The merits that arise from the community approach are many. First of all the human knowledge is captured, is enriched with semantics (i.e. tags) and is organized collaboratively (i.e. folksonomies, wikis) in a mechanically readable way. Instead of a multitude of distinct applications that do not cooperate, the community platform is the World Wide Web, and the community activities and services can be developed using commonly agreed standards and common terminology. Web offers ubiquitous access to the community services, since web 2.0 applications are light and can be accessed by mobiles, PDAs, or even tv-sets. New content (i.e. video blogging or podcasting), requests for advice, patient related information or input to surveys can be attached using the same devices (e.g. patient can select their symptoms from a list and communicated them to the community experts).

The personalization of the community content to the specific needs of each member can be done by selecting the mini-applications (widgets) that fit each patient's needs. Smart alert systems can be developed that will remind patients of their scheduled treatment or that will inform doctors on their patients health status.

All community transactions and communications must be secure and various access levels can be used. Trust inside the community can be guaranteed by a strong administrator organization through the use of proper technologies, validation mechanisms and security structures. Trust can also be developed by using an evaluation and reputation system. In this system, expert users will be able to validate content, and all community members will be able to judge, vote and tag content in order to make it useful for others.

As it is the case with all communities, the administrators should be careful to avoid several dangers. Most of the efforts we mentioned in section 2, are made by individuals, or by a single institute or university and are not supported by a big organization or a medical forum. A centrally co-ordinated effort is necessary for a successful and effective community. Administration should be performed in co-operation with companies and associations. When the community serves for patients or doctors to support other associates, the advices and information exchanged between individuals should be validated. Group moderators need monitoring tools in order to proactively coordinate groups, and would be pleased to have collaborative platforms to support their groups. Validity can be achieved through monitoring, although, it is preferable to replace monitoring with an authorization mechanism. Advices, comments or opinions that are not signed are considered of low quality and consequently invalid. Valid information and services are issued by authorized community members only and are always signed.

The diversity of web 2.0 tools can be confusing to the community members, especially when all novelties are introduced in one step. Changes and new services should be added slowly and training, facilitation and user feedback are advisable.

Another issue that must be considered in a medical community relates to the amount and quality of information offered. The flood of information can be confusing both to patients and doctors and for this reason, information must be filtered and organized. Since anyone is able to publish information and since it is not always easy to see the origin of the information, users could be making decisions on the basis of a source that might not be quality assured. A certification authority is necessary to guarantee the expertise level of every user, control the quality of the published information and build trust among the community members. Even when the information is of high quality, users are not capable to make their own judgments and need support from the experts. Other issues relate to the expertise of all members in handling virtual discussions or providing diagnosis remotely. These issues should be considered in the design phase in order to increase members' participation and improve the quality of the community services.

5 Conclusions

This paper performed an overview of web 2.0 applications and compared their features to traditional web services under the prism of the medical community and its needs. Current attempts in using web 2.0 applications in favor of the medical community are fragmented, so we present a structure that will allow their interconnection. The community will bring together doctors, nurses and volunteers around patients and will provide the tools for requesting and providing medical information, advices and psychological support. Healthcare associations, companies and researchers will be able to join the community, disseminate their instructions, products and findings respectively and undertake crucial tasks such as the quality control of services and information. The use of community services will load the community database with valuable information concerning user feedback, patient needs, treatment suggestions, patient profiles and medical record history. The stockpiled information can be analyzed: by the community administrators who want to improve services, by scientists who perform medical research, by future patients who seek for a quick advice from a fellow-sufferer. The knowledge produced inside the community will be continuously filtered and managed in order to maintain quality.

References

1. Akerkar, S.M., Bichile, L.S.: Doctor patient relationship: Changing dynamics in the information age. Journal of Postgrad Medicine 50, 120–122 (2004)
2. Antonacci, D.M., Modaress, N.: Second Life: The Educational Possibilities of a Massively Multiplayer Virtual World (MMVW). Presented at Southwest Regional Conferences (2005),
   `http://www2.kumc.edu/ir/tlt/SLEDUCAUSESW2005/`
   `SLPresentationOutline.htm` (accessed: 2010-06-25)
3. Apostolakis, I., Kastania, A.N.: Distant teaching in telemedicine: Why and Who we do it. Journal of Management and Health 1(1), 66–73 (2000)
4. Apostolakis, I., Valsamos, P., Varlamis, I.: Decentralization of the Greek National Telemedicine System through the upgrading of the Regional Telemedicine Centers. In: Tan, J. (ed.) Healthcare Information Systems and Informatics: Research and Practices, pp. 278–296. IGI Global (2008)
5. Bang, M., Timpka, T.: Ubiquitous computing to support co-located clinical teams: Using the semiotics of physical objects in system design. International Journal of Medical Informatics, 58–64 (2006)
6. Barsky, E.: Introducing Web 2.0: weblogs and podcasting for health librarians. JCHLA/JABSC (27), 33–34 (2006),
   `http://pubs.nrc-cnrc.gc.ca/jchla/jchla27/c06-013.pdf`
   (accessed: 2010-06-25)
7. Boulos, M.N., Maramba, I., Wheeler, S.: Wikis, blogs and podcasts: a new generation of Web-based tools for virtual collaborative clinical practice and education. BMC Med. Educ. 6, 41 (2006)
8. Clinical Skills Online (CSO) website (2009), `http://www.etu.sgul.ac.uk/cso` (accessed: 2010-06-25)
9. Eysenbach, G.: Medicine 2.0: Social Networking, Collaboration, Participation, Apomediation, and Openness. J. Med. Internet Res. (2008) DOI:10.2196/jmir.1030
10. Eysenbach, G., Kohler, C.: Health-related searches on the Internet. JAMA 291, 2946 (2004)
11. Giustini, D.: How Web 2.0 is changing medicine. BMJ 333(7582), 1283–1284 (2006), doi:10.1136/bmj.39062.555405.80
12. Hartmann, C.W., Sciamanna, C.N., et al.: A Website to Improve Asthma Care by Suggesting Patient Questions for Physicians: Qualitative Analysis of User Experiences. J Med Internet Res 9(1), e3 (2007)
13. Linke, S., Murray, E., Butler, C., Wallace, P.: Internet-Based Interactive Health Intervention for the Promotion of Sensible Drinking: Patterns of Use and Potential Impact on Members of the General Public. J. Med. Internet Res. 9(2), e10 (2007)
14. Linkous, J.D.: Telemedicine: an overview. Journal of Medical Practice Management 18(1), 24–27 (2002)
15. Mathieu, J.: Blogs, Podcasts, and Wikis: The New Names in Information Dissemination. Journal of the American Dietetic Association 107(4), 553–555 (2007)

16. Mclean, R., Richards, B.H., Wardman, J.I.: The effect of web 2.0 on the future of medical practice and education: Darwikinian evolution or folksonomic revolution? Medical Journal of Australia 187, 174–177 (2007)
17. Medical Wiki's list (2009)
    http://davidrothman.net/list-of-medical-wikis/
    (accessed: 2010-06-25)
18. O'Reilly, T.: What Is Web 2.0. Design Patterns and Business Models for the Next Generation of Software. O'Reilly Network, Sebastopol (2005),
    http://www.oreillynet.com/lpt/a/6228 (Retrieved on 1-2-2008)
19. Stott, D.: Attending medical school in virtual reality. Student BMJ 2007 15, 427–470 (2007), http://student.bmj.com/search/pdf/07/12/sbmj431.pdf
    (accessed: 2010-06-25)
20. SLHealthy Home, About Health and Healthcare in Second Life (2009),
    http://slhealthy.wetpaint.com/ (accessed: 2010-06-25)
21. Vallejo, M.A., Jordán, C.M., Díaz, M.I., Comeche, M.I., Ortega, J.: Psychological Assessment via the Internet: A Reliability and Validity Study of Online (vs Paper-and-Pencil) Versions of the General Health Questionnaire-28 (GHQ-28) and the Symptoms Check-List-90-Revised (SCL-90-R). J. Med. Internet Res. 9(1), e2 (2007)
22. Varlamis, I., Apostolakis, I.: Self supportive web communities in the service of patients. In: Proceedings of IADIS International Conference on Web Based Communities 2007, Salamanca, Spain, February 18-20 (2007)
23. Varlamis, I., Apostolakis, I.: Use of virtual communities for the welfare of groups with particular needs. Journal on Information Technology in Healthcare (JITH) 4(6), 384–392 (2006)
24. Varlamis, I., Apostolakis, I.: A Framework for Building Virtual Communities for Education. In: First European Conference on Technology Enhanced Learning (EC-TEL 2006) Joint Workshop on Professional Learning, Competence Development and Knowledge Management (2006)
25. Umefjord, G., Sandström, H., Malker, H., Petersson, G.: Medical text-based consultations on the Internet: A 4-year study. International Journal of Medical Informatics 77(2), 114–121 (2008)
26. Umefjord, G., Hamberg, K., Malker, H., Petersson, G.: The use of an Internet-based Ask the Doctor Service involving family physicians: evaluation by a web survey. Family Practice Apr. 23(2), 159–166 (2006)

Chapter 15
Intelligent Adaptive Monitoring for Cardiac Surveillance

René Quiniou[1], Lucie Callens[2], Guy Carrault[3], Marie-Odile Cordier[4], Elisa Fromont[5], Philippe Mabo[6], and François Portet[7]

[1] INRIA/IRISA Rennes, France
`rene.quiniou@irisa.fr`
[2] INRIA/IRISA Rennes, France
`lucie.callens@irisa.fr`
[3] LTSI, University of Rennes 1, France
`guy.carrault@univ-rennes1.fr`
[4] IRISA, University of Rennes 1, France
`marie-odile.cordier@irisa.fr`
[5] University of Lyon, University of Saint Etienne, France
`Elisa.Fromont@univ-st-etienne.fr`
[6] Dept. of Cardiology, CHU-University of Rennes 1, France
`philippe.mabo@univ-rennes1.fr`
[7] IMAG, Grenoble, France
`francois.portet@imag.fr`

Abstract. Monitoring patients in intensive care units is a critical task. Simple condition detection is generally insufficient to diagnose a patient and may generate many false alarms to the clinician operator. Deeper knowledge is needed to discriminate among the flow of alarms those that necessitate urgent therapeutic action. Overall, it is important to take into account the monitoring context: sensor and signal context (are the signal data noisy or clear?), the patient condition (is the state of the patient evolving or stable? is the condition of the patient critical or safe?), the environmental context (do the external conditions influence the patient condition or not?). To achieve the best surveillance as possible, we propose an intelligent monitoring system that makes use of several artificial intelligence techniques: artificial neural networks for signal processing and temporal abstraction, temporal reasoning, model based diagnosis, decision rule based system for adaptivity and machine learning for knowledge acquisition. To tackle the difficulty of taking context change into account, we introduce a pilot aiming at adapting the system behavior by reconfiguring or tuning the parameters of the system modules. A prototype has been implemented and is currently experimented and evaluated. Some results, showing the benefits of the approach, are given.

1 Introduction

Monitoring means to process incoming data (signals) recorded by sensors in order to recognize alarming conditions. Such devices may generate alarms in huge volume that can overwhelm an operator who has to validate the alarms and take therapeutic actions.

I. Bichindaritz et al. (Eds.): Computational Intelligence in Healthcare 4, SCI 309, pp. 329–346.
springerlink.com

What the operator really needs is a decision support system that could help him decide whether an alarm needs some action or can be skipped safely. In the 1980's the concept of kwnowledge based system emerged with the aim to associate deep knowledge to diagnosis. An intelligent monitoring system integrates such a knowledge-based system into a monitoring system.

The first step of intelligent monitoring is temporal abstraction. This means transforming numerical time series into symbolic event sequences. There is a huge literature in this domain (for surveys see [35,20]), e.g. in the cardiac domain. The second step is devoted to the reasoning task. Among proposals, model-based diagnosis [28,5] has the main avantage of using an explicit model that can be used to diagnose the series of events observed during monitoring as well as giving comprehensible explanations to the operator. As diseases have an important temporal dimension, we have proposed to represent them by sets of events linked by temporal constraints on their occurrences. Such sets of events are called chronicles [11]. They can model (a faulty model, in this case) the evolution of a disease during time or local typical temporal phenomena, e.g. typical wave sequences of an electrocardiogram (ECG) that represent cardiac beats characteristic of some rhythm problem. Their recognition on an input stream is based on efficient processing of temporal constraint networks [6]. This makes chronicles good candidates for monitoring.

One of the main challenge of temporal abstraction in intelligent monitoring systems is to closely couple signal processing tasks and higher level tasks involved in diagnosis. One source of difficulty is that, generally, recorded data are highly dynamic and subject to changes. For example, the patient may move letting some sensor transmit very noisy data. Also, the patient state may evolve quickly due to the effect of some drug or disease evolution. We propose to introduce a central module called a pilot that analyzes continuously the monitoring context, i.e. the nature and quality of signals as well as the hypotheses devised by the diagnosis module. The aim of the pilot is to select the best signal processing algorithms and the right abstraction level for data abstraction. The pilot makes use of decision rules in order to bring high flexibility for taking into account new monitoring conditions or new monitoring domains.

The major bottleneck of knowledge based approaches is knowledge acquisition and maintenance. Machine learning has been advocated for this task. Since monitored diseases have a temporal relational dimension, first order models are good candidates for knowledge representation. This is why we have used Inductive Logic Programming [25] for learning chronicles. Devising decision rules for the pilot could also be tedious and time consuming [26]. We have proposed decision tree learning for inducing decision rules from the performance of algorithms in a representative set of contexts.

This article summarizes the work done during several years as an active collaboration with experts in biological signal processing and the department of cardiology of the local hospital and which led to the implementation of an experimental platform called Calicot. Section 2 we survey some work on intelligent monitoring and self-adaptation. Section 3 describes the medical applicative context. In Section 3, an overall overview of the system architecture is given. In Sections 5 and 6, we present the temporal abstraction and diagnosis methods. In Section 7, a solution to adaptation to context change is detailed. Learning chronicles and decision rules are presented in Section 8. We provide some evaluation results in Section 9 before concluding.

2   Related Work

Stacey and McGregor's survey [35] lists many intelligent monitoring systems that share several objectives and features with ours. To cite a few, RÉSUMÉ [34], VIE-VENT [22] and its successors like ASGAARD [33] have introduced general knowledge representation paradigms for temporal abstraction with a deep integration of domain knowledge. VIE-VENT could process data streams whereas RÉSUMÉ was limited to databases. For efficiency reasons, instead of being general, our work focusses on cardiac knowledge in order to extract rich information from ECG or pressure signals online. From the temporal reasoning and diagnosis point of view, NÉO-GANESH [8] shares the concept of temporal patterns, called scenarios, with our approach. Recent developments have led to knowledge-based temporal abstraction (KBTA) where machine learning techniques are used to extract the most discriminating patterns which can be identified in normal and several pathological states. There is a wide literature about temporal abstraction in medical domains [20,35]. The Calicot system [3], dedicated to cardiac arrhythmias detection, and the one proposed by Guimaraes [13] which is focused to sleep-related respiratory disorders are two examples. Collaborative knowledge discovery approaches exploiting the properties of multi-agent systems (open character, autonomy of its components) have been proposed recently[16] for the exploration of mechanical ventilation asynchronies.

Self-adaptation techniques have been advocated to cope with changes in the environment of the computation. This has been an issue for many years in the monitoring field, especially in the medical domain. With the advent of pervasive and ubiquitous computing, self-adaptive software is becoming a major concern in the field of software engineering (see [21] for an overview).

Two main operational paradigms have been used for self adaptive software: dynamic planning and control theory-like architecture [29]. Dynamic planning has been used for adaptive monitoring or computation in medical systems such as GUARDIAN [19], ASGAARD [32] or in image processing [2]: giving some goals (describing a therapy or a final execution state), a plan is computed by planning or instantiating a plan model. The plan operations are followed until observations contradict plan expectations. Past and actual plan operations can be used to evaluate the execution of the plan. Future plan operations can be used to focus data abstraction to specific processing and to adapt the involved algorithms. As in our approach, these systems provide upwards and downwards control. However, except for GUARDIAN where a knowledge-based approach is advocated, it is not clear how adaptation is implemented in those systems. In our case, a declarative approach based on event action rules is used.

An alternative method consists in viewing adaptation as in control theory: a supervision module analyzes continuously inputs and outputs in order to reconfigure the system by selecting and adapting the processing components. This approach has been adopted for self-adaptive signal processing [17] or self-adapting numerical software application [9], for instance. Like many other approaches in software engineering [21], the burden is put on how to take an optimal advantage of available resources, i.e. machines, softwares, network resources, etc. For instance, there are many attempts for inventing new generic methods for delegating the reconfiguration capabilities to the middleware. In these approaches the knowledge of the high-level application goals is not fully exploited. We think that such knowledge can be used for processing and abstracting input data as well as for guiding the selection and instantiation of high-level goals from input data features. We advocate the use of a central pilot to achieve this task. Some authors [9,19] have advocated distributed adaptation. We think that distributing control knowledge is difficult since high-level and low-level aspects are strongly connected and must often be treated synchronously.

In addition, we have proposed a supervised method to learn such temporal patterns automatically from annotated temporal data. In [17], a self-adaptive software is introduced to modify the processing chain according to some predefined events such as sensor loss. But this approach does not deal with high-level goals as temporal reasoning which is crucial for monitoring evolving systems. In ASGAARD [32], the data abstraction module focusses on specific input sources according to a contextual plan which can be adapted when the processed inputs contradict expected values. However, data abstraction subtasks are scheduled in rigid sequences and diagnosis information is not used for adapting the current system.

3   Application Domain: Monitoring Cardiac Patients

Several areas in medicine require monitoring and management, e.g. temporary paralysis of the respiratory center in the brain, renal damage, surgical anesthesia or myocardial infarction. In this latter domain, our concern, intensive coronary care units (ICCU) were initiated in the late sixties, for monitoring the vital functions of a patient after a serious cardiac attack. Such intensive care units are still active nowadays and have the same main goal i.e. to prevent, detect and control lethal arrhythmias and cardiac sudden events by therapeutic actions. To this end, ECG and arterial pressure signals as well as cardiac rhythm are analyzed in real time and displayed to an operator: the trends of the main parameters, such as the cardiac frequency, are computed and alarms are generated. All this information assists the clinician operator who is in charge of analyzing the situation, validating the alarms and deciding which action to perform.

3.1   Analysis of Cardiac Signals

The electrocardiogram (ECG, EKG) is a non invasive observation technique that can provide may details about the cardiac condition of a patient. As such, it is widely used for cadiac examination as well as in ICCU where it can be analyzed online. The electrocardiogram provides a graphical representation of the cardiac electrical activity which triggers the contractions of the cardiac muscle. The electrical activity is measured by placing sensors at specific locations of the patient body. An ECG is made of several *leads*. A lead displays the electrical signal extracted from the data recorded by one or several sensors.

In normal conditions, the electrical signal, precisely the depolarization wave, propagates from the top of the heart at the sinoatrial (SA) node, goes through the atria then

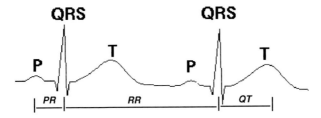

Fig. 1. The main waves of an ECG.

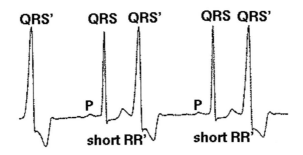

Fig. 2. An example of arrhythmia: bigeminy.

to the bottom of the heart through the atrioventricular (AV) node and the right and left bundle branches and back from the bottom to the top of the right and left ventricles. The cardiac muscular cells located along the propagation path contract themselves at the passage of the depolarization front and this causes the contraction of the atria and the ventricles which in turn provokes the expulsion of the blood in the body. The electrical activity displayed by ECG is generally described by a succession of characteristic waves. In cardiology, these waves are labeled by letters starting from P. The most informative are the *P wave* which can be related to the atria activation, the succession of the Q, R and S waves called the *QRS complex* which can be related to the ventricles activation and the *T wave* which corresponds to the repolarization of the cardiac electrical cells (cf. Fig. 1). Wave shapes and the time elapsed between successive waves are major features from which the heart condition and different cardiac disorders can be inferred. The succession P - QRS - T represents a normal cardiac beat and the succession of normal cardiac beats constitutes a normal ECG.

A *cardiac arrhythmia* occurs when the electrical activity becomes abnormal due, for example, to electrical problems on the propagation path. As a consequence the heart rhythm may become faster, lower or irregular and wave shapes may change or some waves are not present or extra waves appear. As an example, Fig. 2 displays an ECG related to the bigeminy arrhythmia. In this disorder, an extra activation node, called an ectopic node, located in one of the ventricles triggers extra heart contractions also called premature ventricular contractions (PVC). The primed QRS complexes, noted QRS', are related to this kind of extra activations.

The other main signal used for cardiac monitoring is the arterial blood pressure (ABP). It depends on the contraction of the cardiac muscle (and therefore indirectly, also on the propagation of the electrical wave). The heart pumps the blood through the vessels such as the arteries. ABP measures the blood pressure in the largest arteries. The most informative points in an ABP curve are the instants when the pressure is the lowest (the diastole) and when the pressure is the highest (the systole).

3.2   Extracting Observation Information from the ECG

The main task of cardiac monitoring is to process the observed signal data and diagnose pathological states. A monitoring system has generally several stages [24]: signal processing, diagnosis and alarm handling, therapy advising. To tackle these three tasks, intelligent supervision systems appeared in the 90's. Their aim was to integrate several sources of observation (numeric or symbolic) and several types of medical knowledge e.g. surface and deep knowledge. Surface knowledge is related to so-called expert knowledge while deep knowledge corresponds to a complete theory about a particular subject from which all valid statements can be derived.

ECG signals are generally more or less noisy. This is a particular challenge for signal processing, particularly to detect and analize P waves. It turns out that a global approach to data abstraction, i.e. taking into account the particular signal features as well as the context of their occurrence, is preferable to a standalone signal processing approach. This is the way we have followed to design the Calicot cardiac monitoring prototype, the architecture of which is described in the following section.

4   Architecture of the Cardiac Monitoring System Calicot

Calicot has two execution modes: offline and online. The online mode, depicted in Fig. 3, is devoted to monitoring and adopts a pattern-matching approach: multivariate signals are first abstracted in series of symbolic timestamped events and then a matcher attempts to recognize, on the fly, instances of temporal patterns called chronicles in the symbolic event series. A chronicle is associated to some cardiac disease and represent a temporal signature of this disease. More details are given in Section 6 about chronicle representation and chronicle recognition. The offline mode is dedicated to learning and updating the decision rule base and the chronicle base.

Contextual information is of great importance for monitoring. On the one hand, by taking the signal quality (noise) into account one can decide more accurately which is the most relevant signal processing algorithm to use in the current situation. On the other hand, by taking the current state of the patient, as well as his past states, into account one can decide more accurately which are the most expected disorders and, consequently, which are the most relevant chronicles. Moreover, these two decisions are not independent: there are situations in which input signals are so noisy that it is useless to try to detect P-waves, for example. Consequently, chronicles that contain P-wave events cannot be recognized and should be removed from the set of candidates. Also, in the context of a particular disease, some types of event could be absent from the set of candidate chronicles and so it is useless to execute costly signal processing

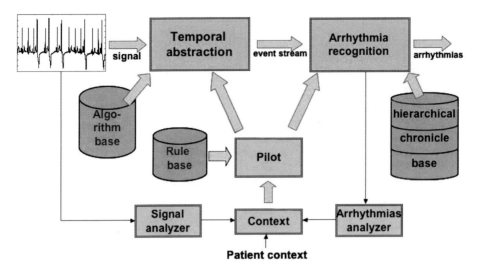

Fig. 3. The architecture of the online part of the adaptive monitoring system Calicot.

algorithms for detecting their related waves. Thus, low (signal processing) and high (chronicle recognition) level computations should be tightly coupled. This is why we opt for an adaptive architecture. On the one hand, a signal processing library containing many signal processing algorithms was built. Their performance have been assessed with many noise and disorder parameter values. Then, these values have been clustered to define abstract contexts that determine when and how to run these algorithms. On the other hand, a chronicle abstraction hierarchy was defined: more abstract chronicles contains less event types and/or less event attributes which makes them more relevant to more noisy contexts. More detailed chronicles are relevant for situations where the detection of specific events could improve the diagnosis accuracy.

The decisions are taken by a central monitor (that we call a pilot) which analyzes continuously the signal and the patient context to determine the best signal processing task and algorithm to execute as well as the related chronicle abstraction level. A centralized control was adopted because it was simpler to specify via decision rules. Figure 3 gives an overview of the architecture.

5   Temporal Data Abstraction

The temporal abstraction step aims at transforming the numerical series into symbolic event sequences that are easier to process by high-level diagnosis. In intensive coronary care units, the main problems come from the presence of different kinds of noise (slow baseline drift, high frequency noise, impulsive noise) and from the great variability of patient dependent patterns and which can change over time. For example, multiform premature ventricular beats (PVC) can combine with permanent or intermittent left or right bundle branch block. The temporal abstraction level achieves two main tasks: QRS complex (ventricular activity) and P wave (auricular activity) detection and QRS classification.

The detection focusses on identifying ventricular and auricular activities on the ECG. Many methods have been proposed for detecting the ventricular activity, i.e. QRSs. Each one fails in specific situations and each reacts differently to the many different QRS waveforms. This is why we retain several algorithms. However, the proposed approach is not to merge the decisions of several algorithms but to select, on line, the most promising one according to its performance in similar to the current situation. Actually, seven algorithms were selected [26].

In this setting, two main problems must be solved:

- devise the activation rules associated to a detector. Decision tree were used to automatically extract these rules. Three main steps were executed i) generate all possible contexts that can be found in an ECG, ii) execute all the QRS detectors in these contexts and iii) select the best detector for a given context.
- define an efficient technique to estimate the current context. Our proposal is based on the observation of several real noisy contexts in order to estimate the covariance matrix and then to apply classical decision rules based upon the covariance matrix and the current observation vector.

Once a QRS has been detected it is classified and a symbolic event is generated. The generation of its attribute values is based on the fact a beat can be efficiently represented by a compactly supported wavelet base [30]. Thus, each QRS is represented by a global extremum at each decomposed level. The QRS classification consists in labeling the beats into two mains classes, normal or abnormal. A probabilistic neural network (PNN) based on radial basis function has been used. A pre-processing step including a principal component analysis was performed in order to reduce the complexity.

P wave detection is very hard because it has a weak amplitude and a variable morphology. P wave detection from the surface ECG signal is generally achieved according to two methodological approaches, window-based search or QRS-T interval cancellation. We retain the QRS-T interval cancellation technique to overcome the limitations of window-based techniques which assumes that a P wave always occurs before some QRS. In particular, such methods have difficulties to detect the P wave in case of arrhythmias with AV dissociation which happen when the AV node blocks the electrical conduction. Our approach [31] mostly relies on: i) QRS-T interval detection and cancellation based on wavelet decomposition, ii) a statistical analysis of the residue for detecting P waves not associated to a QRS, iii) an artificial neural network classifier to reject false detection which frequently occur in P wave detection.

The temporal abstraction module ouputs a sequence of time-stamped events with a shape attribute. For example, below is a sequence of events that could be related to the ECG excerpt of Fig. 2:

```
1   event(p_wave,       5812, normal)
2   event(qrs_complex, 5924, normal)
3   event(qrs_complex, 6315, abnormal)
4   event(p_wave,       7432, normal)
5   event(qrs_complex, 7546, normal)
6   event(qrs_complex, 7882, abnormal)
7   ...
```

where the first argument of event objects is the wave type, the second is a timestamp giving the occurrence time of the events and the third qualifies the wave shape.

6   Diagnosis by Chronicle Recognition

In model-based diagnosis, a model of either normal or faulty behavior is used to detect and identify faults or diseases [28,5]. If a normal behavioral model is used, the values reflecting the patient state are fed into the model and the diagnoser generates an alarm if the model outputs are different from the values observed on the patient. With a faulty causal model, the diagnoser reasons abductively from observations to faults and attempts to generate disease hypotheses that could have produced the actual observations. Sometimes, such a model can be compiled into sets of discriminant patterns that can be efficiently searched for on the input stream. This method is very suited to online monitoring: the input data stream is analyzed continuously and an alarm is emitted in case a set of events that can be related to a disease have been observed in some time window.

In many situations, such as in the case of dynamic systems, time is crucial [4]. The events related to the course of a disease must happen in a specific order and have to respect delay constraints. Moreover, sometimes it is easier to describe a disease by a set of successive or synchronous events respecting temporal constraints than to extract discriminant features from a vector of values recorded by several sensors. This is true in the cardiac domain: the symptom related to some disease, e.g. bigeminy, is described more naturally by the properties of several cardiac beats than by the particular features of a QRS, for instance. Chronicles are particularly suited for the representation of such temporal patterns. Fig. 4 shows the graphical representation of an example of chronicle related to bigeminy and an example of match on two types of signal.

Fig. 5 gives the textual specification of the same chronicle. The syntax is very intuitive. Events are specified by the keyword `event` which have two arguments, the event type with optional attributes enclosed in square brackets and a time variable representing the instant at which the event will occur. Such a variable is instantiated at runtime when an event of the corresponding type is observed on the input stream. Set constraints can be put on attribute variables. Temporal variables can be linked by binary temporal constraints, e.g. in line 4: this constraint says that the delay between the occurrence of a P wave at P1 and the occurence of the following QRS complex at R1 is at least 80 ms and at most 120 ms. All the temporal variables of a chronicle are organized in an STP [6] that can be efficiently processed at runtime. Finally, the overall duration of the episode matched by the chronicle can be specified by a temporal constraint involving the special instants `start` and `end`.

Since input data streams can be huge, recognizing chronicles on the fly must be very efficient. We have used a system called CRS (Chronicle Recognition System) [10] which manages chronicle models, chronicle instances created after detecting events specified in the associated chronicle model and temporal constraints between events belonging to some instance. CRS tries to associate each incoming event with some uninstantiated event of a chronicle instance which satisfies the temporal constraints. It generates also new chronicle instances containing an event that can match the observed

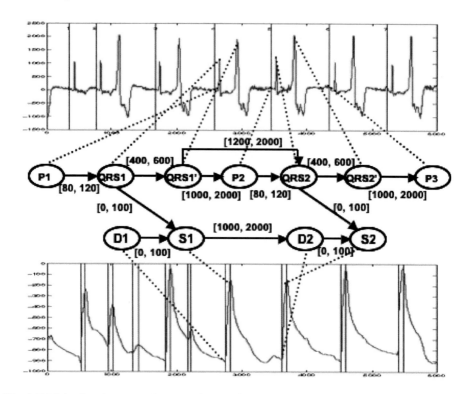

Fig. 4. ECG (top) and pressure (bottom) signals of a bigeminy episode. The graph in the middle shows a bigeminy chronicle model: P stands for a P wave event occurrence, QRS for a QRS complex, D for a diastole, S for a systole. Quoted QRSs represent abnormal ones. Dotted lines indicate possible event matches that satisfy the temporal constraints.

event. Many chronicle instances can be generated in such a way. One strength of CRS is its ability to prune instances, as early as possible, whenever one temporal constraint could not be satisfied by assessing whether an event occurence time has elapsed. This makes it particularly adapted for applications where the detection of critical situations is essential.

7   Adaptation

The architecture of Calicot shares many features with self adaptive systems [29]. Since it is impossible to anticipate every situation and transition, decisions concerning parameter settings and the choice of tasks and algorithms to execute next are postponed to runtime. The goal of this kind of software, is to monitor and control itself. In our case, the system can be viewed as a meta-monitor: a monitoring system, the pilot, monitors a monitoring system. The goal is to obtain the best performance by reconfiguring the system operations, precisely by choosing alternate algorithms and chronicles sets. To each processing module, algorithm or chronicle set, is associated a description which describes the way this module can be used. For example, to a signal processing algorithm

```
1   chronicle bigeminy[]() {
2              event(p_wave[?p1], P1); ?p1 in {normal};
3              event(qrs[?w0], R1); ?r1 in {normal};
4              80<R1-P1<120;
5              event(qrs[?r1_1], R_1); ?r1_1 in {abnormal};
6              noevent(qrs[?], (R1+1, R1_1-1));
7              400<R1_1-R1<600;
8              event(p_wave[?p2], P2); ?p2 in {normal};
9              1000<P2-R1_1<2000;
10             event(qrs[?r2], R2); ?r2 in {normal};
11             80<R2-P1<120; 1200<R2-R1_1<2000;
12             event(qrs[?r2_1], R2_1); ?r2_1 in {abnormal};
13             noevent(qrs[?], (R2+1, R2_1-1));
14             400<R2_1-R2<600;
15             event(p_wave[?p3], P3);?p3 in {normal};
16             1000<P3-R2_1<2000;
17
18             event(diastole[?d1], D1);
19             event(systole[?s1], S1);
20             0<S1-D1<100; 0<S1-R1<100;
21             event(diastole[?d2], D2);
22             1000<D2-S1<2000;
23             event(systole[?s1], S1);
24             0<S2-D2<100; 0<S2-R2<100;
25             0 < end-start < 4000;
26  }
```

Fig. 5. The bigeminy chronicle model.

is associated the task that it can achieve, the objects (types of events) that it can deliver and features describing the contexts in which it should ensure the best performance.

The pilot receives continuously three kinds of contextual information (cf. Fig. 6):

- the line context is mainly related to the signal quality. Noise type and level, the event detection rate and the event distribution are used to estimate the signal quality,
- the arrhythmia context is related to the diagnosis state. The chronicle recognition rate, the types of chronicles recognized so far and their distribution, the expected patient state, etc. are used to estimate the diagnosis quality,
- the patient context is related to historical medical data associated to the patient, i.e. disorders, drugs, etc.

From this contextual information the pilot has to decide whether the context has changed notably and to determine whether a reconfiguration is needed. In this case, the pilot must select the best algorithms and tune their parameters as well as choose the right chronicle abstration level and the set of chronicles to be recognized.

To ensure a maximal flexibility and modularity, the pilot uses expert decision rules to determine when and how to perform reconfigurations. Here follows two examples

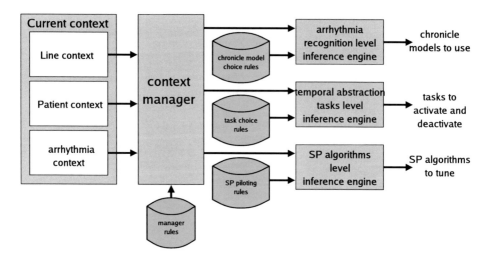

Fig. 6. The pilot architecture for the monitoring system Calicot.

of decision rules. The first one selects a detection algorithm, the second one selects the abstraction level that must be used for chronicles:

if paced **and** noiseType=muscular **and** noiseLevel $\leq$ 0 dB **then** algo df2

if PWaveDetection is active **and** QRSClassification is active **then** abstractionLevel=4

8   Machine Learning

In our approach machine learning is used at two stages: i) for learning chronicles and ii) for learning decision rules for the pilot module. To establish accurate diagnoses efficiently the chronicles should be as discriminating as possible, i.e. they should clearly distinguish the diseases. However, the specification of discriminating chronicles is hard to do manually. Moreover, as first order (temporal) relations are concerned, we have chosen to use a machine learning method that can cope with logical relations and numerical temporal constraints. Inductive logic programming (ILP) satisfies these requirements [25]. From examples describing symbolically signals related to disorder episodes, ILP induces a set of first-order clauses that can discriminate the classes to which the examples belong. Fortunately, one such clause can be translated straightforwardly to a chronicle for CRS. In addition, by varying the language bias, i.e. the description language of examples and clauses, and using related background knowledge, models at different abstraction levels can be learned (see [3]). Furthermore, the model space can be explored efficiently by searching only the most promising parts. In this context, we have proposed a method for learning efficiently from multisource data [12].

The goal of decision rules is to aid the pilot module select the best algorithm and chronicle set according to the current signal and patient context. We have used two approaches to devise such rules. The first one makes use of PCA (Principal Component

Analysis) to determine the most informative context attributes [26] from performance data obtained by executing a set of signal processing algorithms in many situations with different kinds and level of noise and different diseases. Then, decision production rules conditioned by the selected attributes were built manually by an expert. The second, more systematic, method makes use of decision tree learning [27]. From a similar set of performance data, decision trees are learnt. The nodes of such a tree represent a partition of the values of some attribute and the leaves represent a class, here an algorithm. Every path from the root node to some leave can be translated into a decision rule having as conditions the tests in the path nodes and as conclusion the algorithm given in the leave. It is worth-noting that the performance of learnt rules is very close to the performance of expert rules.

9   Evaluation

The Calicot prototype is implemented in Java[1]. Its graphical interface displays monitored signals annotated with complex events related to recognized chronicles (see Fig. 7). Many experiments were conducted in order to assess its monitoring quality and evaluate its performance. Calicot has been evaluated on real clinical data recorded in ICU but, until now, has not been used in clinical routine. This section gives some results concerning the performance of the prototype on QRS detection, with and without piloting.

The context analyser that was implemented is based on a wavelet decomposition-recomposition in three subbands in which the root mean square is computed to obtain the triplet $\langle ls, ms, hs \rangle$ (low, medium, high subbands). This triplet together with the annotated context attributes r, n, SNR (rhythm, noise type, Signal-to-Noise Ratio) forms the context descriptor used by the pilot to decide which algorithm to use. Piloting rules were extracted by decision tree learning from the performance results of 7 QRS detectors taken from the litterature [27]. Three decision trees were induced: D1 (using all attributes: $r \times n \times SNR \times ls \times ms \times hs$), D2 (using a subset of the attributes: $r \times ls \times ms \times hs$) and D3 (using the subbands attributes only: $ls \times ms \times hs$).

Ten ECGs, lasting around 30 minutes each (containing about 18.000 QRSs in total) and including ten various ventricular and supra-ventricular arrhythmic contexts, were extracted from the MIT-BIH Arrhythmia database [23]. Real clinical noise, from 5 dB to -15 dB, was introduced randomly in each ECG with probabilities $P(no\_noise) = P(bw) = P(ma) = P(em) = 1/4$ and $P(5dB) = 1/2, P(-5dB) = 1/3, P(-15dB) = 1/6$ to reproduce difficult clinical ECG situations and to assess the system performance in specific contexts as well as when the context changes. The performance was evaluated from the standard measures: TP (True Positive – correct result), FN (False Negative – missed result) and FP (False Positive – false result) were used to compute the sensitivity $Se = \frac{TP}{TP+FN}$, the positive predictivity $PP = \frac{TP}{TP+FP}$ and the F-measure $FM(\beta) = \frac{(1+\beta^2)*PP*Se}{\beta^2*PP+Se}$, where $\beta = 1$ (same weight for Se and PP).

To estimate the upper bound performance reachable by Calicot with the pilot, the best detector performance (i.e. achieved by the detector with maximal F-measure) for

---

[1] http://www.irisa.fr/dream/Calicot/

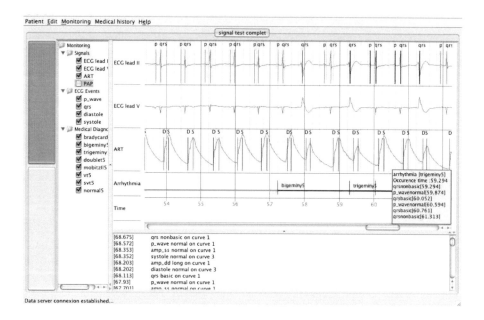

Fig. 7. The graphical interface of Calicot showing the recognition of bigeminy and trigeminy episodes.

each ECG chunck was also kept. These results were used to define the gold standard (bestChoice).

Table 1 synthesizes the results of arrhythmia recognition without the pilot and every QRS detector algorithms, bestChoice (used as gold standard) and the different piloting rule sets. According to the F-measure, pilot D2 outperforms all the other methods. The best non piloted monitoring performance (FM=88.35%) is obtained when using algorithm kadambe for temporal abstraction, followed by af2 (FM=86.67%), and benitez (FM=85.25%). These three algorithms outperform the others with an F-measure greater by 1.73%. The best piloted monitoring performance is obtained by the pilot D2 rule set followed by pilot D1 and pilot D3. pilot D1 performs better than non piloted af2 but worst than non piloted kadambe. The upper bound that can be reached is given by bestChoice with FM=91.71%. This shows that the piloting strategy could be notably improved with more accurate rules (at most by 3.36% on the F-measure).

kadambe associates wavelet analysis with heuristics for self-adapting to the signal, thus, it can be considered as being "piloted". To asses the pilot more fairly, new piloting rules, pilot D1∗, pilot D2∗ and pilot D3∗, were learned excluding kadambe. The best performance of non piloted algorithms was obtained for af2 followed by benitez. The piloted rule sets exibited the best performance: pilot D3∗ with FM = 87.42% outperformed non piloted af2 with FM= 86.67% improving FM by 0.75% which is considered a good improvement in the QRS detection field. The number of switches (column switches) shows that the best possible performance makes 1486 switches. pilot D2 reached good scores with far less switches (294).

Table 1. Recognition results (on 15525 cardiac beats)

detector	sens(%)	P+(%)	FM(1) (%)	switches
af2	92.59	81.47	**86.67**	-
benitez	95.91	76.72	85.25	-
df2	80.64	86.61	83.52	-
gritzali	87.29	75.33	80.87	-
kadambe	94.76	82.74	**88.35**	-
mobd	95.29	68.36	79.61	-
pan	79.66	85.70	82.57	-
bestChoice	92.39	91.04	**91.71**	1486
pilot D1	95.09	82.01	88.06	741
pilot D2	94.74	82.92	**88.43**	294
pilot D3	93.30	81.53	87.02	1478
pilot D1*	91.32	80.74	85.70	443
pilot D2*	92.33	81.38	86.51	343
pilot D3*	94.69	81.20	**87.42**	1642

This is consistent with the fat that this decision tree was learnt from examples described with less attributes, so the decision rules cannot discriminate situations ass prcisely as `pilot D1` or `pilot D3*`. Without using `kadambe`, `pilot D3*` switched 1642 times showing that it uses the available algorithms much more.

Compared to `kadambe`, the advantage of using a pilot is that it uses explicit declarative rules which can be easily updated. This demonstrates the value of using a smart adaptation of QRS detection algorithms according to both signal, patient and diagnosis context.

10   Conclusion and Perspectives

We have presented an approach to intelligent monitoring with self-adaptive capabilities in the cardiac domain. Our proposition associates temporal abstraction, online diagnosis by chronicle recognition, self-adaptation to the monitoring context and automatic knowledge acquisition to learn chronicles and adaptation decision rules. A prototype named Calicot has been implemented.

Efficiency has been a constant concern during the conception and implementation of Calicot, as it was intended to run online. Thus, a temporal abstraction method taking advantage of the domain and data specificities has been proposed. Though they represent complex event, chronicles can be efficiently recognized on multiple data streams, with one or two orders of magnitude less than real time in our case. To enhance the performance we have also proposed an architecture for self-adaptation, featuring a pilot which can reconfigure the processing chain or tune the module parameters when the monitoring context changes. Finally, symbolic machine learning is used, offline, to get discriminating patterns, on the one hand, and adaptation decision rules, on the other hand. Using a symbolic approach for knowledge and (temporal) reasoning makes it possible to provide understandable explanations to the user. This is very important in medicine for letting clinician operators trust such systems.

In our proposal, the adaption functionality relies on a centralized pilot which has to take its decisions *a priori* by analyzing the context. This approach was motivated by limited computing resources. In case of no limitation on computing resources, an *ensemble of detectors* approach could be used [7]. This approach would consist in running all the detectors concurrently and merge their results. Though requiring more computing resources, ensemble methods show good performance and should be assessed for adaptive monitoring. Currently, there is a strong interest in using such methods for change detection [18,1]. We will investigate ensemble methods for self-adaptation in a near future.

We have advocated the use of a supervised learning method, ILP, for learning chronicles. In many situations, collecting labelled examples is difficult and unsupervised learning methods are more relevant. We are investigating data mining methods for discovering temporal patterns containing numerical constraints that could be easily translated to chronicles [14].

Until now Calicot has used a static diagnostic knowledge: decision rules and chronicles are learnt offline and are not modified during monitoring. To perform full self-adaptation Calicot should be able to learn or adapt its diagnostic knowledge online in order to cope with context change or with important changes in the state of the patient. In an other application domain, intrusion detection, we are investigating solutions for dealing with concept change and adaptation [36,15]. These solutions could be tried on patient monitoring as well.

This research could not have been achieved without an active and fruitful collaboration with the medical staff. Working with clinicians in hospital is not always easy for computer scientists: experts are overbooked, getting data is sometimes difficult as protocols for recording data are very strict, especially they should not introduce any risk for the patient or any violation of data privacy. But, confronting ideas and views from different research, knowledge and practice domains is particularly rewarding.

References

1. Bach, S.H., Maloof, M.A.: Paired learners for concept drift. In: ICDM, pp. 23–32. IEEE Computer Society Press, Los Alamitos (2008)
2. Brémond, F., Thonnat, M.: Issues of representing context illustrated by video-surveillance applications. International Journal of Human-Computer Studies Special Issue on Context 48, 375–391 (1998)
3. Carrault, G., Cordier, M.-O., Quiniou, R., Wang, F.: Temporal abstraction and inductive logic programming for arrhythmia recognition from ECG. Artificial Intelligence in Medicine 28, 231–263 (2003)
4. Cordier, M.-O., Dousson, C.: Alarm driven monitoring based on chronicles. In: Safeprocess 2000, pp. 286–291 (2000)
5. de Kleer, J., Mackworth, A., Reiter, R.: Characterizing diagnoses and systems. Artificial Intelligence 56(2-3), 197–222 (1992)
6. Dechter, R., Meiri, I., Pearl, J.: Temporal constraint networks. Artificial Intelligence 49(1-3), 61–95 (1991)

7. Dietterich, T.G.: Ensemble methods in machine learning. In: Kittler, J., Roli, F. (eds.) MCS 2000. LNCS, vol. 1857, pp. 1–15. Springer, Heidelberg (2000)
8. Dojat, M., Pachet, F., Guessoum, Z., Touchard, D., Harf, A., Brochard, L.: Néoganesh: a working system for the automated control of assisted ventilation in ICUs. Artificial Intelligence in Medicine 11(2), 97–117 (1997)
9. Dongarra, J., Bosilca, G., Chen, Z., Eijkhout, V., Fagg, G.E., Fuentes, E., Langou, J., Luszczek, P., Pjesivac-Grbovic, J., Seymour, K., You, H., Vadhiyar, S.S.: Self-adapting numerical software (SANS) effort. IBM Journal of Research and Development 50(2/3), 223–238 (2006)
10. Dousson, C.: Alarm driven supervision for telecommunication networks. ii- on-line chronicle recognition. Annales des Télécommunications 51(9-10), 501–508 (1996)
11. Dousson, C., Gaborit, P., Ghallab, M.: Situation recognition: representation and algorithms. In: Proceedings of the International Joint Conference on Artificial Intelligence (IJCAI), pp. 166–172 (1993)
12. Fromont, E., Quiniou, R., Cordier, M.-O.: Learning rules from multisource data for cardiac monitoring. In: Miksch, S., Hunter, J., Keravnou, E.T. (eds.) AIME 2005. LNCS (LNAI), vol. 3581, pp. 484–493. Springer, Heidelberg (2005)
13. Guimarães, G., Peter, J.-H., Penzel, T., Ultsch, A.: A method for automated temporal knowledge acquisition applied to sleep-related breathing disorders. Artificial Intelligence in Medicine 23(3), 211–237 (2001)
14. Guyet, T., Quiniou, R.: Mining temporal patterns with quantitative intervals. In: 4th International Workshop on Mining Complex Data (December 2008)
15. Guyet, T., Quiniou, R., Cordier, M.-O., Wang, W.: Diagnostic multi-sources adaptatif application la dtection dintrusion dans des serveurs web. In: EGC 2009 (January 2009)
16. Guyet, T., Garbay, C., Dojat, M.: Knowledge construction from time series data using a collaborative exploration system. Journal of Biomedical Informatics 40(6), 672–687 (2007)
17. Karsai, G., Lédeczi, Á., Sztipanovits, J., Péceli, G., Simon, G., Kovácsházy, T.: An approach to self-adaptive software based on supervisory control. In: Laddaga, R., Shrobe, H.E., Robertson, P. (eds.) IWSAS 2001. LNCS, vol. 2614, pp. 24–38. Springer, Heidelberg (2003)
18. Kolter, J.Z., Maloof, M.A.: Using additive expert ensembles to cope with concept drift. In: De Raedt, L., Wrobel, S. (eds.) ICML. ACM International Conference Proceeding Series, vol. 119, pp. 449–456. ACM, New York (2005)
19. Larsson, J.E., Hayes-Roth, B.: GUARDIAN: An intelligent autonomous agent for medical monitoring and diagnosis. IEEE Intelligent Systems 13, 58–64 (1998)
20. Lavrac, N., Zupan, B., Kononenko, I., Kukar, M., Keravnou, E.T.: Intelligent data analysis for medical diagnosis: Using machine learning and temporal abstraction. AI Communications 11, 191–218 (1998)
21. McKinley, P.K., Sadjadi, S.M., Kasten, E.P., Cheng, B.H.C.: Composing adaptive software. IEEE Computer 37(7), 56–64 (2004)
22. Miksch, S., Horn, W., Popow, C., Paky, F.: Utilizing temporal data abstraction for data validation and therapy planning for artificially ventilated newborn infants. Artificial Intelligence in Medicine 8, 543–576 (1996)
23. Moody, G.B.: ECG database applications guide, 9th edn. Harvard-MIT Division of Health Sciences and Technology Biomedical Engineering Center (1997)
24. Mora, F., Passariello, G., Carrault, G., Le Pichon, J.-P.: Intelligent patient monitoring and management systems: A review. IEEE Engineering in Medicine and Biology 12(4), 23–33 (1993)
25. Muggleton, S., De Raedt, L.: Inductive Logic Programming: Theory and methods. The Journal of Logic Programming 19 & 20, 629–680 (1994)
26. Portet, F., Hernández, A.I., Carrault, G.: Evaluation of real-time QRS detection algorithms in variable contexts. Medical & Biological Engineering & Computing 43(3), 381–387 (2005)

27. Portet, F., Quiniou, R., Cordier, M.-O., Carrault, G.: Learning decision tree for selecting QRS detectors for cardiac monitoring. In: Bellazzi, R., Abu-Hanna, A., Hunter, J. (eds.) AIME 2007. LNCS (LNAI), vol. 4594, pp. 170–174. Springer, Heidelberg (2007)
28. Reiter, R.: A theory of diagnosis from first principles. Artificial Intelligence 32(1), 57–96 (1987)
29. Robertson, P., Laddaga, R.: Model based diagnosis and contexts in self adaptive software. In: Babaoğlu, Ö., Jelasity, M., Montresor, A., Fetzer, C., Leonardi, S., van Moorsel, A., van Steen, M. (eds.) SELF-STAR 2004. LNCS, vol. 3460, pp. 112–127. Springer, Heidelberg (2005)
30. Senhadji, L., Carrault, G., Bellanger, J.-J.: Comparing wavelet transforms for recognizing cardiac patterns. IEEE Eng. in Medicine and Biology Magazine 14(2), 167–173 (1995)
31. Senhadji, L., Wang, F., Hernández, A.I., Carrault, G.: Wavelet extrema representation for QRS-T cancellation and P wave detection. In: Computers in Cardiology, pp. 37–40 (2002)
32. Seyfang, A., Miksch, S., Horn, W., Urschitz, M.S., Popow, C., Poets, C.F.: Using time-oriented data abstraction methods to optimize oxygen supply for neonates. In: Quaglini, S., Barahona, P., Andreassen, S. (eds.) AIME 2001. LNCS (LNAI), vol. 2101, pp. 217–226. Springer, Heidelberg (2001)
33. Shahar, Y., Miksch, S., Johnson, P.: The Asgaard project: a task-specific framework for the application and critiquing of time-oriented clinical guidelines. Artificial Intelligence in Medicine 14(1-2), 29–51 (1998)
34. Shahar, Y., Musen, M.A.: Knowledge-based temporal abstraction in clinical domains. Artificial Intelligence in Medicine 8(3), 267–298 (1996)
35. Stacey, M., McGregor, C.: Temporal abstraction in intelligent clinical data analysis: A survey. Artificial Intelligence in Medicine 39(1), 1–24 (2007)
36. Wang, W., Guyet, T., Quiniou, R., Cordier, M.-O., Masseglia, F., Trousse, B.: Adaptive intrusion detection with affinity propagation. In: Theeramunkong, T., Kijsirikul, B., Cercone, N., Ho, T.-B. (eds.) PAKDD 2009. LNCS, vol. 5476. Springer, Heidelberg (2009)

Chapter 16
Computational Intelligence in Cognitive Healthcare Information Systems

Lidia Ogiela

AGH University of Science and Technology
Al. Mickiewicza 30, PL-30-059 Krakow, Poland
logiela@agh.edu.pl

Abstract. This publication presents key problems of cognitive information systems. Cognitive data analysis systems will first be classified, then their genesis and development will be presented, and then their two main classes will be discussed: UBIAS (Understanding Based Image Analysis Systems) and UBMSS (Understanding Based Management Support Systems). The image analysis class is used to analyse the medical significance of lesions of various human organs. UBMSS systems provide automatic support for the strategic and financial decision-making process in enterprises. Due to the subject discussed here, UBMSS systems will be presented as assets supporting the management of medical units.

Keywords: cognitive informatics, pattern understanding, cognitive analysis, computational intelligence, natural intelligence, intelligent systems, cognitive categorization systems.

1 Introduction

The data analysis systems currently in use are increasingly frequently enhanced by adding the functionality for interpreting the meaning of the analysed data. This type of an analysis is made possible, among other elements, by the use of cognitive data interpretation formalisms which include meaning analyses, linguistic descriptions and semantic reasoning.

Traditional information systems used for data analysis are gradually being replaced by cognitive data analysis systems. The classification and functions of cognitive data analysis systems will be presented in subsequent subsections of this publication, along with their main elements distinguishing the analysed decision-support systems from other information systems.

Cognitive data analysis is based on formalisms of meaning-based data interpretation, which in turn are founded in philosophy and psychology. The meaning based interpretation, understanding and analysis are very often similar to human cognitive and decision-making processes, in which information acquisition, storage and transmission are of major importance.

Analysis, interpretation and reasoning processes were used to build and describe new classes of cognitive categorisation systems which are to execute in-depth analyses

I. Bichindaritz et al. (Eds.): Computational Intelligence in Healthcare 4, SCI 309, pp. 347–369.
springerlink.com © Springer-Verlag Berlin Heidelberg 2010

and reasoning processes on the data being interpreted. The main subject of this publication is to present a selected class of cognitive categorisation systems which support analyses of data recorded in the form of images and vectors. Cognitive categorisation systems operate by executing a particular type of thought, cognitive and reasoning processes which take place in the human mind and which ultimately lead to making an in-depth description of the analysis and reasoning process.

The most important element in this analysis and reasoning process is that it occurs both in the human cognitive and thinking process and in the system's information and reasoning process that conducts the in-depth interpretation and analysis of data. It should be added that this process is based on cognitive resonance which occurs during the examination process [16], [28], and which forms the starting point for the process of data understanding consisting in extracting the semantic information and the meaning contained in the analysed type of data that makes reasoning possible [27].

Cognitive analysis and cognitive resonance is an attempt to compare and distinguish certain similarities and differences between the set of analysed data and the set represented by a knowledge base.

The set of data containing the analysed data group is subjected to a process of broadly-understood analysis, which means analysing the form, content, meaning, shape and the like. This analysis makes it possible to extract certain significant features of the analysed data. At the same time, the set of knowledge collected (possessed) by the system is used to generate certain expectations as to the substantive content of the analysed data. These expectations are then compared to the features of the analysed data extracted during the analysis process.

When the features and expectations are compared, cognitive resonance occurs; its essence is that it indicates the similarities that appear between the analysed dataset and the generated set of expectations about the possible results of the knowledge acquired by the system. These similarities are revealed during the comparative analysis conducted by the system, in the course of which the analysed data is subjected to the phenomenon of understanding.

The reasoning process which forms the result of the understanding process is an indispensable factor for the correct data analysis. If it did not occur, it would become impossible to forecast and reason as to the future of the phenomenon being studied. So conducting the analysis without the reasoning process could actually lead to impoverishing the entire analysis process, as it would be limited only to understanding the reasons why the analysed phenomenon occurred, but without a chance of determining its further development.

2   Intelligent Cognitive Information Systems

So-called intelligent information systems were first distinguished within the entire set of information systems in late 1990s. The word 'intelligent' is understood in this case mainly as referring to the ability of these systems to signal their readiness to answer the formulated question in a not fully determined environment, in conditions of uncertainty, when the right behaviour cannot be determined algorithmically. At the same time these systems make success the most likely. In this sense, intelligence is developed on many (intelligence) levels, determined by the computing and storage capacity of the system, automatic data searches and the automatic selection of data processing routines when the system is used to find solutions of problems not fully known at the time of system development, as well as the quality and quantity of information collected in the system (in the sense of both its semantics and quantity resulting from information theory theses).

Intelligent information systems are designed not just to solve indicated problems, but also to foresee changes which may take place in the future in order to anticipate them and take preventive steps. Generally, these systems are characterised by activity aimed at maximising the likelihood that the system will achieve complete success, whereas success may be defined in very different ways depending on the circumstances.

Various grades and types of intelligent information systems are used to achieve different grades and types of success, understood in this case as the measures of the capacity and the efficiency of converting data into information, information into messages, messages into knowledge and finally knowledge into 'wisdom'. The need to built intelligence into information systems is due to the frequent use of these systems to support decision-making. This is because the right decisions are made not when the decision-maker has access only to the data itself, which is indispensable to resolve all dilemmas on the road to the right decision, but when the decision-maker is effectively helped in correctly interpreting that data.

Undoubtedly, a factor which guarantees achieving this success is the correctly defined goal, which directly determines the structure and the tasks of the information system under consideration. The same goal is also used to define the qualitative criterion which determines the degree to which the required success has been achieved, and if it has not been achieved, the degree of its absence. It is good if the information system success is not considered as a binary category (meaning: "success has been achieved or none has been"). The measure of success should be multi-level, as intelligent information systems usually have a well-defined basic level of their operation quality ('acceptable result') and the level of higher success (the highest level). What is more, success should be considered as a time-dependent variable, because the systems considered here most often operate based on achieving a defined goal in stages.

Natural intelligence, just as the brain in which every process controlling the human body begins, is a result of a long process of natural selection. This is where human intelligence has come from and progressed to the current state, and the origin of the well-defined operating principles that have by today been identified to a significant extent. Every intelligence system (natural or artificial) is based on mechanisms that serve to generate desirable behaviours, but every one of these mechanisms stems from individual capacities and capabilities of functions making this system up. What is of immense importance for the correct operation of an intelligent system is the use of basic functions, which include education and development functions as well as the 'instinct'. These functions (Fig. 1) take the same forms as the functions of human intelligence.

Every information system, in particular an intelligent one, must have a function for communicating not just internally, but also between itself and its environment (including with other systems). For information to be transmitted between systems or between the system and its external environment, the information to be sent must first be coded and dispatched to the recipient in that form, secondly the recipient must

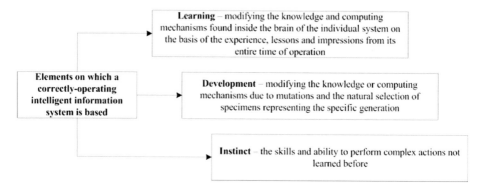

Fig. 1. Components of an intelligent information system
Source: own development

receive and correctly decode it, and thirdly the information recipient must correctly interpret and understand it. Information interpretation and understanding characterise intelligent information system, while the remaining element - data transmission - is characteristic of all information systems.

Intelligent information systems are based on the complexity (calculation) theory, whose foundations consist of, according to James S. Albus and Alexander M. Meystel [1], [15], of perceiving, planning, motivating, training and emotions. However, their most important component is knowledge, whose resources are kept in the human brain. The fundamental computating element and at the same time the main component making up the human brain is a single neuron. Every neuron is a tiny processor containing receptors: synapses on dendrites. Every message is sent to other neurons located inside an axon, whose each branch ends in a synapse on a dendrite or in a human body cell far away from other neuron, or in a stimulated cell, like a muscle or a gland.

Every image, and therefore every piece of information coming from its structure or contents, is sent to the human brain, where it is analysed, classified and understood. This is why all external stimuli sent to the brain in the form of images undergo a whole series of processes which characterise the specific piece of information using symbols assigned to each piece. All known languages, mathematics, science, art, music, dance and theatre are founded on manipulating one or many forms of symbolism, and what is more, industry, business, commerce and warfare could not operate without using symbols. The issue here is the poor understanding of the theory explaining how neurons in the human brain present symbols or execute various types of operations on the representations of symbols.

All over the world, research results concerning the representations of knowledge are very actively studied by informatics and lead to lively discussions in the field of artificial intelligence (AI) and robotics. Scientists elaborating theories describing linguistic trends and representations in the human brain have a strong tendency to depict all symbolism as a form that presents logical theories, expert system or linguistic grammar rules [28]. Many researchers largely or completely ignore the meaning of images as components of knowledge representation.

The circle of artificial intelligence researchers has frequently been criticised in publications by Hubert Dreyfus, John Seale, M. Kickhard and Loren Terveen [16] and many other scientists who pointed out that further manipulations of symbols are not sufficient to understand language and are much less suitable for describing the correct operation of human perception, understanding, behaviours and action.

Nowadays it is noted that to assess the phenomenon taking place, one can refer to the subjective feelings, religious experiences and the free execution of calculations by thought processes inside neurons. There is hope that the brain function mechanism will correctly, suitably and very precisely explain computational theories, although scaled computations of a high difficulty level are nothing else than what has been implemented according to a certain data set.

Today, scientists constructing intelligent information systems pin their hopes on the development of laboratory procedures for their further modification. Around the world, there are whole laboratories dedicated to this subject, which compete with one another to find new, better and better methods of implementing intelligence in information systems, as they are competing for markets to sell those systems in, and their future depends on the innovation of the solutions applied.

Intelligent information systems became the foundation for building cognitive systems whose purpose is not just the simple analysis of data consisting in its recording, processing and interpreting, but mainly an analysis by understanding and reasoning about the semantic contents of the processed data.

Every information system which analyses a selected image or piece of information using certain features characteristic for it keeps in its database some knowledge – indispensable for executing the correct analysis – which forms the basis for generating the system's expectations as to all stages of the interpretation it conducts. As a result of combining certain features found in the analysed image with the expectations - generated using the knowledge - about the analysed semantic contents of the image or information, cognitive resonance occurs [17]-[24], [27]-[33]. In addition, cognitive information systems use methods which determine semantic/structural reasoning techniques serving to match patterns [28]. Consequently, during this analysis the analysed structure of the image (or another form of data) is compared to the structure of the image which serves as such a pattern. This comparison is conducted using strings of derivation rules which enable the pattern to be generated unambiguously. These rules, sometimes referred to as productions, are established in a specially derived grammar, which in turn defines a certain formal language, called an image language. An image (a piece of information) thus recognised is assigned to the class to which the pattern that represents it belongs.

Cognitive analysis used in cognitive information systems very frequently takes advantage of a syntactic approach which employs functional blocks to analyse the meaning and interpret the image [28]. The input image is subjected to pre-processing, which includes image coding with the terminal components of the introduced language, approximating the shapes of analysed objects, as well as filtering and pre-processing the input image.

The completion of these stages represents the image anew in the form of hierarchical structures of a semantic tree and subsequent steps by which this representation is derived from the initial symbol of the grammar [28]. At the stage of data pre-processing, an intelligent cognitive recognition system must (in an overwhelming majority of cases) segment it, identify picture primitives and also determine relations between them. The classification proper (and also machine perception) consists in recognising whether the given representation of input data belongs to the class of images generated by the formal language defined by one of the grammars that can be derived. Such grammars may be sequential, tree or graph grammars, and the recognition with their use takes place during the syntactic analysis conducted by the system [25], [26].

Artificial intelligence techniques are used to support the correct reasoning based on the data sets stored (collected). These techniques, apart from the simple recognition of the data designated for analysis, can also extract significant semantic information supporting the meaning interpretation of that data, that is its complete understanding.

This process applies only to cognitive information systems and is much more complex than just the recognition, as the information flow in this case is clearly two-way. In this model, the stream of empirical data contained in the subsystem whose job is to record and analyse data interferes with the stream of *expectations* generated. A certain type of interference must occur between the stream of expectations generated by the specified *hypothetical* meaning of the information and the stream of data obtained by analysing the image currently under consideration. This interference means that some coincidences (of expectations and features found in the data set) become more important, while others (both consistent and inconsistent) lose importance. It leads to cognitive resonance, which confirms one of the possible hypotheses (in the case of data whose contents can be understood), or justifies a statement that there is a non-removable inconsistency between the data currently perceived and all gnostic hypotheses which have understandable interpretations. The second case means that the attempt at the automatic understanding has failed.

Cognitive information systems work due to cognitive resonance which is characteristic for only these systems and distinguishes them from other intelligent information systems. The use of such systems may be varied, as today's science provides broad possibilities for them. However, the greatest opportunities for using cognitive information systems are currently offered by medicine, which distinguishes more and more disease units in the disease processes afflicting particular human organs, which units are detected and recognised better and better. Medical images belong to the most varied types of data and are characterised by extremely deep and significant (e.g. for the patient's fate) interpretation of their meaning. Cognitive information systems are also used in other fields, particularly in economics, where cognitive systems are deployed to analyse strategic and financial figures of enterprises.

3   Cognitive Data Analysis and Interpretation Systems

The classification of cognitive data analysis systems is aimed at presenting the breakdown of cognitive systems and identifying areas of their application. In addition, cognitive data analysis systems are also categorised, which means that selected classes of decision-support systems are assigned labels, meanings and classifiers which can be used to differentiate between cognitive systems. It is for this reason that a classification of cognitive categorisation systems presented below has been introduced. The following system classes have been distinguished among cognitive data analysis systems:

- decision-support systems – UBDSS systems (*Understanding Based Decision Support Systems*),
- image analysis systems – UBIAS systems (*Understanding Based Image Analysis Systems*),
- economic and strategic data analysis systems – UBMSS systems (*Understanding Based Management Support Systems*),
- person analysis systems – UBPAS systems (*Understanding Based Personal Authentication Systems*),
- signal analysis systems – UBSAS systems (*Understanding Based Signal Analysis Systems*),
- automatic control systems – UBACS systems (*Understanding Based Automatic Control Systems*).

Cognitive categorisation systems can very precisely analyse data, and as the above classification of this group of systems shows, they can do so regardless of the type of data to be analysed. The key to this approach is to select the right grammatical rules based on the linguistic data notation and the meaning analysis of this data, which means interpreting mainly the semantic contents of sets. Semantic contents are usually assessed using information such as:

- the volume of data;
- the size of data sets;
- the type of observable changes:
  - frequency with which these changes occur;
  - type of changes;
  - number of changes;
  - the size (length, width, thickness of changes occurring etc.
- identifying the characteristic features of data sets;
- assessing the importance of changes occurring – prioritizing them.

Cognitive data analysis systems work by prioritizing the changes detected and assigning patterns to the analysed types of data, which patterns allow the variance from the pattern data to be determined. Establishing patterns for all classes of cognitive categorisation systems depends on the type of data analysed and the type of phenomena interpreted.

4   UBIAS Systems for the Cognitive Analysis of Image Data

UBIAS systems used to analyse image data can execute analyses of various types of images, of which the group best developed are medical images. UBIAS systems have been developed for several years and have been used to analyse the data of various kinds of human organs, including images of the central nervous system (the spinal cord), fractures of long bones of upper and lower extremities, of wrist bones and lesions of foot bones. This last example is presented in this chapter.

It has been mentioned above that UBIAS systems have been designed for analysing, understanding and reasoning about a special type of data, namely image-type data. This is why their uses have included cognitive analyses of images of the central nervous system - the spinal cord - and the understanding of long bone fracture images [16]-[24], [27]-[33]. Here we will present an attempt at using them for a new class of medical images: to analyse foot bone images shown further down in this publication.

The cognitive analysis of images showing foot bones has been conducted using formalisms for the linguistic description, analysis and interpretation of data. These include such formalisms as graph grammar. The purpose is to identify and intelligently understand the analysed X-ray images of bones of the foot. In order to perform a cognitive analysis aimed at understanding the analysed data showing foot bone lesions, a linguistic formalism was proposed. It takes the form of an image grammar whose purpose is to define a language describing the possible layouts of foot bones which are within physiological norms and the possible lesions of foot bones.

The aim of this research project was to determine the utility of cognitive analysis methods for this specific class of medical information systems and the analysed images of foot bones. This utility will be measured by the effectiveness of executing a task during which the system detects lesions indicating the presence of selected disease units. The following have been distinguished among these units: fractures, deformations, bone displacements and the appearance of an additional bone. The lesions described can be divided further into various types of foot bone fractures, degenerations leading to the skeleton being deformed, bone displacements,the appearance of an additional bone among foot bones, the appearance of hematomas, calcifications and various irregularities in the structure of foot bones.

Cognitive reasoning and analysis methods were used in this project to detect all the above groups of pathological phenomena related to foot bones. We will prove that the results achieved confirm the suitability of the cognitive approach, although the unanimous identification of all disease units appeared to be extremely difficult. This was due to subtle differences in the input data (images) which were used to take the decision to classify the case under consideration to a specific disease unit.

However, before foot visualisations are analysed, it is necessary to complete a sequence of pre-processing operations. These operations help to extract all bones making up the foot skeleton from the X-ray image. For this purpose it is necessary to segment the image, label the detected bones, and determine their centres of gravity. These centres will then be represented by the apexes of graph descriptions introduced. A special algorithm previously developed for separating wrist bones [19]-[20] was used to segment such images. the characteristic features of wrist and foot bones are similar. Consequently, this algorithm is also suitable for segmenting the individual small bones found in the foot. After the proper segmentation, the image showing bones was subjected to median filtration to smooth out minor irregularities of the contour.

After the necessary pre-processing operations are completed, we get binary images showing the contours of all bones. These pre-processed images will be subjected to further analysis aimed at creating graph representations in the projection considered below.

One example of using the cognitive interpretation of image-type data to analyse data depicting foot bone pathologies is an analysis of images acquired in the lateral projection. We will present solutions for the external lateral projection. For such a projection, the appropriate set of foot bone names was adopted:

- tibia (t),
- fibula (f),
- talus (ta),
- heel (c),
- os naviculare (on),
- os cuboideum (oc),
- os cuneiforme intermedium (oci),
- os cuneiforme tertium (oci).

A linguistic description was also introduced to present the foot bone skeleton (Fig. 2) corresponding to the correct anatomy of this part of the lower extremity.

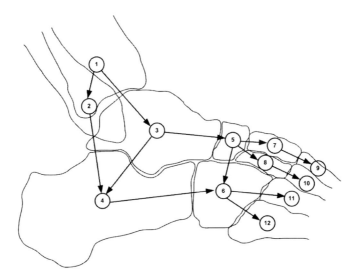

Fig. 2. The definition of a graph describing the foot bone skeleton
Source: own development

In order to analyse X-rays of foot bones in the external lateral projection, it was obligatory to define a graph representation of these bones showing numbers consistent with the neighbourhood relationships of these structures. Such a definition is formulated based on a description of a graph of special topological relationships between particular elements of the graph. A graph of spatial relationships is show in Fig. 3:

Using a graph of spatial relationships to build a graph containing the numbers of adjacent foot bones for an external lateral projection is shown in Fig. 4.

The next stage in conducting a substantively correct cognitive analysis is to define the appropriate formalism for the linguistic analysis and interpretation of

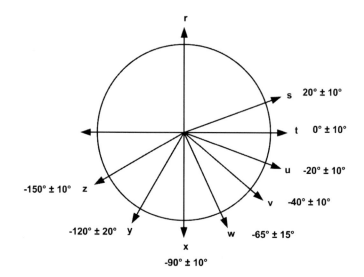

Fig. 3. A graph of relationships
Source: own development

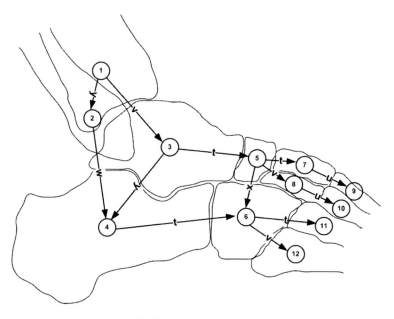

Fig. 4. A graph with numbers of adjacent bones marked based on the graph of special relationships

Source: own development

data. In the case of the external lateral projection, the proposed graph grammar has the following form:

$$G = (N, \Sigma, \Gamma, ST, P)$$

where:

N = {ST, TIBIA, FIBULA, TALUS, CALCANEUS, OS NAVICULARE, OS CUBOIDEUM, OS CUNEIFORME INTERMEDIUM, OS CUNEIFORME LATERALE, M1, M2, M3, M4},

Σ = {s, t, u, v, w, x, y, z, t, f, ta, c, on, oc, oci, ocl, m1, m2, m3, m4}

Γ – the graph shown in Fig. 5

The start symbol S = ST

P – a finite set of productions shown in Fig. 5

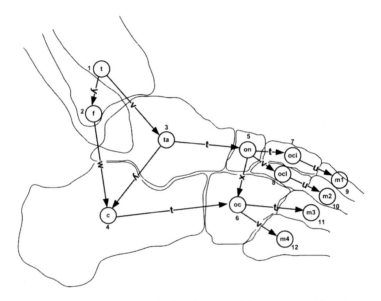

Fig. 5. Interrelations between particular elements of the structure of foot bones
Source: own development

Defining such elements of the grammar is aimed at specifying a set of grammatical rules. Such rules would enable all cases of images showing the correct structure of foot bones to be interpreted. It should be kept in mind that this is a different set of grammatical rules for every projection. Figure 6 shows a set of graphs defining the correct structure of foot bones visible in the external lateral projection.

Determining the correct relationships and the correct structure of foot bones enables UBIAS systems to conduct a meaning analysis. For such projections of foot images, these analyses can generate results of reasoning about and interpreting selected types of fractures and pathological situations. Examples of those situations are shown in Fig. 7.

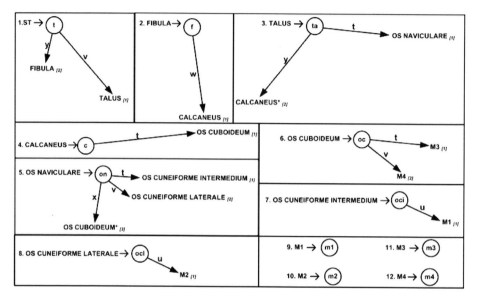

Fig. 6. A set showing the healthy structure of foot bones including their numbers
Source: own development

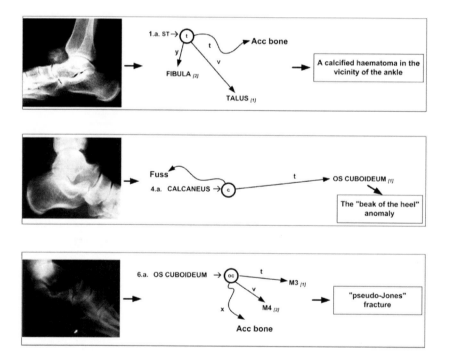

Fig. 7. The automatic understanding of foot bone lesions detected by the UBIAS system
Source: own development

The presented type of automatic understanding of image-type data for interpreting and analysing X-rays of foot bones in the external lateral projection was aimed at detecting various types of fractures and irregularities appearing in the structure of the bone and at detecting lesions - haematomas.

In the cognitive analysis of X-ray images of foot bones aimed at determining the semantics of the analysed foot skeleton data, the interpretation process was applied to images showing such pathologies as bone fractures, deformations and dislocations.

To summarise the above discussions, it can be said that the type of foot projection described above became the basis for introducing definitions of grammars and formal descriptions that are to support the in-depth analysis, interpretation and the semantic description of analysed data in the image form. The analysis and reasoning conducted were not just about the simple identification of the pathology. They were mainly about identifying the type of that pathology, understanding it and presenting the semantics contained in the image. The attempt at the automatic understanding of the analysed data by the UBIAS system was made using the cognitive analysis and interpretation of selected medical images depicting various types of foot bone deformations. Identifying very robust formalisms of the linguistic description and the meaning analysis of data makes it possible to conduct a complete analysis of foot bone images, comprising the semantic reasoning and the indication of the specific type of a pathology. It can also be used to indicate specific therapeutic recommendations in the diagnostic/treatment process conducted by a specialist physician (taking into consideration additional information from the patient's medical history).

The example presented earlier showed the results of the semantic, meaning interpretation of analysed and detected lesions found in the area of foot bones.

The efficacy of applying the cognitive analysis is presented in a table and is aimed at comparing the results obtained by the cognitive analysis with results which can be considered as correct diagnoses (Tab. 1).

Table 1. The efficacy of applying a cognitive analysis for the meaning diagnosis of selected disorders of foot bones

Lesion analysed	Number of images analysed	Number of images (lesions) diagnosed correctly	Cognitive analysis efficacy [%]
Bone fractures	12	10	83,3
Bone displacements	20	18	90,0
Deformations, degenerations	16	16	100,0
Incorrect bone structures	20	18	90,0
Appearance of an additional bone	10	8	80,0
Total	78	70	89,7

Source: own development

These results were achieved by applying a cognitive (semantic) analysis conducted by semantic reasoning modules of parsers in the proposed diagnostic system. Semantics could be identified by defining semantic actions subordinated to structural rules of the introduced graph grammars. It seems that this proposed approach has the characteristics of a scientific novelty, as there are no reports in the literature of similar algorithmic solutions and analyses of highly complex, i.e. multi-object, images. This approach could be applied in practice in medical diagnostic support systems.

The research work conducted to demonstrate the legitimacy of cognitive analysis application in UBIAS systems, image data analysis systems, aims to develop them and broaden their application capabilities. This type of data analysis and interpretation is only possible due to image analysis. It is worth adding that the image analysis process rarely covers the complete image. Very frequently only fragments of the image, important from the perspective of the analysis process carried out, are analysed. Elements acquired from an image by the process of exposing them constitute an important element of the correct process of cognitive data analysis. We need to remember that very frequently, the analysed image contains some (frequently a lot of) interference due to either hardware defects or the lack of skill of the person taking that image. Such cases require special precision in acquiring significant information necessary to carry out the cognitive analysis from the image. If insignificant information were acquired, this could lead to the wrong interpretation of the analysed data. If medical lesions are interpreted, this could threaten the patient's life and health. This could happen during an attempt at the automatic analysis of image data, while in the case of the cognitive analysis of data it should be emphasised that this analysis allows such a hazard to be eliminated. This is because the analysis process itself runs in two trains. An important stage in the process of cognitively analysing the interpreted data is reasoning, based on the semantic (meaning) content, that is e.g. the size of the lesion, its location, length, width, area etc. At the same time, a comparative stage (described here as the cognitive resonance) is carried out, as a result of which expert knowledge is used to compare the information coming from the system with the current database of expert knowledge. It is this structure of the system which helps to minimise mistakes, which can be made during the varied processes of data analysis and interpretation.

At the current stage, the research work allows us to find that the proposed solution works right when analysing and interpreting medical data, in particular foot bone images. It is worth noting that the notion of applying cognitive categorisation processes to analyse image data can be used to analyse other types of images. However, it should be added that such an experiment will require the formal linguistic structures proposed here to be re-established and the correct groups of lesion types to be defined for other medical deformations found in other image groups. It will also be necessary to build an expert database about the lesions analysed.

The research conducted by the author based on analyses of images depicting lesions of foot bones has shown that the cognitive analysis of data in the form of images may significantly enhance the capabilities of modern information systems and systems supporting medical diagnostics. In particular, this research has shown that a correctly built grammar makes it possible to precisely define and then run an analysis and then describe selected diagnostic cases. Then, significant semantic information can be extracted from them about the nature of the processes and lesions occurring in foot bone structures. It is worth emphasising that the results obtained in this research project were due to a cognitive process. This process imitates the way in which a specialist reasons -he/she sees the deformation of the organ revealed in the medical image used and tries to understand the pathological process which caused the observed deformation. He/she does not just make a simple classification whose sole purpose is to identify the pattern most similar to the pathological image. In addition, this research has shown that linguistics based on graph image grammars can be used to try make cognitive analyses of lesions within foot bones [17].

5   UBMSS Systems for the Cognitive Analysis of Economic and Financial Data

UBMSS systems, as cognitive data analysis systems, can be used not just to analyse the economic figures of a company, but can also to supplement the analysis of information from data in the health sector. These systems are thus beginning to support the financial and strategic analysis of health-care providers (hospitals, clinics, medical companies offering various health services). What is characteristic of UBMSS system is that they conduct a financial analysis of a company using elements of cognitive data analysis.

In this paper was presented an example UBMSS system illustrating cognitive data interpretation methods for the efficient management of the investment process. UBMSS systems can be used for the cognitive analysis of economic ratios, particularly financial or macroeconomic ones. UBMSS systems can, for example, conduct analyses using the following ratios:

1. liquidity ratios:
    *   COGS (cost of goods sold),
    *   EBIT (earnings before deducting interest and taxes),
    *   NPV (net present value),
    *   CR (current ratio),
    *   QR (quick ratio),
    *   cash ratio,
    *   inventory turnover,
    *   ACP (average collection period),
2. profitability ratios:
    *   gross margin,
    *   profit margin,
    *   operating margin,
    *   net profitability ratio,
    *   gross profitability ratio,
    *   ROA (return on assets),
    *   ROE (return on equity),
    *   ROI (return on investment),
    *   ROIC (return on invested capital),
    *   ROS (return on sales),
    *   NPM (net profit margin),

- ROCE (return on capital employed),
- RONA (return on net assets),
- IRR (internal rate of return),
- WACC (weighted average cost of capital).

The simplest type of UBMSS systems are those that analyse single ratios characterising a company. The most important of them include systems which analyse the NPV. This type of systems is the simplest type of a UBMSS system, and an example of its operation is presented below.

The formal grammar presented below has been proposed for the suggested UBMSS system conducting an analysis based on the NPV:

$$G_{NPV} = (\Sigma_N, \Sigma_{T,} P, S)$$

where:

Σ_N – the set of non-terminal symbols, Σ_N = {*INVESTMENT, W1, ACCEPT, NO_ACCEPT, A, B, C*}

Σ_T – the set of terminal symbols, Σ_T = {$'a'$, $'b'$, $'c'$}, and the particular elements were defined as follows: $a = \{0\%\}$, $b \in (0\%, 100\%]$, $c \in (-100\%, 0\%)$.

This publication is an attempt at defining a UBMSS system for the cognitive analysis of investments on the basis of key financial indicator, which include NPV – net present value (symbol: W1) (Fig. 8).

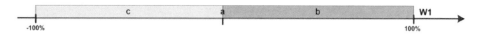

Fig. 8. The set of terminal symbols in grammar G_{NPV}
Source: own development

S – the start symbol, $S \in \Sigma_N$, S = INVESTMENT

P – the set of productions shown below:
1. INVESTMENT→ ACCEPT | NO_ACCEPT
2. ACCEPT→ W1 //*if (w1 = accept) final_decision := accept*
3. NO_ACCEPT → W1 //*if (w1 = not akcept) final_decision := not accept*
4. W1 → A // *w1=decision*
5. A → a // *decision:= accept*
6. B → b // *decision:= accept*
7. C → c // *decision:= not accept*

The analysis of economic ratios conducted in UBMSS systems allows the semantic contents of the analysed data to be used to determine the nature of that data, its impact on the current situation of the company and the extent of changes they cause to the company and its environment taking into account the information currently possessed. Such an analysis is possible due to semantic information contained in the analysed data. Semantic information may relate to:

- The scale (value) of analysed economic ratios,
- The frequency of their changes,
- The manner of their changes,
- The regularity of repetition,
- The number of changes observed,
- The type of changes observed.

The example UBMSS system discussed here can conduct a cognitive analysis of selected financial and economic ratios, which will make it possible to take the best strategic decision for the selected (analysed) company. Figure 9 shows example results of the operation of the UBMSS system proposed for meaning-based analyses and interpretations stemming from understanding the analysed set of financial ratio – the net present value.

Figure 9 shows a situation in which the NPV is positive (0,656). This value of the ratio tells us that the investment project should be undertaken, so this is a fully acceptable situation.

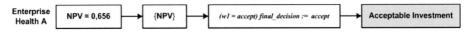

Fig. 9. Example UBMSS system for analysing and assessing the acceptability of an investment based on NPV ratio

Source: own development

Figure 10 shows an example analysis in which the ratio is equal to zero, and in this situation the UBMSS system will also decide that the investment under consideration is acceptable.

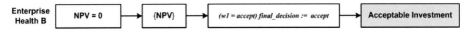

Fig. 10. Example UBMSS systems
Source: own development

Figure 11 shows an example of a UBMSS system conducting an analysis in which the NPV is negative. In this case, the decision to be taken is unacceptable.

The UBMSS system presented above is an example of a very simple cognitive system, but it shows what the interpretation of the meaning of the analysed economic ratio looks like. Every such system can be extended to include other ratios material for the economic and financial analysis conducted. This is why below we present a UBMSS system which interprets several selected economic ratios, including the following: NPV, r_d, IRR.

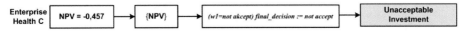

Fig. 11. Example UBMSS system for analysing and assessing the acceptability of an investment

Source: own development

This publication is an attempt at defining a UBMSS system for the cognitive analysis of investments on the basis of three key financial indicators, which include: NPV – net present value (symbol: W1), r – discount rate (W2), IRR – internal rate of return (W3).

For the proposed UBMSS systems, a sequence grammar of the following form has been defined:

$$G_{INV} = (\Sigma_N, \Sigma_T, P, S)$$

where:

Σ_N – the set of non-terminal symbols

Σ_N = {INVESTMENT, W1, W2, W3, WEAK_ACCEPT, ACCEPT, STRONG_ACCEPT, NO_ACCEPT, A, B, C, D, E}

Σ_T – the set of terminal symbols

$\Sigma_T = \{'a', 'b', 'c', 'd', 'e'\}$, and the particular elements were defined as follows:

$a = \{0\%\}$, $b \in (0\%, 15\%]$, $c \in (15\%, 45\%)$, $d \in [45\%, 100\%)$, $e \in (-100\%, 0\%)$ (Fig. 12.)

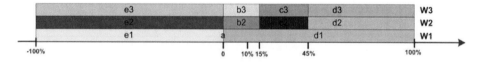

Fig. 12. The set of terminal symbols
Source: own development

S – the start symbol, $S \in \Sigma_N$, S = INVESTMENT

P – the set of productions shown below:

1. INVESTMENT→ WEAK_ACCEPT I ACCEPT I STRONG_ACCEPT I NO_ACCEPT
2. WEAK_ACCEPT→ W1 W2 W3 //if (w1 & w2 & w3 = weak accept) final_decision:= weak accept
3. ACCEPT→ W1 W2 W3 //if (w1 & w2 & w3 = accept) final_decision := accept
4. STRONG_ACCEPT → W1 W2 W3 //if (w1 & w2 & w3 = strong accept) final_decision := strong accept
5. NO_ACCEPT → W1 W2 W3 //if (w1 & w2 & w3 =not akcept) final_decision := not accept
6. W1 → A I B I C I D I E // w1=decision
7. W2 → A I B I C I D I E // w2=decision
8. W3 → A I B I C I D I E // w3=decision
9. A → a // decision:= weak
10. B → b // decision:= weak
11. C → c // decision:= accept
12. D → d // decision:= strong
13. E → e // decision:= not accept

The example UBMSS system discussed here can conduct a cognitive analysis of selected financial and economic ratios, which will make it possible to take the best strategic decision for the selected (analysed) company. Figures 13-15 show example results of the operation of the UBMSS system proposed for meaning-based analyses and interpretations stemming from understanding the analysed set of three financial ratios: the net present value, the discount rate, the internal rate of return.

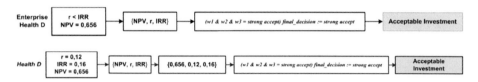

Fig. 13. Example UBMSS system for analysing and assessing the acceptability of an investment based on selected economic ratios
Source: own development

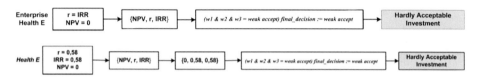

Fig. 14. Example UBMSS system for analysing and assessing the acceptability of an investment
Source: own development

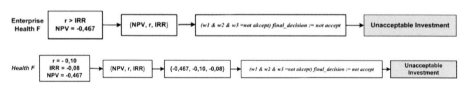

Fig. 15. Example UBMSS systems
Source: own development

Figure 13 shows a situation in which the UBMSS system analyses the economic data of an acceptable investment, in Figure 14 the investment is very good and deserving full acceptance, and in Figure 15 the system analysed ratios describing an unacceptable investment.

All cases of analysed economic and financial ratios demonstrate that it is of utmost importance to determine their impact on and their significance for the decision taken by the system.

Based on the values of the selected economic/financial ratios, the UBMSS system shows what strategic decision is best when it takes the said ratios into the analysis process. This decision is taken by comparing the analysed values with the values, kept by the system in particular knowledge bases, which have been defined based on optimum ratio values assumed by experts.

The above semantic information associated with the analysed economic data presented in the form of financial ratios allows a detailed identification of the type of situation (whether it is pathological or is a phenomenon expected and accepted by the company management with regard to the considered investment) prevailing within the company.

It must be borne in mind that changes taking place inside companies are brought about by various types of situations, phenomena and determinants. These situations may be either external or internal. This is why defining the right patterns applied to UBMSS systems which will be taking strategic and business decisions is very difficult, as it requires analysing a whole range of various factors that can have a significant impact on the decision-making process. It is because of this fact that the UBMSS systems presented in this chapter for supporting the right decision whether to make (or forego) a given investment greatly help choose the best decision and determine whether the investment under consideration is acceptable or not; and if the decision is acceptable, then whether the acceptance is unconditional, or whether there is a certain danger (risk) inherent in implementing it (this situation is illustrated by the minimum permissible values of financial ratios selected for analysing).

UBMSS systems are of great help in understanding the analysed economic, financial and strategic situation with regard to the analysed company, investment and strategy. So they are systems which perform a very important type of analysis – a cognitive, interpretational, reasoning and forecasting analysis based on mechanisms of the linguistic and meaning-based description of data.

6 Conclusions

Artificial intelligence techniques used to analyse complex data and build a new generation of intelligent information systems are discussed assuming a clear dedication to a specific field of application. Due to the legibility and the exceptional character of operations described here when applied to images (which are complex data structures particularly easily penetrated by the human mind), frequent references to image-type data were used in all examples. However, it has also been shown that numerical data can be analysed and its cognitive analysis can be conducted no less effectively if linguistic data recording formalisms are used to do this.

The cognitive information systems considered here, using cognitive data analysis, are diverse, and their diversification results from the broad range of opportunities for applying particular techniques. Data stored in information systems is today subjected to broad analyses to improve this data (e.g. image) quality, to analyse the meaning of this data, to recognise it, understanding it and reason based on the information sets available.

A look at the newest trends in the development of intelligent information systems shows that the pre-processing, analysis and classification (recognition) of the data in question is no longer sufficient. This is why it is proposed to orient these systems towards the automatic understanding of the meaning of the analysed and processed data, e.g. of the semantics of the studied data sets. The human mind has incomparably greater perception skills than even the best programmed computer, which allows the mind to reach the meanings characteristic for the observed objects or analysed data incomparably faster than a machine can. However, machine understanding techniques are also improving, so in time they will be able to execute more complex reasoning by referring to the meaning of the collected data, and not just executer simple analyses of this data. Advanced artificial intelligence techniques are used to make information systems capable of such semantic reasoning about data. Apart from the simple analysis of information and the possible classification (recognition) of data identified for analysing, these techniques also enable extracting significant semantic information from this data, which indicates the interpretation of its meaning. At the present stage, the semantic analysis of data is always rooted in some context assumed up front, as the computer cannot at the same time discover the purpose of the analysis and its result. This means that the cognitive systems being constructed are trying to understand data and reason about it having the purpose of this reasoning specified. This must be contrasted with a human, who encounters a specific novel situation, analyses its many facets, and as a result can draw completely unexpected conclusions which bear witness to the deep mental exploration of this situation, in other words to understanding it fully.

Acknowledgement

This work has been supported by the Ministry of Science and Higher Education, Republic of Poland, under project number N N516 196537.

References

[1]   Albus, J.S., Meystel, A.M.: Engineering of Mind – An Introduction to the Science of Intelligent Systems. A Wiley-Interscience Publication John Wiley & Sons Inc., Hoboken (2001)
[2]   Berners-Lee, T.: Weaving the Web. Texere Publishing (2001)
[3]   Berners-Lee, T., Fensel, D., Hendler, J.A., Lieberman, H., Wahlster, W. (eds.): Spinning the Semantic Web: Bringing the World Wide Web to Its Full Potential. The MIT Press, Cambridge (2005)
[4]   Branquinho, J. (ed.): The Foundations of Cognitive Science. Clarendon Press, Oxford (2001)
[5]   Brejl, M., Sonka, M.: Medical image segmentation: Automated design of border detection criteria from examples. Journal of Electronic Imaging 8(1), 54–64 (1999)
[6]   Burgener, F.A., Kormano, M.: Bone and Joint Disorders. Thieme, Stuttgart (1997)
[7]   Chomsky, N.: Language and Problems of Knowledge: The Managua Lectures. MIT Press, Cambridge (1988)
[8]   Cohen, H., Lefebvre, C. (eds.): Handbook of Categorization in Cognitive Science. Elsevier, The Netherlands (2005)
[9]   Davis, L.S. (ed.): Foundations of Image Understanding. Kluwer Academic Publishers, Dordrecht (2001)
[10] Duda, R.O., Hart, P.E., Stork, D.G.: Pattern Classification, 2nd edn. A Wiley-Interscience Publication/John Wiley & Sons, Inc. (2001)
[11] Jurek, J.: On the Linear Computational Complexity of the Parser for Quasi Context Sensitive Languages. In: Pattern Recognition Letters, vol. 21, pp. 179–187. Elsevier, Amsterdam (2000)

[12] Jurek, J.: Recent developments of the syntactic pattern recognition model based on quasi-context sensitive language. Pattern Recognition Letters 2(26), 1011–1018 (2005)

[13] Kłopotek, M.A., Wierzchoń, S.T., Trojanowski, K.: Intelligent Information Processing and Web Mining. In: Proceedings of the International IIS: IIP WM 2004 Conference Held in Zakopane, May 17-20, Springer, Poland (2004)

[14] Lassila, O., Hendler, J.: Embracing web 3.0. IEEE Internet Computing, May-June 2007, pp. 90–93 (2007)

[15] Meystel, A.M., Albus, J.S.: Intelligent Systems – Architecture, Design, and Control. A Wiley-Interscience Publication John Wiley & Sons, Inc., Canada (2002)

[16] Ogiela, L.: Usefulness assessment of cognitive analysis methods in selected IT systems. Ph. D. Thesis. AGH Kraków (2005)

[17] Ogiela, L.: Cognitive Understanding Based Image Analysis Systems (UBIAS) of the Diagnostic Type. In: IEEE International Workshop on Imaging Systems and Techniques – IST, Krakow, Poland, May 4-5 (2007), CD-ROM

[18] Ogiela, L.: UBMSS (Understanding Based Managing Support Systems) as an Example of the Application of Cognitive Analysis in Data Analysis. In: CISIM 2007, IEEE Proceedings 6th International Conference CISIM 2007 – Computer Information Systems and Industrial Management Applications, Ełk, Poland, June 28-30, pp. 77–80 (2007)

[19] Ogiela, L., Tadeusiewicz, R., Ogiela, M.: Cognitive Analysis In Diagnostic DSS-Type IT Systems. In: Rutkowski, L., et al. (eds.) ICAISC 2006. LNCS (LNAI), vol. 4029, pp. 962–971. Springer, Heidelberg (2006)

[20] Ogiela, L., Tadeusiewicz, R., Ogiela, M.R.: Cognitive Approach to Visual Data Interpretation in Medical Information and Recognition Systems. In: Zheng, N., Jiang, X., Lan, X. (eds.) IWICPAS 2006. LNCS, vol. 4153, pp. 244–250. Springer, Heidelberg (2006)

[21] Ogiela, M.R., Tadeusiewicz, R.: Modern Computational Intelligence Methods for the Interpretation of Medical Images. Springer, Heidelberg (2008)

[22] Ogiela, M.R., Tadeusiewicz, R., Ogiela, L.: Intelligent Semantic Information Retrieval In Medical Pattern Cognitive Analysis. In: Gervasi, O., Gavrilova, M.L., Kumar, V., Laganá, A., Lee, H.P., Mun, Y., Taniar, D., Tan, C.J.K. (eds.) ICCSA 2005. LNCS, vol. 3483, pp. 852–857. Springer, Heidelberg (2005)

[23] Ogiela, M.R., Tadeusiewicz, R., Ogiela, L.: Image languages in intelligent radiological palm diagnostics. Pattern Recognition 39, 2157–2165 (2006)

[24] Ogiela, M.R., Tadeusiewicz, R., Ogiela, L.: Graph image language techniques supporting radiological, hand image interpretations. Computer Vision and Image Understanding 103, 112–120 (2006)

[25] Skomorowski, M.: Use of random graph parsing for scene labeling by probabilistic relaxation. Pattern Recognition Letters 20(9), 949–956 (1999)

[26] Skomorowski, M.: Syntactic recognition of distorted patterns by means of random graph parsing. Pattern Recognition Letters 28(5), 572–581 (2007)

[27] Tadeusiewicz, R., Ogiela, L., Ogiela, M.R.: Cognitive Analysis Techniques in Business Planning and Decision Support Systems. In: Rutkowski, L., et al. (eds.) ICAISC 2006. LNCS (LNAI), vol. 4029, pp. 1027–1039. Springer, Heidelberg (2006)

[28] Tadeusiewicz, R., Ogiela, M.R.: Medical Image Understanding Technology. In: Artificial Intelligence and Soft-Computing for Image Understanding. Springer, Heidelberg (2004)

[29] Tadeusiewicz, R., Ogiela, M.R.: New Proposition for Intelligent Systems Design: Artificial Understanding of the Images as the Next Step of Advanced Data Analysis after Automatic Classification and Pattern Recognition. In: Kwasnicka, H., Paprzycki, M. (eds.) Proceedings 5th International Conference on Intelligent Systems Design and Application - ISDA 2005, Wrocław, September 8-10, pp. 297–300. IEEE Computer Society Press, Los Alamitos (2005)

[30] Tadeusiewicz, R., Ogiela, M.R.: Automatic Image Understanding - A New Paradigm for Intelligent Medical Image Analysis. Bio-Algorithms And Med-Systems 2(3), 5–11 (2006)

[31] Tadeusiewicz, R., Ogiela, M.R.: Why Automatic Understanding? In: Beliczynski, B., Dzielinski, A., Iwanowski, M., Ribeiro, B. (eds.) ICANNGA 2007. LNCS, vol. 4432, pp. 477–491. Springer, Heidelberg (2007)

[32] Tadeusiewicz, R., Ogiela, M.R., Ogiela, L.: A New Approach to the Computer Support of Strategic Decision Making in Enterprises by Means of a New Class of Understanding Based Management Support Systems. In: Saeed, K., Abraham, A., Mosdorf, R. (eds.) CISIM 2007 – IEEE 6th International Conference on Computer Information Systems and Industrial Management Applications, Elk, Poland, June 28-30, pp. 9–13. IEEE Computer Society, Los Alamitos (2007)

[33] Tadeusiewicz, R., Ogiela, M.R.: Automatic Understanding of Images. In: Adipranata, R. (ed.) Proceedings of International Conference on Soft Computing, Intelligent System and Information Technology (ICSIIT 2007), Bali - Indonesia, July 26-27. Special Book for Keynote Talks, Informatics Engineering Department, pp. 13–38. Petra Christian University, Surabaya (2007)

[34] Tanaka, E.: Theoretical aspects of syntactic pattern recognition. Pattern Recognition 28, 1053–1061 (1995)

[35] Zhong, N., Raś, Z.W., Tsumoto, S., Suzuki, E. (eds.): Foundations of Intelligent Systems. 14th International Symposium, ISMIS 2003, Maebashi City, Japan (2003)

Chapter 17

An Advanced Probabilistic Framework for Assisting Screening Mammogram Interpretation

Marina Velikova[1,*], Nivea Ferreira[1], Maurice Samulski[2],
Peter J.F. Lucas[1], and Nico Karssemeijer[2]

[1] Institute for Computing and Information Sciences, Radboud University Nijmegen
6525 ED, Nijmegen, The Netherlands
[2] Department of Radiology, Radboud University Nijmegen Medical Centre
6525 GA, Nijmegen, The Netherlands

Abstract. Breast cancer is the most common form of cancer among women world-wide. One in nine women will be diagnosed with a form of breast cancer in her lifetime. In an effort to diagnose cancer at an early stage, screening programs have been introduced by using periodic mammographic examinations in asymptomatic women. In evaluating screening cases, radiologists are usually presented with two mammographic images of each breast as a cancerous lesion tends to be observed in different breast projections (views). Most computer-aided detection (CAD) systems, on the other hand, only analyse single views independently, and thus fail to account for the interaction between the views and the breast cancer detection can be obscured due to the lack of consistency in lesion marking. This limits the usability and the trust in the performance of such systems. In this chapter, we propose a unified Bayesian network framework for exploiting multi-view dependencies between the suspicious regions detected by a single-view CAD system. The framework is based on a multi-stage scheme, which models the way radiologists interpret mammograms, at four different levels: region, view, breast and case. At each level, we combine all available image information for the patient obtained from a single-view CAD system using a special class of Bayesian networks–causal independence models. The results from experiments with actual screening data of 1063 cases, from which 383 were cancerous, show that our approach outperforms the single-view CAD system in distinguishing between normal and abnormal cases. This is a promising step towards the development of automated systems that can provide a valuable "second opinion" to the screening radiologists for improved evaluation of breast cancer cases.

1 Introduction

According to the International Agency for Research on Cancer (IARC), breast cancer is the most common form of cancer among women world-wide, and evidence show that early detection combined to appropriate treatment is currently

---

* Corresponding author: `marinav@cs.ru.nl`

I. Bichindaritz et al. (Eds.): Computational Intelligence in Healthcare 4, SCI 309, pp. 371–395.
springerlink.com   © Springer-Verlag Berlin Heidelberg 2010

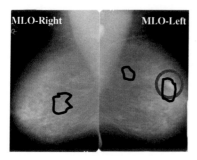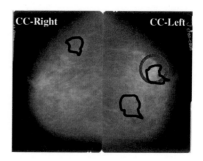

Fig. 1. MLO and CC projections of a left and right breast. The circle represents a lesion and the irregular areas represent regions, true positive and false positive, detected by a single-view CAD system

the most effective strategy on reducing mortality rates. This is the reason why many countries have introduced breast cancer screening programs which target at women of a certain age, usually starting at age of 50 years, aiming to detect the occurrence of breast cancer as early as possible. Breast cancer screening is widely seen as one of the keystone of breast cancer management, and an impressive decrease in breast cancer mortality in the age group invited for breast cancer screening has been shown [1].

The screening process involves carrying out an X-ray examination of the breasts and the reading of the resulting images, or *mammograms*, by trained radiologists. A screening mammographic exam usually consists of four images, corresponding to each breast scanned in two views – mediolateral (MLO) view and craniocaudal (CC) view; see Figure 1. The MLO projection is taken under (approximately) 45° angle and shows part of the pectoral muscles. The CC projection is a top-down view of the breast.

Despite the high level of expertise of radiologists involved in breast cancer screening, the number of misinterpretations in the screening process is still high. For instance, it is not unusual to encounter cases of women which have breast cancer, but have their lesions missed during the reading process. This is due to the fact that diagnosis is subject to one's interpretation: either a lesion representing the cancer is not detected by the radiologist or the lesion is identified but incorrectly evaluated. In other words, mammogram reading is not a straightforward task: image quality, breast density and a vague definition of the characteristics of breast cancer lesions are some of the factors which influence such reading.

In order to support radiologists on their observations, and interpretation, computer-aided detection (CAD) systems are used. Most CAD systems have the purpose of helping avoiding detection errors. However, CAD systems can also be exploited to increase the radiologist's performance by providing some interpretation to mammograms [2].

In reading mammograms, radiologists judge for the presence of a lesion by comparing views. The general rule is that a lesion is to be observed in both views (whenever available). CAD systems, on the other hand, have been mostly developed to analyse each view independently. Hence, the correlations in the lesion characteristics are ignored and the breast cancer detection can be obscured due to the lack of consistency in lesion marking. This limits the usability and the trust in the performance of such systems. That is the reason why we develop a Bayesian network model that combines the information from all the regions detected by a single-view CAD system in MLO and CC to obtain a single probabilistic measure for suspiciousness of a case. We explore multi-view dependencies in order to improve the breast cancer detection rate, not in terms of individual regions of interest but, at a case level.

In detail, the power of our model relies on

- Incorporating background knowledge with respect to mammogram reading done by experts: multiple views are not analysed separately, and the correlation among corresponding regions in different views are preserved as a consequence;
- Analysing beyond the features of given regions: the interpretation is extended up to case level. In the end, an interpretation to whether a given case can, or cannot, be considered as cancerous is our ultimate goal;
- The design itself as representing a step forward on a better understanding of the domain, establishing clearly the qualitative and quantitative information of the relevant concepts in such domain.

Our design of a Bayesian network model in the context of image analysis has important implications with respect to the structure and content of that network, i.e., the understanding of the variables being used, and how those relate to one another. This is seen as one of the major contributions of the present work.

The remainder of the chapter is organised as follows. In the next section we give some introduction on terms of the domain, which will be used throughout this chapter. In Section 3 we briefly review previous research in multi-view breast cancer detection. In Section 4 we introduce basic definitions related to Bayesian networks and in Section 5 we then describe a general Bayesian network framework for multi-view detection. The proposed approach is evaluated on an application of breast cancer detection using actual screening data. The evaluation procedure and the results are presented in Section 6. Finally, conclusions and directions for extension of our model are given in Section 7.

2   Terminology

To get the reader acquainted with the terminology used in the domain of breast cancer and throughout this chapter, we introduce next a number of concepts. By *lesion* we refer to a physical cancerous object detected in a patient. We call a contoured area on a mammogram a *region*. A region can be true positive (for example, a lesion marked manually by a radiologist or detected automatically by a CAD system) or false positive; see Figure 1. A region detected by a CAD system is described by a number of continuous (real-valued) *features* describing, for example, size, density and location of the region. By *link* we denote matching (established correspondence) between two regions in MLO and CC views. The term *case* refers to a patient who has undergone a mammographic exam.

In addition, two main types of mammographic abnormalities are distinguished: microcalcifications and masses. *Microcalcifications* are tiny deposits of calcium and are associated with extra cell activity in breast tissue. They can be scattered throughout the mammary gland, which usually is a benign sign, or occur in clusters, which might indicate breast cancer at an early stage.

According to the BI-RADS [3] definition, "a *mass* is a space occupying lesion seen in two different projections." When visible in only one projection, it is referred as a "mammographic density". However, the density may be a mass, perhaps obscured by overlying glandular tissue on the other view, and if it is characterised by enough malignant features then the patient would be referred for further examination. For instance, many cancerous tumours may be presented as relatively circumscribed masses. Some might be sharply delineated or may be partly irregular in outline, while other cancers (which induce a reactive fibrosis) have an irregular or stellated appearance resulting in a characteristic radiographic feature, so-called spiculation. Masses might vary in size, usually not exceeding 5 cm. In terms of density, they appear denser (brighter on the mammogram) when compared to breast fat tissue.

Masses are the more frequently occurring mammographic type of breast cancer. In the context of screening mammography, there is strong evidence that misinterpretation of masses is a more common cause of missing cancer than perceptual oversight. Furthermore, applications have shown that CAD tends to perform better in identifying malignant microcalcifications compared with masses [4]. Masses are more difficult to detect due to the great variability in their physical features and similarity to the breast tissue, especially at early stages of development. Hence, the prompt of the current CAD comprises not only the cancer but also a large number of false positive (FP) locations-undesired result in screening where the reading time is crucial. Given the challenge in true mass identification, in this work, we focus only on the detection of malignant masses.

3   Previous Research

The rapid development of computer technology in the last three decades has brought unique opportunities for building up and employing numerous automated intelligent systems in order to facilitate human experts in decision making, to increase human's performance and efficiency, and to allow cost saving. One of the domains where intelligent systems have been applied with great success is healthcare [5]. Healthcare practitioners usually deal with large amounts of information ranging from patient and demographic to clinical and billing data. These data need to be processed efficiently and correctly, which often creates enormous pressure for the human experts. Hence, healthcare systems have emerged to facilitate clinicians as intelligent assistants in diagnostic and prognostic processes, laboratory analysis, treatment protocol, and teaching of medical students.

The initial research efforts in this area were devoted to the development of *medical expert systems*. Their main components comprise knowledge base, containing specific facts from the application area, rule-based system to extract the knowledge, explanation module to support and explain the decisions made to the end user, and user interface to provide natural communication between the system and the human expert. One of the early prominent examples is MYCIN, developed in mid-1970s to diagnose and treat patients with infectious blood diseases caused by bacteria in the blood [6]. Up to date, the number of developed medical expert systems has grown up enormously as discussed in [7].

With the extensive use of diagnostics imaging techniques such as X-ray, Magnetic resonance imaging (MRI) and Ultrasound, recently, another promising type of medical intelligent paradigm has emerged, namely *computer-aided detection*, or shortly *CAD*. As its name implies, the primary goal is to assist, rather than to substitute, the human expert in image analysis tasks, allowing him comprehensive evaluation in a short time. One typical application area of CAD systems is the breast cancer detection and diagnosis. In [8], it is presented a general overview of various tasks such as image feature extraction, classification of microcalcifications and masses, and prognosis of breast cancer as well as the related techniques to tackle these tasks, including Bayesian networks, neural networks, statistical and Cox prognostic models. Next, we review some of the recent techniques used for the development of breast cancer CAD systems, and then we discuss a number of previous studies dealing with multi-view dependencies to facilitate mammographic analysis.

3.1   Computer-Aided Detection for Breast Cancer

In some previous research, Bayesian network technology has been used in order to model the intrinsic uncertainty of the breast cancer domain [9,10]. Such models incorporate background knowledge in terms of (causal) relations among variables. However, they use BI-RADS terms to describe a lesion, rather than numerical features automatically extracted from images. This requires the human expert to define and provide the input features a priori, which limits the automatic support of the system. Other research attempt is the expert system for breast cancer detection, proposed in [11]. The main techniques used are association rules for reducing the feature space and neural networks for classifying the cases. Application on the Wisconsin breast cancer dataset [12] showed that the proposed synthesis approach has the advantage of reducing the feature space, allowing for better discrimination between cancerous and normal cases. A limitation of this study, however, is the lack of any clinically relevant application of the proposed method with a larger dataset and an extensive validation procedure.

Automatic extraction of features is applied in [13], where the authors propose a CAD system for automatic detection of microcalcifications on mammograms. The method uses least-squares support vector machines to fit the intensity surface of the digital X-ray image and then convolution of the fitted image with mixture of kernels to detect maximum extremum points of microcalcifications. Experimental results with benchmark mammographic data of 22 mammograms have demonstrated computational efficiency (detection per image in less than 1 second) and the potential reliability of the classification outcome. However, these results required a better validation with a larger dataset in order to provide an insight for the clinical application of the method.

In [14], a logistic generalized additive model with bivariate continuous interactions is developed and applied for automatic mammographic mass detection. The main goal is to determine the joint effect of the minimum and maximum gray level value of the pixels belonging to each detected region on the probability for malignant mass, depending on the type of breast tissue (fatty or dense). The results on a large dataset of detected mammographic regions showed that the breast tissue type plays a role in the analysis of detected regions. Advantage of this method is its insightful nature, allowing interpretation and understanding of the results obtained from the CAD system. However, this approach focuses only on the lesion localisation on a mammogram rather than on the case classification using multiple images.

Despite the potential of these studies some general drawbacks are observed. On the one hand, the methods using descriptors provided by the human expert allow evaluation on a patient level–a desired outcome in screening. However, they are highly dependent on the expertise level and subjective evaluation of the reader, which might lead to high variation in the classification results. On the other hand, the approaches developed to automatically extract features from the mammograms allow more consistent and efficient computer-aided detection. But they tend to analyse independently every image belonging to a patient's examination and prompt localised suspicious regions rather than to use the information from all the images to provide an overall probability for the patient having cancer. To overcome some of the limitations of these single-view CAD systems, a number of approaches that deal with multi-view breast cancer detection have been suggested, as discussed in the next section.

3.2   Multi-View Mammographic Analysis

In [15] Gupta et al. use LDA to build a model that also makes use of BI-RADS descriptors from one or two views. The results of two classifiers, one for MLO and one for CC, are combined in order to improve the classification of the CAD system. However, an overall interpretation of a case-based on its related images is not taken into account. In [16], Good et al. have proposed a probabilistic method for true matching of lesions detected in both views, based on Bayesian network and multi-view features. The results from experiments demonstrate that their method can significantly distinguish between true and false positive linking of regions. Van Engeland et al. develop another linking method in [17] based on Linear Discriminant Analysis (LDA) classifier and a set of view-link features to compute a correspondence score for every possible region combination. For every region in the original view the region in the other view with the highest correspondence score is selected as the corresponding candidate region. The proposed approach demonstrates an ability to discriminate between true and false links.

In [18], Van Engeland and Karssemeijer extend this matching approach by building a cascaded multiple-classifier system for reclassifying the level of suspiciousness of an initially detected region based on the linked candidate region in the other view. Experiments show that the lesion-based detection performance of the two-view detection system is significantly better than that of the single-view detection method. Paquerault et al. also consider established correspondence between suspected regions in both views to improve lesion detection ([19]). LDA is used to classify each object pair as a true or false mass pair. By combining the resulting correspondence score with its one-view detection score the lesion detection improves and the number of false positives reduces. Other studies on identifying corresponding regions in different mammographic views have also used LDA and Bayesian artificial neural networks, in order to develop classifiers for lesions [20,21]. The aim is, once again, identifying a lesion rather than giving an overall interpretation of the case based on its related images.

In [22], the authors proposed a neural network approach to compute the likelihood of paired regions on MLO and CC views, which are within similar distance from the nipple (a common landmark, used by radiologists for finding correspondence between view regions). Their system keeps the same case-based sensitivity (true detection rate) while reducing significantly the case-based false positives. In another study [23], some of the previous authors examined further the effect of three methods for matching regions on both views on the performance of the CAD system. The matching was based on different search criteria for corresponding region on the other view. Results showed that the straight strip method required a smaller search area and achieved the highest level of CAD performance.

In recent study [24], Wei et al. extended a previous dual system for mass detection trained with average and subtle masses, with a two-view analysis to improve mass detection performance. Potential links between the mass candidates detected independently on both views are established using regional registration technique and similarity measure is designed using paired morphological and texture features to distinguish between true and false links. Using a simple aggregation strategy of weighting the similarity measure with the cross-correlation of the object pair, the authors obtained two-view score for malignancy, which is further combined using Linear Discriminant Analysis (LDA) with the single-view score to obtain the final likelihood for malignant mass. Experimental results showed that the two-view dual system achieves significant better performance than the dual and the single-view system for average masses and improves upon the single-view system only for subtle masses, which are by default more difficult to classify.

All these studies dedicated their attention on establishing whether a region in one view corresponds to a region in the other view and demonstrate improvement in the localised detection of breast cancer, mostly for prompting purposes.

Hence, in these approaches the likelihood for cancer in a case is often determined by the region with the maximum likelihood. However, while the correct detection and location of a suspicious region is important, in breast cancer screening the crucial decision based on the mammographic exam is whether or not a patient should be sent for further examination. Furthermore, most of these approaches are based on black-box models such as LDA and neural networks, and thus they lack explanatory power and capability to interpret the classification results. Therefore, in contrast to previous research, in the current study we aim at building a probabilistic CAD system, using Bayesian networks, in order to (i) discriminate well between normal and cancerous cases by considering all available information (in terms of regions) in a case and (ii) provide an insight in the automatic mammographic interpretation.

4   Bayesian Networks

4.1   Basic Definitions

Consider a finite set of random variables X, where each variable X_i in X takes on values from a finite domain $dom(X_i)$. Let P be a joint probability distribution of X and let S, T, Q be subsets of X. We say that S and T are conditionally independent given Q, denoted by $S \perp\!\!\!\perp_P T \mid Q$, if for all $s \in dom(S)$, $t \in dom(T)$, $q \in dom(Q)$, the following holds:

$$P(s \mid t, q) = P(s \mid q), \text{ whenever } P(t, q) > 0.$$

In short, we have $P(S \mid T, Q) = P(S \mid Q)$.

Bayesian networks, or BNs for short, are used for modelling knowledge in various domains, from bioinformatics (e.g., gene regulatory networks), to image processing and decision support systems. A Bayesian network [25] is defined as a pair BN $= (G, P)$ where G is an acyclic directed graph (ADG) and P is a joint probability distribution. The graph $G = (\mathbf{V}, \mathbf{A})$ is represented by a set of nodes $\mathbf{V}$ corresponding one to one to the random variables in X and a set of arcs $\mathbf{A} \subseteq (\mathbf{V} \times \mathbf{V})$ corresponding to direct causal relationships between the variables. Independence information is modelled in an ADG by blockage of paths between nodes in the graph by other nodes.

A path between a node u and a node v in an ADG is *blocked* by a node w if the node w does *not* have two incoming arcs, i.e., $\cdot \longrightarrow w \longleftarrow \cdot$, which is called a *v-structure*. If there is a v-structure for w on the path from u to v then the path is *unblocked* by w or by one of the descendants of w, i.e., nodes that have a directed path to w. Let U, V, and W be sets of nodes, then if any path between a node in U and a node in V is blocked by a node in W (possibly the empty set), then U and V are said to be *d-separated* given W, denoted by $U \perp\!\!\!\perp_G V \mid W$. The reader should observe the association of the subscript G with the relation $\perp\!\!\!\perp$. The idea is that the nodes in the sets U and V are unable to 'exchange' information as any communication path between the nodes in these sets is blocked. If the sets U and V are *not* d-separated given W, then U and

V are said to be *d-connected* given W. This implies that the sets can exchange information.

As the graphical part of a Bayesian network is meant to offer an explicit representation of independence information in the associated joint probability distribution P, we need to establish a relationship between $\perp\!\!\!\perp_G$ and $\perp\!\!\!\perp_P$. This is done as follows. We say that G is an *I–map* of P if any independence represented in G by means of d-separation is satisfied by P, i.e.,

$$U \perp\!\!\!\perp_G V \mid W \quad \Longrightarrow \quad X_U \perp\!\!\!\perp_P X_V \mid X_W,$$

where U, Z and W are sets of nodes of the ADG G and X_U, X_V and X_W are the sets of random variables corresponding to the sets of nodes U, V and W, respectively. This definition implies that the graph G is allowed to represent more dependence information than the probability distribution P, but never more independence information.

A Bayesian network is a I–map model whose nodes represent random variables, and where missing arcs encode conditional independencies between the variables. In short, it allows a compact representation of independence information about the joint probability distribution P in terms of *local conditional probability distributions* (*CPDs*), or, in the discrete case, in terms of *conditional probability tables* (*CPTs*), associated to each random variable. This table describes the conditional distribution of the node given each possible combination of values of its parents. The joint probability can be computed by simply multiplying the CPTs.

In a BN model the *local Markov property* holds, i.e., each variable is conditionally independent of its non-descendants given its parents:

$$X_v \perp\!\!\!\perp X_{\mathbf{V}\backslash de(v)} \mid X_{pa(v)} \quad \text{for all } v \in \mathbf{V}$$

where $de(v)$ is the set of descendants of v. The joint probability distribution defined by a Bayesian network is given by

$$P(X_{\mathbf{V}}) = \prod_{v \in \mathbf{V}} P(x_v \mid X_{pa(v)})$$

where $X_{\mathbf{V}}$ denote the set of random variables in the given model, x_v is a variable in such set and $X_{pa(v)}$ represents the parent nodes of the variable x_v. BN is a Bayesian network model with respect to G if its joint probability density function can be written as a product of the individual density functions, conditional on their parents.

Bayesian networks are commonly used in the representation of causal relationships. However, this does not have to be the case: an arc from node u to node z does not require variable x_z to be causally dependent on x_u. In fact, considering its graphical representation, it is the case that in a BN,

$$u \longrightarrow z \longrightarrow w \quad \text{and} \quad u \longleftarrow z \longleftarrow w$$

are equivalent, i.e., the same conditional independence constraints are enforced by those graphs.

Inference in Bayesian network refers to answering probabilistic queries regarding the (random) variables present in the model. For instance, when a subset of the variables in the model are observed – the so-called *evidence* variables – then inference is used in order to update the probabilistic information about the remaining variables. In other words, once the state of some variables became known, the probabilities of the other variables (might) change and distributions need to be coherently revised in order to maintain the integrity of the knowledge encoded by the model. This process of computing the posterior distribution of variables given evidence is called *probabilistic inference* in which essentially three computation rules from probability theory are used: marginalisation, conditioning, and Bayes' theorem.

Next we present two specific Bayesian network architectures where the notion of independence is used to represent compactly the joint probability distribution.

4.2   Naive Bayes

A naive Bayesian (NB) classifier is a very popular special case of a Bayesian network. These network models have a central node, called the *class* node Cl, and nodes representing feature variables F_i, $i = 1, \ldots, n$, $n \geq 1$; the arcs are going from the class node Cl to each of the feature nodes F_i [26]. A schematic representation of a naive Bayes model is shown in Figure 2.

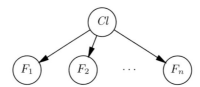

Fig. 2. A schematic representation of a naive Bayes model

The conditional independencies that explain the adjective 'naive' determine that each feature F_i is conditionally independent of every other feature F_j, for $j \neq i$, given the class variable Cl. In other words,

$$P(F_i \mid Cl, F_j) = P(F_i \mid Cl).$$

The joint probability distribution underlying the model is:

$$P(Cl, F_1, \ldots, F_n) = P(Cl) \prod_{i=1}^{n} P(F_i \mid Cl),$$

and the conditional distribution over the class variable Cl can be expressed as

$$P(Cl \mid F_1, \ldots, F_n) \propto P(Cl) \prod_{i=1}^{n} P(F_i \mid Cl).$$

In many practical applications, parameter estimation for naive Bayes models uses the method of maximum likelihood estimates. Despite their naive design and apparently over-simplified assumptions, naive Bayes classifiers often demonstrate a good performance in many complex real-world situations.

The naive Bayes classifier combines the above naive Bayesian network model with a *decision rule* [27]. A common rule is choosing most probable hypothesis–a maximisation criterion. In this case, the classifier is defined by the function:

$$\text{NB}(f_1, \ldots, f_n) = \underset{c}{\text{argmax}} \; P(Cl = c) \prod_{i=1}^{n} P(F_i = f_i \mid Cl = c). \qquad (1)$$

4.3 Causal Independence

It is known that the number of probabilities in a CPT for a certain variable grows exponentially in the number of parents in the ADG. Therefore, it is often infeasible to define the complete CPT for variables with many parents. One way to specify interactions among statistical variables in a compact fashion is offered by the notion of *causal independence* [28], where multiple causes (parent nodes) lead to a common effect (child node). The general structure of a causal-independence model is shown in Figure 3 and below we give a brief description of the notion following the definitions in [29].

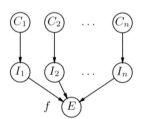

Fig. 3. Causal-independence model

A causal-independence model expresses the idea that causes $C_1, \ldots, C_n$ influence a given common effect E through intermediate variables $I_1, \ldots, I_n$. We denote the assignment of a value to a variable by lower-case letter, e.g., i_k stands for $I_k = \top$ (*true*) and $\bar{i}_k$ otherwise. The *interaction function* f represents in which way the intermediate effects I_k, and indirectly also the causes C_k, interact. This function f is defined in such way that when a relationship between the I_k's and $E = \top$ is satisfied, then it holds that $f(I_1, \ldots, I_n) = e$; otherwise, it holds that $f(I_1, \ldots, I_n) = \bar{e}$. Furthermore, it is assumed that if $f(I_1, \ldots, I_n) = e$ then $P(e \mid I_1, \ldots, I_n) = 1$; otherwise, if $f(I_1, \ldots, I_n) = \bar{e}$, then $P(e \mid I_1, \ldots, I_n) = 0$. Using information from the topology of the network, the notion of causal independence can be formalised for the occurrence of effect E, i.e. $E = \top$, in terms of probability theory by:

$$P(e \mid C_1, \ldots, C_n) = \sum_{f(I_1, \ldots, I_n) = e} \prod_{k=1}^{n} P(I_k \mid C_k).$$

Finally, it is assumed that $P(i_k \mid \bar{c}_k) = 0$ (absent causes do not contribute to the effect); otherwise, $P(I_k \mid C_k) > 0$.

An important subclass of causal-independence models is obtained if the deterministic function f is defined in terms of separate binary functions g_k; it is then called a *decomposable* causal-independence model [28]. Usually, all functions $g_k(I_k, I_{k+1})$ are identical for each k. Typical examples of decomposable causal-independence models are the noisy-OR [30] models, where the function f represents a logical OR. A simple example for the application of the logical OR in the domain of breast cancer is given in the Appendix, motivating the use of noisy-OR models in the general theoretical framework presented in the next section.

5   Bayesian Multi-View Detection

The inputs for the proposed multi-view detection scheme are the regions detected by a single-view CAD system presented in [17] and for completeness it is briefly described here.

5.1   Single-View CAD System

As its name implies, the single-view CAD system analyses independently each mammographic view of each breast. Figure 4 depicts a schematic representation of the single-view system used in this study. It consists of the following four main steps:

1. *Mammogram segmentation* into background area, breast, and for MLO, the pectoral muscles.
2. *Local maxima detection* based on pixel-based locations. For each location in the breast area a number of features are computed that are related to

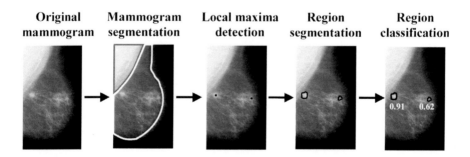

Fig. 4. Stages in the single-view CAD system

tumour characteristics such as presence of spicules (star-like structure) and focal mass. Based on these features, a neural network (NN) classifier is then employed to compute the region likelihood for cancer. The locations with a likelihood above certain threshold are selected as locations of interest.

3. *Region segmentation* with dynamic programming using the detected locations as seed points. For each region a number of continuous features are computed based on breast and local area information, e.g., contrast, size, location.

4. *Region classification* as "normal" and "abnormal" based on the region features. A likelihood for cancer is computed based on supervised learning with a NN and converted into *normality score* (NSc): the average number of normal regions in a view (image) with the same or higher cancer likelihood. Hence, the lower the normality score the higher the likelihood for cancer.

Based on the single-view CAD system the likelihood for cancer for a view, breast or case is computed by taking the likelihood of the most suspicious region within the view, breast or case, respectively. Although this system demonstrates good detection rate at a region level, its performance deteriorates at a case level. One of the main reasons is that the single-view processing fails to account for view interactions in computing the region likelihood for cancer. To overcome this limitation, we consider the problem of multi-view breast cancer detection, presented in the next section, and subsequently we propose a Bayesian network framework to model this problem.

5.2   Multi-View Problem Description

The objective of mammographic multi-view detection is to determine whether or not the breast and respectively the patient exhibits characteristics of abnormality by establishing correspondences between two-dimensional image features in multiple breast projections. Figure 5 depicts a schematic representation of multi-view detection.

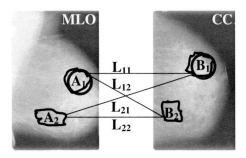

Fig. 5. Schematic representation of mammographic multi-view analysis with automatically detected regions

A lesion projected in MLO and CC views is displayed as a circle; thus, the whole breast and the patient is cancerous. An automatic single-view system detects regions in both views and a number of real-valued features are extracted to describe every region. In the figure regions A_1 and B_1 are correct detection of the lesion, i.e., these are true positive (TP) regions whereas A_2 and B_2 are false positive (FP) regions. Since we deal with projections of the same physical object we introduce links (L_{ij}) between the detected regions in both views, A_i and B_j. Every link has a class (label) $L_{ij} = \ell_{ij}$ defined as follows

$$\ell_{ij} = \begin{cases} true & \text{if } A_i \text{ } \mathbf{OR} \text{ } B_j \text{ are } \mathbf{TP}, \\ false & \text{otherwise.} \end{cases} \tag{2}$$

This definition allows us to maintain information about the presence of cancer even if there is no cancer detection in one of the views. In contrast to the clinical practice, in the screening setting the detected lesions are usually small and due to the breast compression they are sometimes difficult to observe in both views. A binary class C, with values of $true$ (presence of cancer) and $false$, for region, view, breast and patient is assumed to be provided by pathology or a human expert.

In any case, multiple views corresponding to the same cancerous part contain correlated characteristics whereas views corresponding to normal parts tend to be less correlated. For example, in mammography an artefactual density might appear in one view due to the superposition of normal tissue whereas it disappears in the other view. To account for the interaction between the breast projections, in the next section we present a Bayesian network framework for multi-view mammographic analysis.

5.3   Model Description

The architecture of our model for two-view mammographic analysis is inspired by the way radiologists analyse images, where several levels of interpretation are distinguished. At the lowest image level, radiologists look for regions suspicious for cancer. If suspicious regions are observed on both views of the same breast, then the individual suspiciousness of these regions increases implying that a lesion is likely to be present. As a result, the whole breast as well as the exam and patient is considered suspicious for cancer; otherwise, the breast, exam and patient is considered normal.

From a CAD point of view the first step–identifying suspicious regions–have already been tackled by the single-view CAD systems developed by our group. Furthermore, in [31,32] we proposed a two-step Bayesian network framework for multi-view detection using the regions from the single-view system. Here, we extend this system to create an unified framework to model the following stages in the mammographic analysis as described above. Figure 6 represents the new advanced framework.

At first we compute the probability that a region in one view is classified as $true$ given its links to the regions in the other view. A straightforward way to

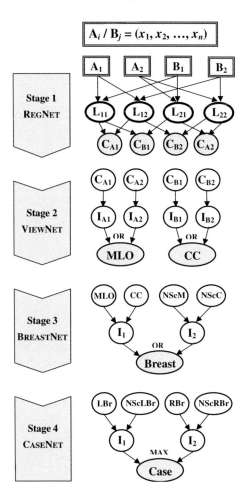

Fig. 6. Bayesian network framework for representing the dependencies between multiple views of an object

model a link L_{ij} is to use the corresponding regions A_i and B_j as causes for the link class, i.e., creating the so-called *v-structure* $A_i \longrightarrow L_{ij} \longleftarrow B_j$, defined in Section 4.1. Since the link variable is discrete and the regions are represented by a vector of real-valued features $(x_1, x_2, \ldots, x_n)$ extracted from an automatic detection system, we apply logistic regression to compute $P(L_{ij} = true | A_i, B_j)$:

$$P(L_{ij} = true | A_i, B_j) = \frac{\exp\left(\beta_0^{\ell_{ij}} + \beta_1^{\ell_{ij}} x_1 + \cdots + \beta_k^{\ell_{ij}} x_k\right)}{1 + \exp\left(\beta_0^{\ell_{ij}} + \beta_1^{\ell_{ij}} x_1 + \cdots + \beta_k^{\ell_{ij}} x_k\right)}$$

where β's are the model parameters we optimise and k is the total number of features of regions A_i and B_j. Logistic regression ensures that the outputs $P(L_{ij} = true | A_i, B_j)$ lie in the range $[0, 1]$ and they sum up to one. Next we compute the probabilities $P(C_{A_i} = true|L_{ij} = true)$ and $P(C_{B_j} = true|L_{ij} = true)$ where C_{A_i} and C_{B_j} are the classes of regions A_i and B_j, respectively. Given our class definition in (2), we can easily model these relations through a causal independence model using the logical OR. The Bayesian network `RegNet` models this scheme.

At the second stage of our Bayesian network framework we combine the computed region probabilities from `RegNet` by using a causal independence model with the logical OR to obtain the probability for cancer of the respective view. Thus we represent the knowledge that the detection of at least one cancerous region is sufficient to classify the whole view as cancerous whereas the detection of more cancerous regions will increase the probability of the view being cancerous. We call this Bayesian network `ViewNet`.

At the third stage, we combine the view probabilities obtained from `ViewNet` into a single probabilistic measure for the breast as a whole. As additional inputs we use the likelihoods for cancer (NSc) for each view computed by the single-view CAD system, which are already indicators for the level of suspiciousness of the view. To explicitly account for the view dependences we model the probabilities obtained from `ViewNet` and the single-view measure by two v-structures, whose outputs are combined using the logical OR function. We refer to this Bayesian network model as to `BreastNet`.

In the last, fourth, stage, we compute the probability for a case being cancerous using two combining schemes. Since in the screening programs breast cancer occurs mostly in one of the breasts then the first simple combining technique is to take the maximum of both breast probabilities obtained from `BreastNet`. As a second more advanced scheme we use a causal independence model and the MAX function to combine the breast probabilities from `BreastNet` and the single-view likelihoods for cancer for each breast. We refer to the latter as to `CaseNet` and to the whole multi-view detection scheme as to `MV-CAD-Causal`.

6   Application to Breast Cancer Data

6.1   Data Description

The proposed model was evaluated using a data set containing 1063 screening exams from which 383 are cancerous. All exams contained both MLO and CC views. The total number of breasts were 2126 from which 385 had cancer. All cancerous breasts had one visible lesion in at least one view, which was verified by pathology reports to be malignant. Lesion contours were marked by, or under supervision of, a mammogram reader.

For each image (mammogram) we selected the first 5 most suspicious regions detected by the single-view CAD system. In total there were 10478 MLO regions and 10343 CC regions. Every region is described by 11 continuous features automatically extracted by the system, which tend to be relatively correlated across the views. These features include the neural network's output from the single-view CAD and lesion characteristics such as spiculation, focal mass, size, contrast, linear texture and location coordinates. Every region from MLO view was linked with every region in CC view, thus obtaining 51088 links in total. We added the link class variable with binary values *true* and *false* following the definition in equation (2). Finally to every region, view, breast and case, we assigned class values of *true* (presence of cancer) and *false* according to the ground-truth information provided by pathology reports.

6.2 Evaluation

To train and evaluate the proposed multi-view CAD system, we used a stratified two-fold cross validation: the dataset is randomly split into two subsets with approximately equal number of observations and proportion of cancerous cases. The data for a whole case belonged to only one of the folds. Each fold is used as a training set and as a test set. At every level (region, view, breast and case) the same data folds were used. Although we use the results from the single-view CAD system, we note that the random split for the multi-view CAD system is done independently. This follows from the fact that the current framework uses only a subset of the data (cases without CC views have been excluded).

The Bayesian networks at all stages of our `MV-CAD-Causal` model have been built, trained and tested by using the Bayesian Network Toolbox in Matlab ([33]). The learning has been done using the EM algorithm, which is typically used to approximate a probability function given incomplete samples (in our networks the OR-nodes are not observed).

We compare the performance of our `MV-CAD-Causal` model with the performance of the single-view CAD system (`SV-CAD`). As additional benchmark methods for comparison at the breast and case level, we use the naive Bayes classifier (`MV-CAD-NB`) and the logistic regression (`MV-CAD-LR`). Both classifiers use the same inputs as `MV-CAD-Causal` at both levels. The model comparison analysis is done using Receiver Operating Characteristic (ROC) curve ([34]) and the Area Under the Curve (AUC) as a performance measure. The significance of the differences obtained in the AUC measures is tested using the ROCKIT software ([35]) for fully paired data: for each patient we have a pair of test results corresponding to `MV-CAD-Causal` and the benchmark systems.

6.3 Results

Classification accuracy. Based on the results from `ViewNet`, Figure 7 presents the classification outcome with the respective AUC measures per MLO and CC view, respectively.

The results clearly indicate an overall improvement in the discrimination between suspicious and normal views for both MLO and CC projections. Such an improvement is expected as the classification of each view in our multi-view system takes into account region information not only from the view itself but also from the regions in the other view. To check the significance of the difference between the AUC measures we test the hypothesis that the AUC measures for `MV-CAD-Causal` and `SV-CAD` are equal against the one-sided alternative hypothesis that the multi-view system yields higher AUCs for MLO and CC views. The

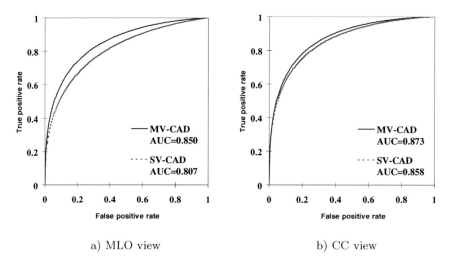

a) MLO view   b) CC view

Fig. 7. ROC analysis per a) MLO and b) CC view

p-values obtained are: 0.000 for MLO view and 0.035 for CC view, indicating a significant improvement in the classification accuracy at a view level.

Furthermore, we observe that for both MV-CAD and SV-CAD the performance for CC view in terms of AUC is better than that for the MLO view. This can be explained by the fact that the classification of CC views is generally easier than that of MLO views due to the breast positioning. At the same time our multi-view system improves considerably upon the single-view CAD system in better distinguishing cancerous from normal MLO views whereas for CC views this improvement is less.

While the view results are very promising, from a radiologists' point of view it is more important to look at the breast and case level performance. In Tables 1 and 2 the AUCs from the multi-view and single-view systems are presented as well as the corresponding p-values and 95% confidence intervals obtained from the statistical tests for the differences between the AUC measures for MV-CAD-Causal and the benchmark methods.

Table 1. AUC and std.errors obtained from the single- and multi-view systems at a *breast* level with the one-sided *p*-values and 95% confidence intervals for the differences

Method	BREAST		
	AUC± std.err	*p*-value	Confidence interval
MV-CAD-Causal	0.876±0.011	–	–
MV-CAD-LR	0.869±0.011	2.9%	$(0.000, 0.009)$
MV-CAD-NB	0.867±0.012	1.3%	$(0.004, 0.011)$
SV-CAD	0.849±0.012	0.1%	$(0.007, 0.032)$

Table 2. AUC and std.errors obtained from the single- and multi-view systems at a *case* level with the one-sided *p*-values and 95% confidence intervals for the differences

Method	CASE		
	AUC± std.err	*p*-value	Confidence interval
MAX			
MV-CAD-Causal	0.833±0.013	–	–
MV-CAD-LR	0.835±0.013	41%	$(-0.007, 0.005)$
MV-CAD-NB	0.826±0.014	21%	$(-0.004, 0.010)$
SV-CAD	0.797±0.014	1.1%	$(0.003, 0.040)$
TRAIN			
MV-CAD-Causal	0.847±0.013	–	–
MV-CAD-LR	0.835±0.014	1.3%	$(0.002, 0.026)$
MV-CAD-NB	0.833±0.014	0.1%	$(0.005, 0.022)$
SV-CAD	0.797±0.014	0.1%	$(0.009, 0.043)$

The results show that MV-CAD-Causal significantly outperforms SV-CAD at both breast and case level. With respect to the two multi-view benchmark methods, our causal model is superior at a breast level and a case level using training as a combining scheme (CaseNet). As expected the case results for MV-CAD-Causal using the maximum (MAX) out of two breast probabilities has less satisfactory performance than using training in the causal independence model. This shows that combining all available information in a proper way is beneficial for accurate case classification.

Although MV-CAD-NB and MV-CAD-LR are overall less accurate than the last two stages of the multi-view causal model, it is clear that all three MV-CAD models achieve superior performance with respect to SV-CAD. This result follows naturally from the explicit representation of multi-view dependences at a region and view level of the multi-view model and it clearly indicates the importance of incorporating multi-view information in the development of CAD systems.

To get more insight into the areas of improvement at a case level we plotted ROC curves for all systems. For all the plots we observed the same tendency of an increased true positive rate at low false positive rates (< 0.5)–a result ultimately desired at the screening practice where the number of normal cases is considerably larger than the cancerous ones; Figure 8 presents the ROC plot for the best performing models.

Evaluation of the multi-view model fitness. To have a closer look at the quality of classification for the three multi-view models, we compute the average log-likelihood (ALL) of the probabilities for different *units*–link, region, MLO/CC view, breast and case–by:

$$ALL(Cl) = \frac{1}{N} \sum_{i=1}^{N} -\ln P(Cl_i | \mathcal{E}_i), \tag{3}$$

where N is the number of records for a unit, Cl_i and $\mathcal{E}_i$ is the class value
and the feature vector of the i-th observation, respectively. Thus, the value of
$ALL(Cl)$ indicates how close the posterior probability distribution is to reality:
when $P(Cl_i|\mathcal{E}_i) = 1$ then $\ln P(Cl_i|\mathcal{E}_i) = 0$ (no extra information); otherwise
$-\ln P(Cl_i|\mathcal{E}_i) > 0$.

The log-likelihood results are given in Table 3. The lowest $ALL(C)$ is achieved
for the links meaning that the estimated probabilities best fit the link probability
distribution. A possible explanation is that in our Bayesian network framework
the links are directly dependent on the original region features and thus they are
better fitted. On the other hand, the rest of the units are based on combining
estimated probabilities from previous levels where noise could play a role. The
MV-CAD-Causal and MV-CAD-LR obtain comparable results for all units whereas

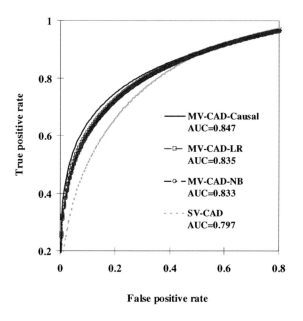

Fig. 8. ROC analysis per case

Table 3. Average log-likelihood of the class based on the multi-view scheme for different units

Unit	Method		
	MV-CAD-Causal	MV-CAD-LR	MV-CAD-NB
Link		0.19	
Region		0.38	
MLO/CC		0.34/0.31	
Breast	0.300	0.235	0.553
Case-MAX	0.482	0.483	0.790
Case-TRAIN	0.476	0.477	0.543

`MV-CAD-NB` leads to considerably larger average log-likelihoods, especially at a case level using the MAX combining scheme. The latter can be explained by the nature of the naive Bayes classifier, which assumes independence of the views and leads to less accurate breast probabilities as indicated in Tables 1 and 2. With the TRAIN combining scheme, the case probabilities computed by `MV-CAD-NB` are better fitted to the truths.

7   Discussion and Conclusions

In this work, we proposed a unified Bayesian network framework for automated multi-view analysis of mammograms, which is an extension of the work presented in [31,32]. The new framework is based on a multi-stage scheme, which models the way radiologists interpret mammograms. More specifically, using causal independence models, we combined all available image information for the patient obtained from a single-view CAD system at four different levels of interpretation: region, view, breast and case. In comparison to our previous work, where the breast and case classification were done using logistic regression, the new scheme allowed a better representation of the multi-view dependencies and handling uncertainty in the estimation of the breast/case probabilities for suspiciousness.

Furthermore, based on experimental results with actual screening data, we demonstrated that the proposed Bayesian network framework improved the detection rate of breast cancer at lower false positive rates in comparison to a single-view CAD system. This improvement is achieved at view, breast and case level and it is due to a number of factors. First, we built upon a single-view CAD system that already demonstrates relatively good detection performance. By applying a probabilistic causal model we linked the original features extracted by the single-view CAD system for all the regions in MLO and CC views and we combined all the links for one breast to obtain a single measure for suspiciousness of a view, breast and case. Another factor for the improved classification is that our approach incorporated domain knowledge. Following radiologists' practice, we applied a straightforward scheme to account for multi-view dependencies such that (i) correlations between the regions in MLO and CC views are considered per breast as whole and (ii) the classification of breast/case as "suspicious" is employed through the logical OR. Thus the proposed methodology can be applied to any domain (e.g., fault detection in manufacturing processes) where similar definitions and objectives hold.

We also note important advantages of our probabilistic system in comparison to previous approaches for automated mammographic analysis. On the one hand, most Bayesian network-based systems for breast cancer detection require that radiologists provide categorical description of the findings a priori to classification. In contrast, our causal approach is completely automated and it is entirely based on the image processing results from the single-view CAD system. This implies that in screening setting, where time is a crucial factor, the proposed multi-view approach has more realistic application and it can be of great help to the human expert. On the other hand, fully automated approaches based on LDA and neural networks fail to account for uncertainty and an explicit representation of view dependences, as done in our probabilistic approach. In addition, the former approaches aimed mostly in improving the detection of the breast cancer at a regional level, whereas we focused on modelling the whole image and breast context information for better distinction between cancerous and normal patients–the ultimate goal of a breast cancer screening program.

Although we demonstrated that the proposed framework has the potential to assist screening radiologists in the evaluation of breast cancer cases, a number of issues can be addressed for extending the proposed multi-view approach. Currently, we consider only cases where both MLO and CC views are present. However, in practice, for half of the patients taking subsequent mammographic exams, only MLO views are available. The question then is to modify the system such that cases with missing CC views can also be analysed. Another interesting direction for extension is with respect to the region linking. Instead of linking all regions from MLO view to all regions from CC view of the same breast, as currently done, it would be natural to consider only the potential true links and avoid a large number of false positive links. To do so, an important piece of domain knowledge used by radiologists in mammogram analysis is that a cancerous lesion projected on MLO and CC views is located on approximately the same distance from the nipple. Thus, links to regions that clearly violate this rule can be ignored and the system can become more precise.

In conclusion, we emphasise that in the coming years, the development and practical application of computer-aided detection systems is likely to expand considerably. This trend is expected to be most observed in the screening programs where the mammograms are to be digitised, the breast cancer incidence rates are very low, the workload is tremendous and the detection of breast cancer is difficult due to the small and subtle changes observed. By providing a "second opinion" in the image analysis, CAD can help radiologists increase cancer detection accuracy at an earlier stage. This can create both health and social benefits by saving women's lives, increasing families' well-being, reducing unnecessary check-up costs and compensating the shortage of radiologists. To create reliable and widely applied CAD, however, it is crucial to integrate the knowledge and the working principles of radiologists in the CAD development. The multi-view CAD system described in this chapter is a promising step forward in this direction.

Acknowledgement

This research is funded by the Netherlands Organisation for Scientific Research under BRICKS/FOCUS grant number 642.066.605.

Appendix

Figure 9 depicts an example of a causal-independence model for breast cancer prediction. We have two binary cause variables *mass* (MASS) and *microcalcifications* (MCAL), which are the two main mammographic indicators for the

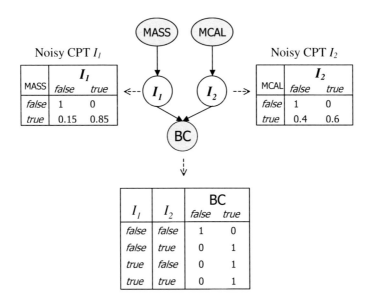

Fig. 9. Example of a noisy-OR model for breast cancer prediction

patient having *breast cancer* (BC), the so-called effect variable. It is also known that masses are more frequent occurring sign, which is reflected in the noisy probability distributions $P(I_1|\text{MASS})$ and $P(I_2|\text{MCAL})$. Finally, the domain knowledge suggests that the combined occurrence of both signs increases the probability for having breast cancer, which is modelled by the logical OR as an interaction function $f(I_1, I_2)$ for the effect BC.

Then the probability of having breast cancer given the states of MASS and MCAL is computed as follows:

$$P(\text{BC} = true|\text{MASS}, \text{MCAL}) =$$

$$= \sum_{f(I_1, I_2) = true} P(\text{BC} = true|I_1, I_2)P(I_1|\text{MASS})P(I_2|\text{MCAL})$$

$$= P(I_1 = true|\text{MASS})P(I_2 = true|\text{MCAL}) +$$
$$P(I_1 = true|\text{MASS})P(I_2 = false|\text{MCAL}) +$$
$$P(I_1 = false|\text{MASS})P(I_2 = true|\text{MCAL}).$$

For example, given the evidence of MASS = *true* and MCAL = *false* then the probability for breast cancer is:

$$P(\text{BC} = true|\text{MASS}, \text{MCAL}) = 0.85 \cdot 0 + 0.85 \cdot 1 + 0.15 \cdot 0 = 0.85.$$

Now suppose that MASS = *true* and MCAL = *true*. Then we obtain

$$P(\text{BC} = true|\text{MASS}, \text{MCAL}) = 0.85 \cdot 0.6 + 0.85 \cdot 0.4 + 0.15 \cdot 0.6 = 0.94,$$

indicating the combined influence of both causes on the probability of having breast cancer.

References

1. Otten, J.D., Broeders, M.J., Fracheboud, J., Otto, S.J., de Koning, H.J., Verbeek, A.L.: Impressive time-related influence of the Dutch screening programme on breast cancer incidence and mortality, 1975-2006. International Journal of Cancer 123(8), 1929–1934 (2008)
2. Engeland, S.V.: Detection of mass lesions in mammograms by using multiple views. PhD Thesis (2006)
3. BI-RADS: Breast Imaging Reporting and Data System. American College of Radiology, Reston (1993)
4. Morton, M.J., Whaley, D.H., Brandt, K.R., Amrami, K.K.: Screening mammograms: interpretation with computer-aided detection-prospective evaluation. Radiology 239, 375–383 (2006)
5. Sardo, M., Vaidya, S., Jain, L.C.: Advanced Computational Intelligence Paradigms in Healthcare, vol. 3. Springer, Heidelberg (2008)
6. Buchanan, B.G., Shortliffe, E.H.: Rule-Based Expert Systems: The MYCIN Experiments of the Stanford Heuristic Programming Project. Addison-Wesley, Reading (1984)
7. Liebowitz, J.: The Handbook of Applied Expert Systems. CRC Press, Boca Raton (1997)
8. Jain, A., Jain, A., Jain, S., Jain, L.: Artificial Intelligence Techniques in Breast Cancer Diagnosis and Prognosis. World Scientific, Singapore (2000)
9. Burnside, E.S., Rubin, D.L., Fine, J.P., Shachter, R.D., Sisney, G.A., Leung, W.K.: Bayesian network to predict breast cancer risk of mammographic microcalcifications and reduce number of benign biopsy results. Journal of Radiology (2006)
10. Kahn, C.E., Roberts, L.M., Shaffer, K.A., Haddawy, P.: Construction of a bayesian network for mammographic diagnosis of breast cancer. Computers and Biology and Medicine 27(1), 19–30 (1997)
11. Karabatak, M., Ince, M.C.: An expert system for detection of breast cancer based on association rules and neural network. Expert Systems with Applications: An International Journal 36(2), 3465–3469 (2009)
12. Wolberg, W.H., Street, W.N., Mangasarian, O.L.: Machine learning techniques to diagnose breast cancer from fine-needle aspirates. Cancer Letters 77, 163–171 (1994)
13. Ye, J., Zheng, S., Yang, C.: SVM-based microcalcification detection in digital mammograms. In: Proceedings of the 2008 International Conference on Computer Science and Software Engineering, vol. 6, pp. 89–92 (2008)
14. Roca-Pardiñas, J., Cadarso-Suárez, C., Tahoces, P.G., Lado, M.J.: Assessing continuous bivariate effects among different groups through nonparametric regression models: An application to breast cancer detection. Computational Statistics & Data Analysis 52(4), 1958–1970 (2008)
15. Gupta, S., Chyn, P., Markey, M.: Breast cancer CADx based on bi-rads descriptors from two mammographic views. Medical Physics 33(6), 1810–1817 (2006)
16. Good, W., Zheng, B., Chang, Y., Wang, X., Maitz, G., Gur, D.: Multi-image cad employing features derived from ipsilateral mammographic views. In: Proceedings of SPIE, Medical Imaging, vol. 3661, pp. 474–485 (1999)

17. Engeland, S.V., Timp, S., Karssemeijer, N.: Finding corresponding regions of interest in mediolateral oblique and craniocaudal mammographic views. Medical Physics 33(9), 3203–3212 (2006)
18. Engeland, S.V., Karssemeijer, N.: Combining two mammographic projections in a computer aided mass detection method. Medical Physics 34(3), 898–905 (2007)
19. Paquerault, S., Petrick, N., Chan, H., Sahiner, B., Helvie, M.A.: Improvement of computerized mass detection on mammograms: Fusion of two-view information. Medical Physics 29(2), 238–247 (2002)
20. Yuan, Y., Giger, M., Li, H., Luan, L., Sennett, C.: Identifying corresponding lesions from CC and MLO views via correlative feature analysis. In: Krupinski, E.A. (ed.) IWDM 2008. LNCS, vol. 5116, pp. 323–328. Springer, Heidelberg (2008)
21. Gupta, S., Zhang, D., Sampat, M.P., Markey, M.K.: Combining texture features from the MLO and CC views for mammographic CADx. Progress in biomedical optics and imaging 7(3) (2006)
22. Zheng, B., Leader, J.K., Abrams, G.S., Lu, A.H., Wallace, L.P., Maitz, G.S., Gur, D.: Multiview-based computer-aided detection scheme for breast masses. Medical Physics 33(9), 3135–3143 (2006)
23. Zheng, B., Tan, J., Ganott, M.A., Chough, D.M., Gur, D.: Matching breast masses depicted on different views a comparison of three methods. Academic Radiology 16(11), 1338–1347 (2009)
24. Wei, J., Chan, H., Sahiner, B., Zhou, C., Hadjiiski, L.M., Roubidoux, M.A., Helvie, M.A.: Computer-aided detection of breast masses on mammograms: dual system approach with two-view analysis. Medical Physics 36(10), 4451–4460 (2009)
25. Pearl, J.: Probabilistic Reasoning in Inteligent Systems: Networks of Plausible Inference. Morgan Kaufmann, San Francisco (1988)
26. Jensen, F., Nielsen, T.: Bayesian Networks and Decision Graphs. Springer, Heidelberg (2007)
27. Domingos, P., Pazzani, M.: On the optimality of the simple Bayesian classifier under zero-one loss. Machine Learning 29, 103–130 (1997)
28. Heckerman, D., Breese, J.S.: Causal independence for probability assessment and inference using Bayesian networks. IEEE Transactions on Systems, Man and Cybernetics, Part A 26(6), 826–831 (1996)
29. Lucas, P.J.F.: Bayesian network modelling through qualitative pattern. Artificial Intelligence 163, 233–263 (2005)
30. Diez, F.: Parameter adjustment in Bayes networks: The generalized noisy or-gate. In: Proceedings of the Ninth Conference on UAI. Morgan Kaufmann, San Francisco (1993)
31. Velikova, M., Lucas, P., de Carvalho Ferreira, N., Samulski, M., Karssemeijer, N.: A decision support system for breast cancer detection in screening programs. In: Proceedings of the 18th biennial European Conference on Artificial Intelligence (ECAI), vol. 178, pp. 658–662 (2008)
32. Velikova, M., Samulski, M., Lucas, P., Karssemeijer, N.: Improved mammographic CAD performance using multi-view information: A Bayesian network framework. Physics in Medicine and Biology 54(5), 1131–1147 (2009)
33. Murphy, K.: Bayesian Network Toolbox for Matlab, BNT (2007), http://www.cs.ubc.ca/~murphyk/Software/BNT/bnt.html
34. Hanley, J.A., McNeil, B.J.: The meaning and use of the area under a Receiver Operating Characteristic (ROC) curve. Radiology 143, 29–36 (1982)
35. Metz, C., Wang, P., Kronman, H.: A new approach for testing the significance of differences between ROC curves measured from correlated data. In: Information Processing in Medical Imaging, Nijhoff (1984)

Chapter 18
Pattern Classification Techniques for Lung Cancer Diagnosis by an Electronic Nose

Rossella Blatt, Andrea Bonarini, and Matteo Matteucci

Politecnico di Milano, Dipartimento di Elettronica e Informazione,
Via Ponzio 34/5 20133 Milan, Italy
rblatt@iit.edu, {Bonarini,Matteucci}@elet.polimi.it

Abstract. Computational intelligence techniques can be implemented to analyze the olfactory signal as perceived by an electronic nose, and to detect information to diagnose a multitude of human diseases. Our research suggests the use of an electronic nose to diagnose lung cancer. An electronic nose is able to acquire and recognize the volatile organic compounds (VOCs) present in the analyzed substance: it is composed of an array of electronic, chemical sensors, and a pattern classification module based on computational intelligence techniques. The three main stages characterizing the basic functioning of an electronic nose are: acquisition, preprocessing and pattern analysis. In the lung cancer detection experimentation, we analyzed 104 breath samples of 52 subjects, 22 healthy subjects and 30 patients with primary lung cancer at different stages. In order to find the best classification model able to discriminate between the two classes *healthy* and *lung cancer* subjects, and to reduce the dimensionality of the problem, we implemented a genetic algorithm (GA) that can find the best combination of feature selection, feature projection and classifier algorithms to be used. In particular, for feature projection, we considered Principal Component Analysis (PCA), Fisher Linear Discriminant Analysis (LDA) and Non Parametric Linear Discriminant Analysis (NPLDA); classification has been performed implementing several supervised pattern classification algorithms, based on different k-Nearest Neighbors (k-NN) approaches (classic, modified and fuzzy k-NN), on linear and quadratic discriminant functions classifiers and on a feed-forward Artificial Neural Network (ANN). The best solution provided from the genetic algorithm has been the projection of a subset of features into a single component using the Fisher Linear Discriminant Analysis and a classification based on the k-Nearest Neighbors method. The observed results, all validated using cross-validation, have been excellent achieving an average accuracy of 96.2%, an average sensitivity of 93.3% and an average specificity of 100%, as well as very small confidence intervals. We also investigated the possibility of performing early diagnosis, building a model able to predict a sample belonging to a subject with primary lung cancer at stage I compared to healthy subjects. Also in this analysis results have been very satisfactory, achieving an average accuracy of 92.85%, an average sensitivity of 75.5% and an average specificity of 97.72%. The achieved results demonstrate that the

I. Bichindaritz et al. (Eds.): Computational Intelligence in Healthcare 4, SCI 309, pp. 397–423.
springerlink.com © Springer-Verlag Berlin Heidelberg 2010

electronic nose, combined with the appropriate computational intelligence methodologies, is a promising alternative to current lung cancer diagnostic techniques: not only the instrument is completely non invasive, but the obtained predictive errors are lower than those achieved by present diagnostic methods, and the cost of the analysis, both in money, time and resources, is lower. The introduction of this cutting edge technology will lead to very important social and business effects: its low price and small dimensions allow a large scale distribution, giving the opportunity to perform non invasive, cheap, quick, and massive early diagnosis and screening.

1   Introduction

In the last decades, attention on electronic noses has considerably increased and research in the analysis of olfactory signal has become very lively; this is mainly due to the wide variety of problems that this innovative technology is potentially able to solve. Electronic noses have been successfully applied to a vast range of applications, from cosmetic productions to food and beverages manufacturing, from chemical engineering to environmental monitoring, passing through mines and explosives detection as well as medical diagnosis. The latter application plays a crucial role in social environment and health care monitoring, providing diagnostic clues, guide to laboratory evaluation and affecting the choice of immediate therapy.

One of the diseases with the highest mortality rate is lung cancer, which causes 3000 deaths each day in the world and is the leading cause of cancer death among both men and women. The diagnosis in an advanced stage represents the main cause of the therapeutic failure: the surviving rate after five years of treatment, if lung cancer is diagnosed in stage IV, is around 2%; this percentage increases to more than 50% if the cancer is discovered in its earliest stage. These considerations highlight the relevance of performing massive accurate diagnosis and, in particular, early diagnosis. Chest x-rays screening have proven ineffective, and spiral Computed Tomography (CT) trials are on-going. However, imaging tools are expensive and their accuracy is limited by false positive findings. Less invasive and more accurate techniques are necessary to identify lung cancer in its early stages.

A possible solution to this task can be found in the fundamental principle of clinical chemistry, according to which every pathology changes people chemical composition, modifying the concentration of some chemicals in the human body. This happens also in lung cancer: it has been demonstrated that the presence of lung cancer alters the percentage of some volatile organic compounds (VOCs) in the human breath [8,9]. These VOCs can thus be considered as lung cancer markers; the analysis of the olfactory signal of patients' breaths and the recognition of these VOCs in them, through the appropriate multivariate pattern analysis algorithms, can be the tools key to detect lung cancer.

2   Methodology

The experimentation has been developed in collaboration with the Thoracic Surgery Unit of the Istituto Nazionale Tumori (INT - National Cancer Institute), Milan. The study involved a total of 52 volunteers, of which 22 healthy and 30 suffering from different types of primary lung cancer. Patients were enrolled from who underwent tumor resection at the Thoracic Surgery Unit of INT and they were eligible to participate if they were more than 18 years old, could understand the breath collection procedure and could give written informed consent. The healthy volunteers were recruited from the candidates of a randomized study with multislice spiral CT, named Multicentric Italian Lung Detection (MILD) trial for early lung cancer detection promoted by INT from 2005. Control people have no pulmonary disease or respiratory symptoms and have negative chest CT scan. All volunteers were assessed for their eligibility and asked to sign a consent form to participate in the study, including a detailed information sheet. A tobacco smoking history was obtained from all subjects. All volunteers were asked to sign a written consent form, and the study was approved by the Ethical Committee of the INT.

The breath acquisition has been made by inviting all volunteers to blow into a nalophan bag of approximately $500cm^3$ of volume. Considering that the breath exhaled directly from lung is contained only in the last part of exhalation, using a spirometer to evaluate each volunteer exhalation capacity, we diverted the flow at the end of the exhalation into the bag in order to collect only the final portion of forced expiratory volume and analyze only a portion of alveolar air. Finally, the air contained in the bag has been input to the electronic nose and analyzed. Before connecting the bags to the electronic nose, it has been necessary to define the parameters of the instrument: in particular we chose a sample frequency of 1 Hz with a flow equal to $150cm^3$ per minute and the total duration of a measure has been set to 8 minutes (of which one minute and a half for stimulus acquisition). From each bag we took two measures, obtaining a total of 104 measurements, of which 44 correspond to the breath of healthy people and 60 to patients breath.

3   Basic Functioning of the Electronic Nose

An electronic nose is an instrument able to detect and recognize odors, namely the volatile organic compounds present in an analyzed substance [2]. Its functioning is strongly inspired by the biological olfactory system (Figure 1). In human olfaction, odor sensations are induced by the interaction of odorants with specialized receptors in the olfactory epithelium in the top of the nasal cavity; this interaction creates signals that are transmitted to the olfactory bulb and, ultimately, to the brain, which analyzes the received signals and performs the classification or recognition of the odor. Following the same principles, the electronic nose is composed of three fundamental modules (Figure 2):

1. Acquisition of the olfactory stimulus
2. Preprocessing of the olfactory signal
3. Pattern analysis of the preprocessed olfactory signal

The first component regards the gas acquisition system, which is done by a sensor array that measures a given physical or chemical quantity; the second module concerns the preprocessing and dimensionality reduction phase which is aimed at converting the response of the odor sensors into an electrical signal and at transforming it in a more suitable form for subsequent multivariate pattern analysis through analog conditioning and digital processing. The last module has the task of identifying the most significative components for the considered problem and to solve the prediction problem: classification, regression or clustering.

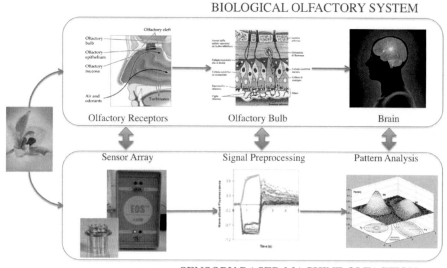

Fig. 1. Parallel between the human biological olfactory system and the sensory based machine olfaction mechanism: in the same way the odor is perceived by specialized olfactory receptors in the olfactory epithelium, in the electronic nose, the olfactory signal is acquired through a sensor array, that sends its response to a signal conditioning and preprocessing module, that corresponds to the olfactory bulb operations. Finally, in humans, signals are elaborated in the brain, that is able to perform different tasks, such as recognition of the odor, classification or concentration analysis. The same tasks are faced and solved from the pattern analysis module, that implements several artificial intelligence techniques to extract the desired information for classification, clustering or regression.

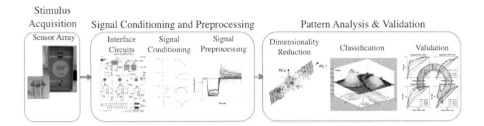

Fig. 2. Block scheme representing the basic functioning of a sensory based machine olfaction: the gas is acquired by means of a sensor array, which response represents the input for the signal conditioning and preprocessing module. Here the response is converted into an electrical signal by means of interface circuits and the signal information is enhanced through analog conditioning. Digital preprocessing aims at transforming the multidimensional signal into the most suitable form for further pattern analysis module. The first computational operation of the last module is dimensionality reduction, performed through feature selection and/or projection; the classifier will then partition the new obtained feature space in c regions (where c is the number of classes), maximizing an objective function evaluated through the validation block.

4   Sensor Array

Gas acquisition in an electronic nose is performed by an array of non specific sensors able to convert a chemical information into an electrical signal. Each sensor reacts in a different way to the analyzed substance providing multidimensional data that can be considered as an olfactory blueprint of the substance itself. According to the physical principles on which the sensor array is based, it is possible to group the different sensor technologies used for electronic noses into four categories: chemoresistors, piezoelectric sensors, MOSFET sensors and optical sensors [3].

Chemoresistors. Chemoresistors, that are based on the conductivity change that occurs when exposed to volatile organic compounds, are the simplest and most used sensors for gas and odor measurements. There are two type of conductivity sensors: Metal Oxide Semiconductors (MOS) and organic polymers. The advantages of the first type stay in their low cost, wide commercial availability and high sensitivity (1-100 ppm or 10-1000 ppm if thin or thick film respectively is employed), while the main disadvantage regards the need to operate at high temperature, the prone to drift and poisoning and the sensitivity to humidity (that can strongly impact the quality of the olfactory signal). The second type of conductivity sensors, based on organic polymers, are also commonly used in electronic nose systems thanks to their high sensitivity (10-100 ppm, sometimes up to 0.1 ppm), the fact that they operate at ambient temperature (they do not need heaters and, thus, are easier to make) and the fact that their electronic interface is straightforward, making them suitable for portable instruments. On the other hand, their response time is inversely proportional to the polymer

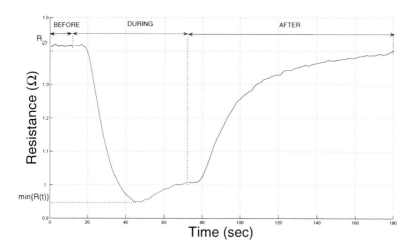

Fig. 3. Example of a MOS sensor response. Each measure consists of three main stages: before each measure the instrument inhales the reference air, showing in its graph a relatively constant curve; after this short period it inhales the analyzed gas, producing a change of the sensor resistance; finally the instrument returns to the reference line, ready for a new measure.

thickness and is usually longer than MOS response time; moreover they suffer of response drift over time and their response is more susceptible to humidity than MOS sensors are.

The electronic nose we have used in this research is composed of an array of six MOS sensors. This choice is due to the fact that, as previously mentioned, MOS sensors are characterized by high sensitivity, low cost, high speed response and a relatively simple electronics. The first aspect takes on great importance if we consider that most of the VOCs markers of lung cancer are present in the diseased subject breath in very small quantities, varying from parts per million to parts per billion. A typical response of a MOS sensor is shown in Figure 3.

Piezoelectric sensors. The piezoelectric family of sensors can measure temperature, mass change, pressure, force and acceleration, but in the electronic nose they are configured as mass change sensing devices. There are two main types of piezoelectric sensors used in electronic noses: Quartz Crystal Microbalance (QCM) and Surface Acoustic-Wave (SAW). The measured variable in both devices is the resonant frequency, that changes according to mass. A drawback of both QCM and SAW devices is a more complex electronics than the electronics needed by chemoresistors sensors as well as the need for frequency detectors, whose resonant frequencies can drift over time. Even if SAW sensors operate at higher frequencies than QCM (and thus generate larger changes in frequency), their measure of mass change is of the same order of magnitude (1.0 ng mass change). SAW sensors are usually characterized by a poor long-term stability and a high sensitivity to humidity.

MOSFET sensors. Metal-Oxide-Silicon Field-Effect-Transistor (MOSFET) odor sensing devices are based on the principle that VOCs in contact with a catalytic metal can produce a reaction in the metal that can diffuse through the gate of a MOSFET to change the electrical properties of the device. MOSFET sensors have been investigated for numerous applications, but, to date, few have been used in commercial electronic nose systems because of a dearth of sensor variants. The advantage of MOSFETs is that they can be made with IC fabrication processes; the disadvantage is that the catalyzed reaction products (e.g., hydrogen) must penetrate the catalytic metal layer. Moreover they suffer of baseline drift and their sensitivity is lower (order of ppm) then other odor sensors.

Optical-fiber sensors. In optical-fiber sensors, the active material contains chemically active fluorescent dyes immobilized in an organic polymer matrix, which polarity is altered as VOCs interact with it. The reaction is a shift of the fluorescent emission spectrum. The advantage of these sensors is their low cost, but the complexity of the instrumentation control system increases the production cost. They have a limited lifetime due to photobleaching, but the exploitation of an array of fiber can provide a wide ranging sensitivity.

5   Signal Conditioning and Preprocessing

The second fundamental module of an odor-sensing instrument consists in the signal conditioning and preprocessing phase, that consists in converting the acquired sensor response in the most appropriate form for the further multivariate pattern analysis module, minimizing the effects of noise and of all those effects (e.g. baseline drift, humidity) that negatively affect the quality of the signal. This task can be distinguished in three main steps:

1. Conversion of the odor sensors response into an electrical signal by means of interface circuits
2. Enhancement of signal information through analog conditioning (e.g. filtering), as well as sampling and analog to digital conversion
3. Digital processing of the sampled signal to make it suitable for further multivariate pattern analysis

5.1   Interface Circuits

The first stage of any electronic instrumentation is the conversion of sensors response (e.g., resistance change) into an electrical signal; this operation is made by means of interface circuits and varies according to the specific technology on which sensors are based. In chemoresistors sensors, for example, interface circuits are relatively simple since they only involve measuring resistance changes; on the contrary, electronics instrumentation for piezoelectric sensors are more complex, as they involve AC signals for high frequency. In [4] an extensive overview of interface circuits theory is provided.

5.2   Signal Conditioning

The electrical signals generated by sensor interface circuits are often not adequate for acquisition into a computer and must be further processed by a number of analog signal conditioning circuits. The main objective of these operations consists in:

- *Buffering*, required to isolate different electronic stages and avoid impedance loading errors
- *Amplifying*, in order to bring the signal of the interface circuits to a level suitable for the dynamic range of the subsequent analog-to-digital converter and filtering
- *Filtering*, to remove unwanted frequency components from the sensor signals

For more details on signal conditioning refer to [4].

5.3   Signal Preprocessing

The first computational stage after the sensor array data have been acquired is signal preprocessing, which aims mainly at extracting the relevant information from the sensor responses and to prepare data for further multivariate pattern analysis minimizing those effect (e.g., baseline drift) that can affect the quality of the signal. During this phase, three main operations are executed:

1. Baseline manipulation
2. Feature extraction
3. Normalization

Baseline manipulation. Baseline manipulation is performed for the purposes of drift compensation, contrast enhancement and scaling. The three most common techniques, all based on a manipulation of the sensor response with respect to its baseline are:

- *Differential.* The baseline $x_s(0)$ is subtracted from the sensor response $x_s(t)$:

$$y_s(t) = (x_s(t) + \delta_a) - (x_s(0) + \delta_a) = x_s(t) - x_s(0) \tag{1}$$

  This allows to compensate any additive noise or drift δ_A that may be present in the sensor signal.
- *Relative.* The sensors response $x_s(t)$ is divided by the baseline $x_s(0)$:

$$y_s(t) = \frac{x_s(t)(1 + \delta_M)}{x_s(0)(1 + \delta_M)} = \frac{x_s(t)}{x_s(0)} \tag{2}$$

  This allows to compensate any multiplicative noise or drift δ_M that may be present in the sensor signal. It provides dimensionless response.

– *Fractional.* This approach combines the differential and relative manipulation, substracting the baseline $x_s(0)$ from the sensor response $x_s(t)$ and dividing the modified sensors response by the baseline $x_s(0)$:

$$y_s(t) = \frac{x_s(t) - x_s(0)}{x_s(0)} \tag{3}$$

It is important to highlight that fractional manipulation provides not only dimensionless, but also normalized measurements.

The choice of baseline manipulation is strongly related to the specific sensor technology and the particular application; for MOS sensors chemoresistors it has been shown [7] that the fractional change in conductance provides the best pattern recognition performance.

Feature extraction. The second stage in preprocessing consists in identifying a number of descriptors able to condense all the response information in few features. This new data will represent the olfactory blueprint of the analyzed substance. This is a very crucial step, since all further pattern analysis will be performed on these data: the lack of information must therefore be avoided. In most electronic nose works the feature extraction operation is performed by keeping one single parameter (usually the steady-state, i.e., the final, maximum or minimum value reached during the response to the stimulus). However this approach is very reductive since the useful information could be elsewhere: transient analysis could indeed provide significant information and thus improve the final performance. In this perspective there are several approaches to detect features in the transient and steady-state response [5]:

– *Sub-sampling methods*: sampling the sensor response and/or its derivative at different times during the acquisition of the analyzed gas
– *Parameter extraction methods*: extracting a number of features able to capture the information contained in the response curve (e.g., integral, maximum or minimum in certain time intervals, rise time, slope etc.)
– *System identification methods*: fitting a theoretical model (e.g. exponential or autoregressive) to the experimental transient and use the model parameters as features

As demonstrated in [5,4], the consideration of the transient, besides the steady-state, in the feature extraction operation, can lead to many advantages, such as an improvement of classification performance (if the discriminative information is in the transient), as well as a potentially better parameters repeatability w.r.t. static descriptors, as exhibited in some cases [6]. Moreover if the discriminative information is in the transient there will be no need to reach the steady-state of the response, allowing a reduction of measurement time and, consequently, an increase of sensor life time.

In the lung cancer diagnosis application, we extracted the features using all the three approaches and taking into consideration both the steady-state and the transient information. The ten descriptors that we extracted from the sensor responses were based on:

- the steady-state value, expressed as the minimum or maximum value reached during the measurement;
- the variation of resistance from the baseline to the maximum or minimum point reached during the transient, expressed in terms of both difference and ratio;
- the derivative of the transient, evaluated as sampling and difference values measured among several points of the transient;
- the integral of the transient;
- the Fast Fourier Transform (FFT).

It is important to highlight that the features extracted computing a value relative to the baseline compensate the potential sensor drift effects.

Data normalization. Once features have been extracted, it is necessary to normalize the obtained dataset to minimize sample-to-sample variations, sensor drift and differences in sensors scaling. According to the considered data, two general approaches can be outlined: local methods and global methods. The first family of methods aims at compensating for sample-to-sample variations due to analyte concentration and sensor drift and is therefore applied to the sensor array of each individual measurement. The most widely used local method is vector normalization, in which the feature vector of each individual measurement is divided by its norm and, as a result, forced to lie on a hypersphere of unitary radius. This approach is suitable when each sample has a unique concentration, but discrimination has to be performed on the basis of odor quality. On the other hand, this method should not be used if the discriminative information is somehow related to the odor intensity, as it forces all the vectors on the hypersphere to have unitary length. Global methods operate across the entire dataset for a single sensor and are generally employed to compensate differences in sensor scaling, allowing sensor magnitudes to be comparable. The two most widely global methods employed in electronic nose systems are:

- *sensor autoscaling*, where the distribution of values of each sensor across the entire dataset is forced to have zero mean and unitary standard deviation:

$$y_s^k = \frac{x_s^k - mean[x_s]}{std[x_s]} \tag{4}$$

  where x_s^k is the response of sensor s to the kth sample.
- *sensor normalization*, where the range of value of each individual sensor is set to $[0,1]$:

$$y_s^k = \frac{x_s^k - min_{\forall k}[x_s^k]}{max_{\forall k}[x_s^k] - min_{\forall k}[x_s^k]} \tag{5}$$

It must be noted that both methods can amplify noise, since all sensors are equally weighted, but sensor autoscaling is more robust to outliers. As a consequence of this consideration, in the electronic nose system for lung cancer diagnosis, we have chosen to normalize the dataset employing the sensor autoscaling global method.

6 Pattern Analysis Module

The multivariate response obtained from the array of chemical gas sensors with broad and partially overlapping selectivities will be utilized as an olfactory blueprint to characterize the considered odors. Besides compensate sensor drift and noise, the preprocessing module is aimed at preparing data in the most suitable form for the further pattern analysis module. The latter has indeed the objective of identifying the most significative components for the considered problem and of to solve the prediction problem: classification, regression or clustering [10].

Classification addresses the problem of recognizing an unknown sample as belonging to one of a predefined and learned set of classes; in regression tasks, the objective is to predict a set of properties (e.g. concentration) for an analyte; finally, in clustering tasks the goal is to learn the structural relationship among different odorants. The task of recognizing a breath belonging to a lung cancer patient with respect to a healthy breath, belongs to the classification family tasks. Before analyzing data for classification, the feature matrix need to be treated in order to reduce the dimensionality of the problem and to maximize the discriminative information of its components. Indeed, after preprocessing, the feature matrix is typically characterized by high dimensionality and redundancy. Besides the obvious issues of high complexity and computational cost, the problem of high dimensionality is related to the more important curse of dimensionality, which implies that the number of training examples must grow exponentially with the number of features in order to learn an accurate model. This means that after a certain dimensionality of the feature space, the performance of the classifier decreases: fixed the number of training data, the optimal number of feature dimensions must be found. Redundancy, that appears when two or more features are collinear, leads the covariance matrix of the entire dataset to be singular (and thus noninvertible), which leads, in turn, to numerical problems in various statistical approaches. These considerations call for the implementation of some dimensionality reduction technique; there are two main dimensionality reduction approaches:

- *Feature selection*: the objective is to find the optimal or a suboptimal subset of features starting from the initial feature set
- *Feature projection*: the objective is to project features into a lower dimensional space able to maximize the discriminative information or some defined objective function

6.1 Feature Selection

The goal of feature selection is to find an optimal subset of M features from the initial N dimensional feature set (with $M \leq N$) that maximizes the objective function. Given a feature set $X = \{x_i, i = 1, .., N\}$, we want to find a subset $Y_M = \{x_{1i}, x_{12}, ..., x_{iM}\}$ with $M \leq N$, that optimizes an objective function $J(Y)$ in some way related to the probability of correct classification. The objective function, that evaluate the goodness of the feature subset, can be related to the predictive accuracy, according to the wrapper approach, or computed from the information content of the subset itself (e.g., inter-class distance, correlation or information theoretic measures), according to the filters approach. With feature selection selected features maintain their original physical interpretation, which can be useful to understand the physical process that generates patterns. Moreover it may lead to a reduction of measurement and/or computational cost (only the selected features will need to be computed) and, if the feature selection operation selected a smaller subset of sensors than the initial one, this may lead to a potential saving in the production process. On the other hand, the process of finding the best feature subset can be computationally very expensive, and it could be necessary to settle for a suboptimal solution. In order to find the best subset several search strategies can be adopted [10]:

- *Best firsts* ranks each feature according to the chosen objective function, and then keeps only the first M features. Unfortunately, this simple approach fails quite always because it does not consider features with complementary information.
- *Exhaustive search* considers all the possible combinations of feature subsets. Although this is the only approach that can guarantee to find the optimal subset, it is rarely used since it is unfeasible even with moderate M and N values.
- *Exponential algorithms* evaluate a number of subsets that grows exponentially with the dimensionality of the search space. Among these, the branch & bound technique is very popular as it guarantees to find the best feature subset if the monoticity assumption of the objective function is verified. The monoticity assumption implies that the addition of a new feature always improves the information content of the subset; unfortunately, in practical problems, this is rarely verified.
- *Sequential algorithms* are a greedy strategy that reduces the number of states to be visited during the search by applying local search. In sequential and backward feature selection, an individual feature is respectively added or removed sequentially evaluating the objective function of the new subset obtained adding or removing that feature (and not of individual features as in the best first approach). The performance may be improved by means of sequential floating feature selection with backtracking capabilities.
- *Randomized algorithms* incorporate randomness into the search procedure in order to attempt to overcome the computational cost of exponential methods and the tendency of sequential methods to fall into local minima. Among these techniques, the random generation plus sequential selection is widely used; another popular randomized approach is the simulated annealing, that is based on the annealing process of thermal systems and performs a stochastic search on a single solution. Another very powerful randomized method is based on genetic algorithms, that are an optimization technique that mimics the evolutionary process of survival of the best; taking inspiration by the process of natural selection, it performs a global random search on population of solutions. In this work a genetic algorithm has been implemented not

only to perform feature selection, but to define the best model for the considered classification problem; the model included feature selection, feature projection and classifier. More details on how we implemented this powerful technique to find the best model for lung cancer diagnosis are provided in Section 8.

6.2 Feature Projection

Feature projection creates new features based on transformations or combinations of the original dataset: given a feature space $x_i \in R^N$ find a mapping $y = f(x) : R^N \to R^M$ with $M \leq N$. The transformed features (a linear or not linear combination of original features) may provide better discrimination ability than the best subset of initial features provided by feature selection, but they may not have clear physical meaning, leading to a potential lack of interpretation. The transformation matrix is found maximizing an objective function related to the discrimination capabilities with signal classification methods, or to the information contained in the structure of data (e.g., variance) in signal representation methods. The first approach is thus preferred for pattern classification problems, while the latter is more suitable when the goal is exploratory data analysis.

The most widely used feature projection techniques are: Linear Discriminant Analysis (LDA), which is based on a signal classification approach, and Principal Component Analysis (PCA), based on a signal representation approach. LDA uses the category information associated with each pattern for linearly projecting data into a lower dimensional space maximizing class separability. This is done generating projections able to maximize the interclass distances and to minimize the intraclass distances. These projections are estimated according to the Fisher criterion and are thus defined by the first eigenvectors of the matrix $S_W^{-1} S_B$ where S_W and S_B are respectively the within-class and between-class covariance matrices. It has to be noted that under the unimodal gaussian assumption this method is optimal. The assumption of gaussianity can be removed by the Non Parametric Linear Discriminant Analysis (NPLDA) [11], that is a generalization of LDA; this is obtained by computing the between scatter-matrix S_B using local information and the k nearest neighbors rule. As a result of this, the matrix S_B is full-rank, allowing to extract more than $c - 1$ features (where c is equal to the number of considered classes) and the projections are able to preserve the structure of the data more closely.

Principal component analysis (PCA), or Karhunen-Loòve expansion, transforms data in a linear fashion projecting features into the directions with maximum variance, which are defined by the first eigenvectors of the covariance Σ_x of feature matrix x. It is important to notice that PCA is an unsupervised approach, that is, it does not consider category labels: this means that the discarded directions could be exactly the most suitable for classification purpose. Anyway it is optimal under the unimodal gaussian assumption. For non-gaussian distributions additional techniques may be more appropriate, including kernel PCA,

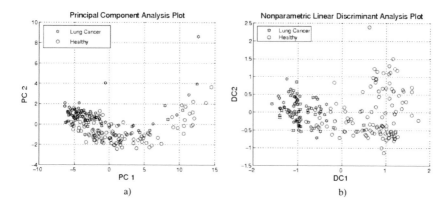

Fig. 4. The results of dimensionality reduction by Principal Component Analysis (PCA), in a), and Non Parametric Linear Discriminant Analysis (NPLDA), in b). As evident, the discrimination problem between the two classes *healthy subject* versus *lung cancer patient* is better solved by NPLDA. This is probably due to the fact that NPLDA is a supervised approach that takes into account the class membership of each training sample and projects data in a way that maximizes the interclass distance and minimizes the intraclass one; the approach is very different from PCA, which, as unsupervised method, does not consider membership labels and projects the components that maximize the variance information. On the other side, PCA plot is very useful because it allows an exploration of data structure, emphasizing it and possible sensor drift.

feed-forward neural network (usually multi-layer perceptrons), Kohonen Self Organizing Maps (SOM), Independent Component Analysis (ICA) and Sammon's maps [10].

In the lung cancer diagnosis by the electronic nose application we evaluated projection based both on PCA, LDA and NPLDA. As evident from Figure 4, NPLDA is able to separate the projected features more clearly than PCA, which plot shows a more evident samples overlap, due to the fact that PCA preserves the original structure of the data, which includes odor variance and sensor drift, without maximizing the class separability.

7 Classification

The objective of classification is to predict the class of an unknown input vector. There are two main families of classification approaches: supervised and unsupervised. The basic idea of supervised methods is to train the classifier providing it a series of examples and the corresponding known classes, in order to learn the relationship between feature data and classes. In unsupervised methods, the classifier learns to separate the different classes from the response vectors routinely, without having any prior information on class membership.

The main issue of defining a classifier system concerns the learning method to adopt. In general, a decision rule which optimally partitions the measurement space into K regions, one for each class C, must be detected; the boundaries between regions are called decision boundaries. In the lung cancer diagnosis by the electronic nose task, we considered three families of classifiers: a number of different versions of the k-Nearest Neighbors classifiers (k-NN) (classic, modified and fuzzy k-NN), Linear and Quadratic Discriminant function classifiers (respectively LD and QD) and an Artificial Neural Network (ANN). In the following a brief overview of these algorithms and of other computational intelligence techniques used in olfactory signal analysis is provided.

K-Nearest Neighbors method. The basic idea behind this simple and powerful algorithm is to assign the input sample to the class to which belongs the majority of the k closest samples in the training set. This method is able to do a nonlinear classification starting from a small number of samples. The algorithm is based on a measure of the distance (e.g., the Euclidean one) among features and it has been demonstrated [12], that the k-NN is formally a non parametric approximation of the Maximum A Posteriori (MAP) criterion. The asymptotic performance of this algorithm, is almost optimal: with an infinite number of training samples and setting $k = 1$, the minimum error is never higher than twice the Bayesian error (that is the theoretical lower bound reachable) [10]. One of the most critical aspects of this method regards the choice of parameter k when having a limited number of samples: if k is too large, then the problem is too much simplified and the local information loses its relevance. On the other hand, a too small k leads to a density estimation too sensitive to outliers. A small variation of the classic k-NN is the modified k-NN, where k represents the number of closest neighbors to look for (as in the classic k-NN), but all belonging to the same class. This dynamically modifies the neighborhood according to the noise in the dataset.

Discriminant Functions classifiers (DF). Classification based on discriminant functions represents a geometric approach where the feature space is divided in c decision regions each one corresponding to a particular class. The classifier is represented as a family of discriminant functions $g_i(x)$ with only one output that minimizes a given cost function. In DF analysis it is assumed that the data are distributed as a multivariate Gaussian. In our work, we considered two types of discriminant functions: the linear (LD) and the quadratic one (QD). A classifier based on a linear discriminant function divides the feature space by planes and it is therefore optimum when the problem is linearly separable. However, this technique is able to produce good performance also when the problem is not linearly separable. We implemented the Minimum Distance to Means (MDM) approach, in which the representatives of each class are calculated as the mean value of samples belonging to that class. This approach is very simple and leads to good generalization; the drawback is that it compresses all the information in only one representative value. If the problem is not linearly separable, a quadratic discrimination function might be more suitable, as it has been verified also in this work.

Artificial Neural Networks (ANNs). Artificial Neural Networks (ANN) are non-linear statistical modeling tools able to model complex relationships between inputs and outputs by means of a training procedure during which they adapt themselves to the data. They consist of massively parallel interconnected and adaptive processing elements. From this perspective they are very attractive in olfactory signal analysis, since, to some extent, they mimic the olfactory system: the processing elements represent the biological olfactory cells or neurons, while their interconnections correspond to the synaptic links. In ANN, the processing elements are organized in three distinct groups of elements: input, hidden and output layer neurons. The input layer corresponds to the input data (the feature matrix), while the output neurons correspond to each of the considered classes; the hidden layers have computational tasks, and the number of hidden layers, as well as the number of neurons in each layer must be determined experimentally. Each neuron sums its weighted inputs and performs a nonlinear transform through to the output layer. The learning process in ANNs starts providing them with a number of sample inputs with their corresponding outputs (supervised learning). During the learning phase, the weights are adjusted to minimize the difference between the obtained output and the actual one. Once the network is trained, it can be used to predict the membership of new samples. It can be demonstrated that an ANN, given a sufficient number of sigmoidal neurons in the hidden levels, is able to approximate any nonlinear function on a compact set. Moreover ANNs asymptotically (with an infinite number of examples) approximate the a-posteriori probability as with the Bayesian classifiers [13]. The issue of generalization must be addressed and early stopping and weight decay can be interesting solutions [13]. One of the main drawbacks of ANN regards the impossibility to decide a priori the best architecture and parameters to use, which must be determined experimentally and will strongly affect the success of the training process, in terms of a fast rate of convergence and good generalization. A possible solution, later discussed in details, consists of using a Genetic Algorithm (GA) to determine automatically a suitable network architecture and the best set of parameters to be used. The interconnection topology and learning rules of the neurons determine the type of a particular network and its performance. In particular the most used ANN topology in electronic noses are feed-forward neural networks, in which the information moves only in a forward direction, from the input nodes, through the hidden nodes (if any) and to the output nodes. There are no cycles or loops in the network. According to the specific architecture, a number of feed-forward neural networks can be outlined:

- *Multy-Layer Perceptrons (MLP)*: MLP are the most popular and simplest type of feed-forward neural networks with one or more layers of neurons between the input and output neurons. The hidden units are connected to either the inputs or outputs by weighted connections. A MLP is able to learn complex nonlinear regression by adjusting the weights in the network by a gradient descent technique known as back-propagation. This is the model used in this work; in particular, the implemented MLP has one hidden layer and the output is a single neuron assuming the value 1 if lung cancer is detected and 0 otherwise. All neurons have a sigmoidal function as activation function. The net has been trained using the resilient back-propagation algorithm, based on the gradient descent approach, in which only the sign of the derivative is used to determine the direction of the weights update. This choice is due to the fact that this algorithm was able to offer the best compromise between the error on the validation set and convergence. Finally, we set the number of neurons in the hidden layer equal to three; this value has been obtained by training a set of networks with increasing number of hidden neurons and picking the smallest one with a good validation error. Since ANN results depend on the values of the initialization, we trained the net 20 times and we chose the best configuration (according to the early stopping error) to evaluate the test set.

- *Radial Basis Functions (RBF)*: RBF is a method to approximate nonlinear functions; they are feed-forward architectures consisting of a hidden layer of radial kernels and an output layer of linear neurons. Each hidden neuron in a RBF is tuned to respond to a local region of feature space by means of a radially symmetric function such as the Gaussian one. The output units linearly combine the hidden units to predict the output variable in a similar fashion to MLPs. After selecting the radial basis centers using c-means clustering [10], the spreads are determined from the average distance between neighboring cluster centers or the sample covariance of each cluster. Finally, the radial basis activations are used as regressors to predict the target outputs. There are several possible learning processes for a RBF network depending on how the centers of the hidden layer are defined. Because of its functioning, the different layers of a RBF network perform different tasks. From a geometrical point of view, RBF network decision boundaries are hyperellipsoids.

- *Self-Organizing Map (SOM)*: SOM or Kohonen maps are an unsupervised learning algorithm that provides a method to represent multidimensional data in a smaller dimensional space. In practice, they map the input vector of dimension M into a smaller space of dimension N (with $N \leq M$). They are a specific topology of feed-forward neural network where each neural unit is connected only to all input units and not to other units. The SOM does not need any output target and can thus be considered as a clustering algorithm for exploratory data analysis. The SOM consists of a regular, typically two-dimensional grid of processing neurons, called map units, that is iteratively trained. Each area reacts to a specific stimulus; the observation of the activation patterns allow to infer some input properties. The accuracy and the generalization capability of a SOM depend on the number of used map units.

- *Learning Vector Quantization (LVQ)*: LVQ is a supervised variant of SOM and can be considered as a special case of artificial neural network where the winner-takes-all Hebbian learning-based approach is applied. The network has three layers: an input layer, a Kohonen classification layer, and a competitive output layer. After the network is given by prototypes, it adapts the weights of the network in order to classify the data correctly. For each data point, a winner neuron is detected as the one closest to the desired value and the weights of its connections are consequently adapted. The main advantage of LVQ is that it creates prototypes that are easy to interpret for experts in the field.

- *Probabilistic Neural Networks (PNN)*: PNN is a parallel implementation of the Bayes statistical technique and is a four layer feed-forward MLP. By replacing the sigmoid activation function with an exponential function (Gaussian), a PNN can compute nonlinear decision boundaries that approach the Bayes optimal. The decision requires an estimate of the probability density function (pdf) for each class. The only adjustable parameter in PNN is the kernel width, which determines the degree of interpolation that occurs in determining the pdf. The main drawback of PNN is that it is limited to applications involving relatively small datasets; large datasets would indeed lead to large network architectures and would increase the rate of misclassification.

Support Vector Machine (SVM). SVM are linear classifiers in high dimensional spaces. The basic idea behind the SVM paradigm is that, if we define a map (usually nonlinear) from the input space to a feature space H, the sample S can be separated by a hyperplane in H even if a separating hyperplane does not exist in X. In the subset of all the S-separating hyperplanes the optimal separating hyperplane must be detected: it is the hyperplane which maximizes the distance between the hyperplane and the closest between the positive and the negative cluster. A hyperplane in the feature space is the image of a nonlinear function in the input space, whose shape depends on the kernel function. Determining the optimal separating hyperplane is a quadratic programming problem. However, mapping the input space to a feature space may make this problem computationally hard. The important advantage of the support vector classifier is that it offers a possibility to train generalizable, nonlinear classifiers in high-dimensional spaces using a small training set. Moreover, since a quadratic programming problem is convex, every local solution is also global (unique if the Hessian is positive definite). On the other hand, the training phase of a SVM can be computationally intensive, but it is also amenable to parallelization and always yields the optimal solution.

Fuzzy logic. Fuzzy logic is a form of multi-valued logic derived from fuzzy set theory conceived by Lotfi Zadeh [14]. It provides a generalization of the traditional forms of logic and set membership. In contrast with binary sets having binary logic, also known as crisp logic, in fuzzy set theory the set membership values can be between 0 and 1, that is, the degree of truth of a statement can range between 0 and 1 and is not constrained to the two truth values $\{true(1), false(0)\}$ as in classic propositional logic. Indeed, in classical set theory an object either belongs to a set or it does not. Probability explains how events occur in random space, while fuzzy logic includes situations where there is imprecision due to vagueness rather than randomness. Probability deals with the likelihood of an outcome, while fuzzy logic deals with the degree of ambiguity, that is expressed as membership value. A probability of 1 indicates that the event is certain to occur. The membership function value, on the contrary, measures the degree to which objects satisfy imprecisely defined properties. An important difference w.r.t. classical set theory is that the sum of fuzzy membership functions can be different from one, in contrast with the sum of mutually independent probabilities of a system in classical set theory that must add to one. An important advantage in fuzzy logic, is that fuzzy membership functions can be developed using a wide range of techniques including probability density functions. Fuzzy logic provides a simple way to define a precise conclusion based upon vague, ambiguous, imprecise, noisy, or missing input information. The input information and the output decision can be combined by means of a rule-based approach, even based on linguistic relationships. This approach to control problems mimics how humans make decisions. Thanks to the ability of fuzzy logic to deal with vague and noisy input, it has been widely used in the olfactory signal analysis. In the following a brief overview of its main application is provided.

– *Fuzzy k-NN*: Fuzzy k-NN, a variation of the classic k-NN based on a fuzzy logic approach, assigns a fuzzy class membership to each sample and provides an output in a fuzzy form [15]. In particular, the membership value of unlabeled sample x to i^{th} class is influenced by the inverse of the distances from neighbors and their class memberships:

$$\mu_i(x) = \frac{\sum_{j=1}^{k} \mu_{ij}(\|x - x_j\|)^{\frac{-2}{m-1}}}{\sum_{j=1}^{k}(\|x - x_j\|)^{\frac{-2}{m-1}}} \tag{6}$$

where μ_{ij} represents the membership of labeled sample x_j to the ith class. This value can be crisp or it can be calculated according to a particular fuzzy rule: in our work we defined a Gaussian membership function with maximum value at the average of the class and standard deviation related to the minimum and maximum values of it. In this way, the closer the sample j is to the average point of class i, the closer its membership value μ_{ij} will be to 1 and vice-versa. Of course other types of membership function may be defined, e.g., according to the lung cancer stage or to the confidence assigned to the target labels. The parameter m determines how heavily the distance is weighted when calculating each neighbor contribution to the membership value; we chose $m = 2$, but almost the same error rates have been obtained on these data over a wide range of values of m.

– *Fuzzy Adaptive Resonance Map (FAM)*: FAM is a specific case of Adaptive Resonance Theory (ART) networks, devised by Grossberg [16]. Adaptive resonant theory networks were introduced as a theory of human cognition in information processing, and are systems capable of adapting autonomously in real time to changes in the environment. Their basic idea takes inspiration from the fact that a human brain can learn new events without necessarily forgetting events learnt in the past. They have indeed been designed to solve the stability-plasticity dilemma and so are stable enough to incorporate new information without destroying the memory of previous learning. They have a stable memory structure even with fast on-line learning that was capable of adapting to new data input, even forming totally new category distinctions. The most advanced model of the ART family is Fuzzy ARTMAP which was developed for supervised slow learning. Unlike traditional MLP neural networks the architecture of FAM is selforganising according, as previously mentioned, to the plasticity-stability dilemma: the network is able to retain learned patterns (stability) while remaining able to learn new ones (plasticity). In a standard MLP network used for pattern classification an output neuron is assigned to each class of objects that the network is expected to learn, and must be trained off-line. In FAM the network dynamically assesses the assignment of output neurons to categories by competitive learning. Two ART modules are interconnected by an associative memory and internal control structures; the first module handles input patterns while the second one handles the class patterns. The network is able to perform real time learning without losing previously learnt patterns by using an incremental weight update procedure known as slow recoding. The main drawback of FAM is its architecture complexity; this limit is partially overcome by the Simplified Fuzzy ARTMAP (SFAM) network that reduces the complexity of the network architectures. It must be noticed that, removing the redundancies in FAM, SFAM are able to train much faster.

8   Finding the Predictive Model by a Genetic Algorithm

The choice of the most suitable pattern analysis algorithms is not trivial. The decision is strongly dependent from the specific problem domain and available data, in terms of quantity and distribution; moreover the performance of a specific classifier is affected to the previous feature extraction, selection and projection operations, that is, different classifiers can have different best feature subset and projection. Thus, each single operation of the pattern analysis module should not be considered as a separate step, independent from the others. If there is no specific reason to choose one approach w.r.t. others, as in the olfactory signal analysis usually happens, one should, in theory, evaluate all the possible combinations of feature selection, projection and classifier. Of course a similar approach is unfeasible. A possible solution, adopted in this work, is provided by Genetic Algorithms (GAs).

GAs are heuristic search algorithms based on the mechanics of natural selection; as optimization technique, they mimic the evolutionary process of survival of the best taking inspiration by the Darwinian process of natural selection. They perform a global random search on population of potential solutions (chromosomes), which allow the technique to be massively parallel in operation. In particular, at each generation the best potential solutions are selected with a certain probability and used to generate new solutions. These latter are produced mixing the parents information (crossover) and introducing few random changes in the new chromosomes (mutation) to avoid local minima and allowing a more extensive exploration of the solution space. The goodness of a solution is evaluated through the so called fitness function, that is the objective function to maximize.

This process leads to the evolution of populations of individuals that are better suited to their environment than the individuals from which they were created, mimicking natural adaptation. GAs, if properly coded, can be used to solve a wide range of problems, such as optimization (e.g., circuits layout, job shop scheduling), prediction (e.g., weather forecast, protein folding), classification (e.g., fraud detection, quality assessment), economy (e.g., bidding strategies, market evaluation), ecology (e.g., biological arm races, host-parasite coevolution) and automatic programming. In the electronic nose field they have been widely used, in particular to perform feature selection, to find the best classifier parameters and to indentify the best architecture and topology for the specific algorithm.

In our work, we implemented a genetic algorithm to find the best combination of feature selection, feature projection, classifier and its parameters. As previously mentioned, the quality of a classifier depends on the feature matrix on which it is applied, and different classifiers may have different optimal feature matrices, that is, different optimal feature subsets and projections. The implemented genetic algorithm was binary coded, and each chromosome included information about the specific features to keep, the projection algorithm to be applied (choosing among LDA, NPLDA and PCA), the classifier to adopt (choosing among k-NN, modified k-NN, Fuzzy k-NN, linear discriminant function, quadratic discriminant function and a feed-forward artificial neural network) and the corresponding parameters (e.g., k value, number of hidden layers, etc.). The population was composed of 100 chromosomes. At each generation, the best solutions were chosen according to the roulette wheel selection rule and the reproduction operation was performed by means of a scattered crossover and a Gaussian mutation. Elitism was adopted in order to improve the avoidance of local minima and to assure a monotonic fitness function of the best chromosomes at each generation. The fitness function was evaluated as a function proportional to the product of the mean squared error and the variance obtained performing the classification with the feature subset, the projection and the classifier encoded in the considered chromosome.

The best model provided by the GA, was a subset composed of four features, projected into a single component using the Linear Discriminant Analysis (LDA) and finally classified by means of the the k Nearest Neighbours (k-NN) method, with $k = 9$.

9   Validation

The previous sections have briefly reviewed a number of pattern analysis techniques used in the olfactory signal analysis and, more in specific, in the lung cancer diagnosis by an electronic nose application. This section addresses the issue of evaluating the performance of the considered pattern classification module. Indeed, it is very common to run into overestimated performance, in most cases due to overfitting. This is a very critical issue in model validation and refers to the lack of generalization of the classifier. This means that the classifier has, in some way, adapted too much to the specific dataset used to train the model and, providing it with unknown samples, fails or performs a bad classification: the performance of a pattern analysis module must be evaluated on novel and untrained samples.

Much attention must be paid to the procedure of estimating the real error rate. A first possible approach to overcome these issues may be to randomly partition the complete dataset into two subsets: a training set and a test set. The first one is used to train the pattern classification module and, thus, to find the best model, while the test set is used to estimate its accuracy. This simple approach works well if the dataset is significantly large, otherwise it would provide unreal performance estimations. Indeed it is strongly affected by the specific properties of the chosen training and test set, that is, changing training and test sets different performance would probably occur. To overcome this, one solution could be the use of bootstrapping, that is a statistical technique that generates multiple training-test partitions by resampling the original dataset with replacement.

Another possible solution is to adopt a cross-validation approach, that is based on the idea of performing multiple partitions of the dataset and averaging the performance of the model across partitions. K-fold cross-validation performs K data partitions, in a way that each data subset will be the test set in one of the K partitions and part of the training set in the remaining ones. In this way, each sample is used both for training and testing, assuring the most reliable estimation of the error rate. Indeed, classifier performance in cross-validation is estimated by averaging the errors obtained at each of the K iterations. A specific case of K fold cross-validation is leave-one-out, where K is equal to the number of data samples and the test set is composed at each iteration by only one measure of the dataset. This is the approach adopted in the presented work. However a little variation had to be done, transforming the leave-one-out approach to a leave-one-subject-out approach. Since, as previously mentioned, we acquired two samples for each subject breath, we needed to guarantee that none of the two measures could belong to the training set while using the other one in the test set. In the leave-one-subject-out cross-validation, each test set was thus composed by the pair of measurements corresponding to the same person, instead of a single measure as would be in the normal leave-one-out method. At each iteration of the leave-one-subject-out cross-validation, we evaluated a confusion matrix from which we extracted the corresponding performance indexes. At the end of the process the mean and the variance of the performance indexes were estimated. Being *TruePositive* (TP) a sick sample classified as sick, *TrueNegative* (TN) a healthy sample classified as healthy, *FalsePositive* (FP) a healthy sample classified as sick and *FalseNegative* (FN) a sick sample classified as healthy, the performance indexes are defined as:

- *Accuracy (Non Error Rate NER)*: the probability of doing a generic correct classification.

$$NER = \frac{TP + TN}{TP + FP + TN + FN} \tag{7}$$

- *Sensitivity (True Positive Rate TPR)*: the probability to classify a person as sick when this is true.

$$TPR = \frac{TP}{TP + FN} \tag{8}$$

- *Specificity (True Negative Rate TNR)*: the probability of classifying a person as healthy when this is true.

$$TNR = \frac{TN}{TN + FP} \tag{9}$$

- *Precision w.r.t. diseased people (PREC_{POS})*: the probability that, having assigned a sample to the class of diseased people, it actually belongs to that class.

$$PREC_{POS} = \frac{TP}{TP + FP} \tag{10}$$

- *Precision w.r.t. healthy people (PREC_{NEG})*: the probability that, having assigned a sample to the class of healthy people, it actually belongs to that class.

$$PREC_{NEG} = \frac{TN}{TN + FN} \tag{11}$$

To obtain indexes able to describe completely the performance of the algorithms, the corresponding confidence intervals must be evaluated:

$$\bar{X} - t_{\frac{\alpha}{2}} \frac{\sigma}{\sqrt{n}} \leq \mu_x \leq \bar{X} + t_{\frac{\alpha}{2}} \frac{\sigma}{\sqrt{n}} \tag{12}$$

where $\bar{X}$ is the estimated index value, n is the number of the degrees of freedom, σ is the standard deviation and $t_{\frac{\alpha}{2}}$ is the quantile of the t-Student distribution corresponding to $n - 1$ and a probability of α.

10   Lung Cancer Diagnosis by an Electronic Nose: Results

The goal of the implemented genetic algorithm was to identify the best combination of feature subset and the considered feature projection and classification algorithms. The obtained solution suggested that the best fitness function (proportional to the classification accuracy and its variance) was reached keeping four of the initial hundreds of features, projecting them into one dimension by means of Linear Discriminant Analysis (LDA) and classifying the new feature samples using a k-Nearest Neighbors rule, with $k = 9$. The achieved results, all validated using leave-one-subject-out cross-validation, are shown in Table 1, where the corresponding performance indexes and confidence intervals are provided. These results confirmed a previous pilot study where we achieved an average accuracy

Table 1. Confusion matrix and corresponding performance indexes obtained classifying the dataset with the model proposed by the Genetic Algorithm (projection of the four features subset into one dimension by LDA and classification by k-NN with $k = 9$). Results have been obtained performing a leave-one-subject-out cross-validation and confidence intervals have been computed for a probability of 95%. Positive samples correspond to diseased subjects, while negative samples represent healthy volunteers.

CONFUSION		TRUE LABELS		Accuracy	$96.15\% \pm 5.41\%$
MATRIX		Positive	Negative	Sensitivity	$93.33\% \pm 9.3\%$
ESTIMATED	Positive	56	0	Specificity	$100\% \pm 0\%$
LABELS	Negative	4	44	Precision$_{POS}$	$100\% \pm 0\%$
Total		60	44	Precision$_{NEG}$	$91.66\% \pm 11.57\%$

of 92.6%, sensitivity of 95.3% and specificity of 90.5% (on 58 control subjects and 43 lung cancer subjects) [1]. A very interesting consideration regards the fact that three of the four found best features are extracted from the same sensor, meaning that those two sensors are enough to diagnose lung cancer with the excellent performance indexes showed in Table 1. Evaluating the performance reached keeping the features extracted only by one sensor (the one corresponding to the best three features) results have been very satisfactory, reaching an average accuracy of 90.38%, sensitivity of 83.33% and specificity of 100%. All the four best features were derived from the transient response, being its integral, its derivative, the difference between the baseline and the steady-state and the ratio between the baseline and the steady-state. This confirms the theory that the transient response contains useful information related to the dynamics of the phenomenon. The best component projected by means of LDA is shown in Figure 5, where the discrimination between the two classes *lung cancer patient* and *healthy subject* is evident. Finally the best classifier has turned out to be the k-NN with k=9. However, performing a Student's t-test between all pair of considered models, no significative differences emerged, suggesting that all computational intelligence methods that we have applied provided satisfying results. It has to be noticed that two of the four misclassified samples correspond to a subject which diagnosis by PET failed too. This suggests that some singular physiological parameters could be present in that patient.

We also investigated the possibility of performing early diagnosis, training the model to distinguish among the class *stage I lung cancer patient* and *healthy subjects*. The followed approach has been the same used for the classification between *lung cancer* (all the stages) versus *healthy subjects*: the genetic algorithm searched the best combination of feature subset, feature projection and classifier and provided a new subset of features (composed of 7 features) and the same projection and classification algorithms (LDA and k-NN with $k = 9$) as in the lung cancer diagnosis task. Results are showed in Table 2. Although these results are relatively satisfactory, their confidence intervals are not that compact and, anyway, are larger than those achieved in the *lung cancer* vs *healthy* classification.

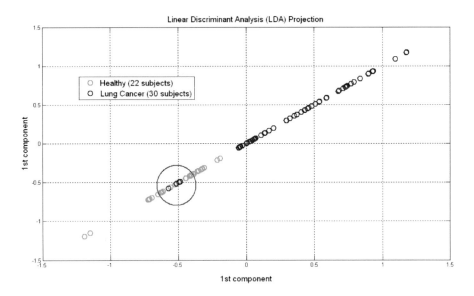

Fig. 5. The results of dimensionality reduction through linear discriminant analysis (LDA) into one component. As evident the separability between the two classes *healthy subject* and *lung cancer patient* is very satisfactory. Samples in the red circle are the misclassified four lung cancer patients erroneously assigned to the healthy class.

Table 2. Confusion matrix and corresponding performance indexes obtained classifying the dataset with the model proposed by the Genetic Algorithm (projection of the seven features subset into one dimension by LDA and classification by k-NN with $k = 9$). Results have been obtained performing a leave-one-subject-out cross-validation and confidence intervals have been computed for a probability of 95%. Positive samples correspond to stage I lung cancer patients, while negative samples represent healthy subjects. Performance are lower than those achieved in the classification *lung cancer patients* (all stages) versus *healthy subjects*, but this is probably due to the small available dataset regarding the positive class and the imbalance between the two classes.

CONFUSION		TRUE LABELS		Accuracy	$92.86\% \pm 8.51\%$
MATRIX		Positive	Negative	Sensitivity	$75\% \pm 34.31\%$
ESTIMATED	Positive	9	1	Specificity	$97.73\% \pm 4.57\%$
LABELS	Negative	3	43	Precision$_{POS}$	$90\% \pm 40.15\%$
Total		12	44	Precision$_{NEG}$	$93.48\% \pm 13.39\%$

This could be due both to the small available dataset (only 12 subjects affected by stage I lung cancer) and to the imbalance of the dataset (12 stage I lung cancer versus 44 healthy subjects). Regardless this analysis, the achieved results suggest that the discrimination between *stage I lung cancer patient* and *healthy subjects* (and thus early diagnosis) is possible and that, with a larger and more balanced dataset, the trained model might achieve even higher performance.

11   Conclusions

A brief overview of pattern analysis algorithms used in the electronic nose field has been provided, focusing on a specific case study of the use of an electronic nose based on an array of MOS sensors to detect lung cancer. Many research directions that are the frontier of sensor based machine olfaction must still be explored, such as the development of hybrid arrays and the implementation of ensemble methods where the outputs of different predictors are combined to produce an overall output. Another cutting edge issue is the development of a transforming mapping among different devices or sensors in order to transfer the predicted model from one device to another. Moreover, converting these potential markets to commercial reality has yet to be achieved: many issues such as requirement for robustness (in particular when dealing with health of patients), variability of samples, the large number of environmental and habitual factors that can affect the measurement, just to mention some, must be faced and solved. Enormous potential exists for the use of the electronic nose technology in a wide range of applications and the medical one, as cancer detection, plays a crucial role among them. A very interesting future development regards the detection of other type of cancers with the electronic nose. Concerning with lung cancer diagnosis, the achieved results demonstrate that an instrument as the electronic nose, combined with the appropriate computational intelligence methodologies, is a promising alternative to current lung cancer diagnostic techniques: the obtained predictive errors are lower than those achieved by present diagnostic methods, and the cost of the analysis, both in money, time and resources, is lower. Moreover, the instrument is completely non invasive. Current diagnostic techniques (e.g., CT, PET) are invasive, very expensive, have radiation risks and a not so good accuracy; moreover, results on early detection and treatment, in last decades, have been very poor and unsatisfying. This calls for the necessity of a non invasive, accurate and cheap diagnostic technique, able to identify the presence of lung cancer in its early stages, as the electronic nose demonstrated to be. Early detection is a major challenge to decrease lung cancer mortality: results achieved in the early detection analysis are very promising and suggest further experimentations and analysis. The introduction of this cutting edge technology will lead to very important social and business effects: its low price and small dimensions allow a large scale distribution, giving the opportunity to perform non invasive, cheap, quick, and massive early diagnosis and screening.

References

1. Blatt, R., Bonarini, A., Calabró, E., Della Torre, M., Matteucci, M., Pastorino, U.: Pattern Classification Techniques for Early Lung Cancer Diagnosis using an Electronic Nose, Frontiers in Artificial Intelligence and Applications. In: 18th European Conference on Artificial Intelligence (ECAI 2008) - 5th Prestigious Applications of Intelligent Systems (PAIS 2008), vol. 178, pp. 693–697 (2008)

2. Gardner, J.W., Bartlett, P.N.: Electronic noses. Principles and applications. Oxford University Press, Oxford (1999)
3. Osuna, R.G., Nagle, H.T., Shiffman, S.S.: The how and why of electronic nose. IEEE Spectrum, 22–34 (September 1998)
4. Pearce, T.C., Nagle, H.T., Shiffman, S.S., Gardner, J.W.: Handbook of machine olfaction. Electronic nose technology. Wiley-VHC, Chichester (2003)
5. Osuna, R.G.: Pattern Analysis for Machine Olfaction: a review. IEEE sensors Journal 2(3), 189–202 (2002)
6. Llobet, E., Brezmes, J., Vilanova, X., Correig, X., Sueiras, J.E.: Qualitative and quantitative analysis of volatile organic compounds using transient and steady-state responses of a thick-film tin oxide gas sensor array. Sensors and Actuators B: Chemical 41(1), 13–21 (1997)
7. Gardner, J.W., Hines, E.L., Tang, H.C.: Detection of vapours and odours from a multisensor array using pattern-recognition techniques Part 2. Artificial neural networks, Sensors and Actuators B: Chemical 9, 9–15 (1992)
8. Gordon, S.M., Szidon, J.P., Krotoszynski, B.K., Gibbons, R.D., O'Neill, H.J.: Volatile organic compounds in exhaled air from patients with lung cancer. Clinical chemistry 31(8), 1278–1282 (1985)
9. Phillips, M.D., Cataneo, R.N., Cummin, A.R.C., Gagliardi, A.J., Gleeson, K., Greenberg, J., Maxfield, R.A., Rom, W.N.: Detection of lung cancer with volatile markers in the breath. Chest 123(6), 2115–2123 (2003)
10. Duda, R.O., Hart, P.E., Stork, D.G.: Pattern classification, 2nd edn. Wiley-Interscience, Hoboken (2000)
11. Fukunaga, K., Mantock, J.M.: Nonparametric discriminant analysis. IEEE Transactions on pattern analysis and machine intelligence PAMI 5(6), 671–678 (1983)
12. Fukunaga, K.: Introduction to statistical pattern recognition, 2nd edn. Academic Press, San Diego (1990)
13. Bishop, C.M.: Neural networks for pattern recognition. Oxford University Press, Oxford (1996)
14. Zadeh, L.: Fuzzy Sets. Information and control 8, 338–353 (1965)
15. Keller, J.M., Gray, M.R., Givens, J.A.: A fuzzy k-Nearest neighbor algorithm. IEEE Transactions on systems, man and cybernetics 15(4), 580–585 (1985)
16. Grossberg, S.: Adaptive pattern classification and universal recoding II: feedback, expectation olfaction and illusions. Biol. Cybern 23, 187–202 (1976)

Chapter 19
A Portable Wireless Solution for Back Pain Telemonitoring: A 3D-Based, Virtual Reality Approach

Fotios Spyridonis and Gheorghita Ghinea

School of Information Systems, Computing and Mathematics, Brunel University,
UB8 3PH, Uxbridge, UK
{Fotios.Spyridonis,George.Ghinea}@brunel.ac.uk

Abstract. Over the years, an increasing number of the adult population suffers from some form of back pain during their lifetime, something that consecutively has a very important impact on a country's health, as well as economic systems. Traditional methods of diagnosing and treating such problems normally involve the collection and gathering of medical information regarding the type and location of pain, and its visualization on a 2D representation of the human body using various monochrome symbols. However, these 2-dimensional pain drawings have usually limited abilities in accurately recording and representing pain, making them in that way difficult and time consuming for both patients and doctors to use. As a result, in this work we propose an alternative interactive environment for back pain information collection and diagnosis, based on a wireless-enabled solution that encompasses a virtual reality user interface. Our proposed approach uses questionnaire methods to collect the appropriate back pain information, and via a 3-dimensional representation of the human body which can be marked in color, it could visualize and record this information, overcoming the aforementioned limitations.

1 Introduction

It is estimated that as the population ages, an increasing number of patients will need help in managing complex, long term medical conditions over time. Examples of such chronic diseases include but are not limited to asthma, diabetes, arthritis, heart failure, chronic obstructive pulmonary disease, dementia and a range of disabling neurological conditions [8]. Unfortunately, if not properly treated, chronic conditions can affect the lives of millions of people and cause thousands of premature deaths, depending on the condition. Quite apart from their impact on physical health, these diseases also disrupt the social and working lives of the people affected by them and have important implications for families, friends, carers, employers and health services [10].

Currently, 80 percent of GP consultations relate to long term conditions, with such patients using over 60 percent of hospital bed days in UK. In addition, treating these conditions is likely to cost the healthcare system of a country a considerable amount of its budgeted resources. Evidence from the US shows that the care of people with

I. Bichindaritz et al. (Eds.): Computational Intelligence in Healthcare 4, SCI 309, pp. 425–461.
springerlink.com   © Springer-Verlag Berlin Heidelberg 2010

chronic conditions consumes about 78 percent of all healthcare spending [8]. Moreover, by examining the allocation of costs in UK healthcare services given by the Department of Health report [9] we can identify that, over the last 3 years there has been an impressive increase in costs for treatment of *long-term conditions*, with the figure reaching 14,353 million in 2006/07 as compared to 6,455 million in 2004/05, which is more than 50 percent increase in two years.

1.1 Back Pain as a Chronic Medical Condition

However, in addition to the ones aforementioned, there are more chronic conditions that could affect most of healthcare stakeholders, with one of the most important ones being back pain. The diagnosis and treatment of Low Back Disorders (LBDs), and specifically of back pain is a major health problem that research in medical as well as in biodynamic areas is currently dealing with. It is that enormous the impact of this disability that back pain alone cost the UK industry about 9090 million pounds in 1997 and 1998, with between 90 and 100 million days of sickness and invalidity benefit paid out per year for back pain complaints, as it is characteristically stated by [47].

Back-pain: Magnitude of problem. According to past studies, it is estimated that 60-80% of the population is suffering by some form of back pain during their life [53], with that percentage remaining the same in 2008, based on a study performed by Backcare where an estimated 80% of people in the UK are affected, with four in five adults experiencing it. Generally speaking, back pain is considered to be a worldwide experience, since based on the literature it appears to be a problem for most of the western and industrialized societies. According to [5], the lifetime prevalence of back pain is more than 70% in most industrialized countries, affecting 20% of the population in the United States per year, whereas the relative numbers in Britain, based on a Department of Health survey, reach 40% of the adult population, 5% of which have to take time off to recover [15]. Specifically, the prevalence of back pain in the general population is estimated to be between 60% and 90%, with most people experiencing it at some time in their lives usually beginning between ages of the 30 and 40 years, and with men and women being affected approximately equally [23]. Moreover, studies around Europe have also shown that back pain does not affect only the adult population, but it is also very common in children with about 50% experiencing back pain at some time in their lives [47].

Back-pain Costs. Moreover, besides being uncomfortable and affecting a major percentage of the human population, back pain has also a considerable effect on health budgets and national economies of countries. Treating such chronic conditions is likely to cost the healthcare system of a country a considerable amount of its budgeted resources. Evidence from the US shows that the care of people with chronic conditions consumes about 78 percent of all healthcare spending [8]. Specifically, in 2008, the figures as published by Backcare [3] indicate that the National Health Service in the UK spends more than £1 billion on back pain related costs per year, which include:

Table 1. Break down of back pain related costs in UK spend in a per year basis

£512 million on hospital costs for back pain patients.
£141 million on GP consultations for back pain.
£150.6 million on physiotherapy treatments for back pain.
In the private health care sector £565 million is spent on back pain every year.
This brings the health care costs for back pain to a total of £1.6 billion per year.
In addition there are other (indirect) costs. The Health and Safety Executive estimates that musculoskeletal disorders, which includes back pain costs UK employers between £590 million and £624 million per year.
The total costs of back pain correspond to between 1% and 2% of gross national product (GDP). Recent reviews suggest that spinal pain utilises between 1-2% of Gross National Product in OECD countries [48].
Other European countries report similar high costs; back pain related costs in The Netherlands in 1991 were more than 4 billion euro. For Sweden in 1995 this was more than 2 billion euro

Accordingly, in the United States, based on the American Chiropractic Association [2], in 2008 the relative figures rose to 31 million Americans experiencing back pain at any given time, and at least $50 billion are spend each year for back pain related costs, a more than 50 % increase as opposed to 1990 costs.

Back-pain: Work Impact. In addition to the impact back pain has in a country's population and economy, it also seems to be a feature influencing a patient's ability to work, with nearly 5 million working days to be lost as a result of back pain in 2003-04, constituting back pain as the number 2 reason for long term sickness in much of the UK, based on Backcare [3]. Finally, back pain can have a significant impact on people's lives by affecting day to day activities on a personal level, something that reduces life quality, as well as social relationships. Without proper diagnosis, treatment and monitoring, back pain can prevent patients from doing essential daily activities (such as collecting water, harvesting, and carrying heavy objects, including children) central in maintaining their homes and livelihoods, specifically for people in developing countries [48]. To this end, back pain is considered to be the second only to the cold as the most common disease in humans, and together with heart disease, arthritis or other joint disease, backache is one of the most common causes of morbidity, disability, and perceived threat to health [23].

Back-pain Causes. Unfortunately, according to [53], the available medical information only provides partial success in diagnosis and treatment of back pain with only
15% of the patients obtaining an accurate diagnosis of their problem. This partial
success is due to the complexity of the back, where its main causes could result from
various reasons, as well as several other external factors.

Having said that, evidence from the literature about the biomechanics of back pain,
suggests that in essence the causes of back pain remain unclear. However, studies in
the field [55] have shown that the most common causes of back pain can be divided in
three major categories, namely *Musculoskeletal, Systemic*, and *Visceral*. Furthermore,
analysis of these studies has shown that 98% of the cases are musculoskeletal in etiology, with the remaining 2% being due to systemic conditions, referred visceral pain,
or psychological and social factors. Specifically, "most musculoskeletal injuries leading to LBP are likely attributable to sprained paraspinous tendons or muscle spasm,
but there are no objective tests to confirm these diagnoses [55]. A more detailed
analysis of the aforementioned factors that affect the development of the disease, as
well as a more detailed categorization of back pain causes, could be found in [28] and
[12] respectively. Accordingly, although the real causes of back pain remain unclear,
[1] suggest that the joints and the spinal discs are the leading sources of back pain
with pain originating from the joints accounting for some 10-15% of patients, and
pain coming from spinal discs to cause more than 40% of the cases.

However, considering the fact that back pain is really difficult to be accurately diagnosed due to the multi-factorial nature of the disease, the logical attitude that each
individual should adopt towards the avoidance of developing such a disorder, is trying
to prevent it. In overall though, whatever the underlying cause is, specific procedures
need to be followed in order for back pain to be thoroughly understood, diagnosed,
and treated, as it is going to be discussed in more detail in the following section.
Based on these procedures, ways that this phenomenon and chronic conditions in
general, could be more effectively managed will be identified.

In spite of what has been discussed so far however, the assessment of this medical
complaint remains notoriously difficult. Despite the huge amount of money spent and
resources lost, it is estimated that only a small percent of success in treating back pain
exists, showing in that way not only the considerable negative impact on the health
budgets and national economies of countries, but also the importance and need of
identifying the best and most effective ways to combat this phenomenon specifically,
and long term conditions in general, which affect a huge percentage of the population.
Improving healthcare and services for people also suffering from long term conditions
therefore will definitely have a beneficial impact on care, waiting lists, demand, workforce, hospital admissions, costs, and prescribing [8].

1.2 Current Back-Pain Assessment Practices

One of the first steps that is traditionally undertaken by patients in a back pain clinic
is the completion of a medical questionnaire, which is intended to identify the location and type of pain being experienced, normally in paper format. In most cases, the
only visual aid to assist medical staff with their assessment is "pain drawings." Traditional pain drawings are 2-D figures of the human body on which the patient is asked
to mark the type and distribution of the pain being suffered. Notwithstanding their
advantages, 2-D pain drawings have their limitations, as they do not capture the 3-D

nature of the human body. Thus, patients are unable to visually express the pain that they are experiencing, as statements of the form "*I have a pain on the inside of my thigh*" are not easily captured in a 2-D pain drawing.

While recent inventions of medical imaging techniques such as computerized tomography and magnetic resonance imaging have revolutionized radiology, the development of 3-D imaging has not yet been ported across the world of pain drawings.

Finally, it is natural that the patient wants to be regularly informed of their health situation, and the doctors on their part to be able to monitor their patients' medical situation, therefore to both have easy and relatively fast access to such health information, avoiding situations such as hospital queues. Thus, in overall, there are appear to be several limitations in the current back pain assessment practices that had led researchers to consider ways of improving the effectiveness of these techniques.

1.3 A Statement of the Problem

To this end, the purpose of this work is therefore, to establish whether the improvement of the existing back pain assessment techniques has an impact on the ways in which back pain patients are treated. If these improvements can be shown as an effective way of also improving the quality of their treatment, then this could be a significant finding, given the large numbers of back pain sufferers in worldwide and the amount of money and resources spend to deal with this chronic condition.

Consequently, the questions arising from this problem identified is what impact does the improvement of the current back pain assessment techniques have on the ways in which back pain patients are treated? Does it comprise an effective way of improving the quality of their treatment?

Therefore, in its broadest form, this work aims to develop a prototype solution that will be introduced as an effective improvement to the existing back pain measurement methods and limitations, as well as identify if, and how this improvement in the current diagnosis methods changes the way in which back pain patients are treated.

1.4 Summary

So, the focus of this work will be the augmentation of the traditional 2-D pain drawing with a novel, computer-based, 3-D version—in the anticipation that electronic 3-D pain drawings shall increase the ease with which patients record their own pain, as well as providing a tool for pain data collection and monitoring for back pain clinicians. Moreover, we will port the developed 3-D pain drawing to a personal digital assistant (PDA) platform, and implement a wireless solution for mobile medical data collection.

Accordingly, the structure of this chapter is as follows. Section 2 provides a more detailed overview of back pain assessment, while Section 3 describes the proposed design, and consecutively the implementation of our prototype, and lastly, evaluations as well as conclusions are drawn in Sections 4 and 5 respectively.

2 Back Pain Monitoring-A Review of the Literature

In the previous section we have already reviewed some relevant literature in the process of outlining the background, significance, and importance of this proposed work.

The review of the literature that follows considers the existing back pain monitoring process, and examines more thoroughly whether this process is indeed adequate in providing patients with the best quality treatment.

2.1 Back Pain Visualization

The diagnosis of the patient suffering from some form of back pain is considered to be so complex that many clinicians in various disciplines still struggle to deal with. Based on the literature [36],[42] a practical and common approach to diagnosis is to begin with a comprehensive patient history and physical examination, subsequently including secondary diagnostic procedures such as medical imaging, neurologic, and psychosocial tests to supplement the initial diagnostic examinations, if necessary. The final step after finishing the above process is to identify and implement a treatment plan that will be based on the final diagnosis.

To this end, the aforementioned practical approach is ideally summarized and further explained by [27], in what is described in their study as *the S.O.A.P. (Subjective testing, Objective testing, Assessment, and Planning)* process. According to their work, this process consists of four distinct and sequentially connected phases (fig. 1), and it is very common amongst clinicians for back pain management.

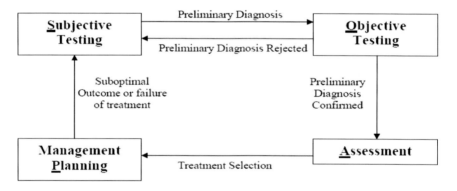

Fig. 1. The S.O.A.P process

Moreover, they argue that of great importance in this process is the accuracy of the *subjective* testing phase, which has significant impact on the following assessments, and on the final treatment plan in a way that service quality could be diminished affecting the patient's well-being.

2.2 Subjective Phase

As has just been mentioned, the back pain diagnosis process initiates with the subjective testing phase, where the clinician normally collects medical information related to *patient history* and *clinical information* [27]. According to the literature [29], there are several pain measurement methods available that have been tested by many authors, and who concluded that they could be used in back pain patients' medical information collection. These pain measurements have been categorized as follows:

- *Self-report measures.* Using this method, the clinician records pain measurements such as the worst pain or the least pain, as perceived by the patient reporting it.

- *Observational measures.* This kind of measures includes the clinician observing the patient regarding aspects such as behavior or activity performance, as related to pain.

- *Physical-functional performance tests.* Finally, this kind of tests is a method of measuring the performance of a patient in functional tests, in order to prove back pain effects in functional activities.

Although all of the aforementioned methods are considered to be valuable and necessary in order to identify and measure a patient's medical information, in reality authorities recognize *self-report* measures to be the gold standard of the intended purpose, because of its consistency with the definition of pain, and which is why it is widely used. Therefore, the most prominent way used to collect back pain related information is usually self-reports, which are typically in the form of *questionnaire* [29]. Moreover, according to [27], this questionnaire normally consists of question items specifically designed to collect information regarding the pain's description, location(s), activation, severity, frequency, symptoms, as well as previous medical problems and/or treatments, all based on the patient's responses. Specifically, the former aspects mentioned (pain description, location(s), activation, severity, frequency, and symptoms) are indicators of a patient's *current clinical information*, whereas the latter (previous medical problems and/or treatments) are part of the *patient's history*.

Patient Medical History. Usually, as the name implies, a patient's medical history includes information regarding previous medical problems and/or their treatment, as well as some information concerning the patient's current situation. To this end, several question forms exist and are used in the literature as a way of collecting such patient medical history information. As an example, to simply illustrate the method, [33] in their study about evaluating patients with chronic back disability, they have used the questionnaire shown in figure 2 to collect the patient's medical history information.

Therefore, in overall, knowledge of a patient's medical history could prove of a great value in the diagnosis process, since it could certainly provide the clinician with such information (e.g. previous admission to hospital, surgery, treatment, etc.) that would be used as indicators to where the subsequent test and measurements should be performed. Moreover, [17] further support the usefulness of a patient's history, by citing in their review study examples which illustrate that besides the classical clinical symptoms that need to be identified, history may also add valuable information to a comprehensive picture of the patient's pain situation and diagnosis.

Patient Clinical Information. The next step after establishing an initial understanding of the patient's medical history is to proceed with the collection of an individual's clinical information regarding his or her current condition. According to [27], such information concerns the basic understanding of the pain description, location(s), activation, severity, frequency, and symptoms. Thus, several tools that address pain *intensity (*how much a person hurts including severity and frequency*), pain affect*

Name _____ RLAH # _____ Rancho Los Amigos Hospital
                                                    Problem Back Treatment Center
Age _____   COUNTY OF LOS ANGELES DEPARTMENT OF HEALTH SERVICES

PATIENT HISTORY FORM

1. How long have you had the present pain? _____ weeks _____ months _____ years
2. How long have you had any trouble with your back, legs, or neck? _____
3. How long have you been off work or unable to do normal housework? _____
4. Did your pain begin: _____ gradually _____ suddenly _____ from an injury
                         _____ while lifting _____ while twisting _____ at work
5. My pain is: (check appropriate box)   Better   Worse   Unchanged
        a.   when I awake in the morning   □   □   □
        b.   bending forward to brush teeth   □   □   □
        c.   with cough or sneeze   □   □   □
        d.   sitting down at a table   □   □   □
        e.   sitting in an automobile   □   □   □
        f.   during the middle of the day   □   □   □
        g.   just before bed time   □   □   □
        h.   during the middle of the night   □   □   □
        i.   lying on my back   □   □   □
        j.   lying on my stomach   □   □   □
        k.   lying on my side with knees bent   □   □   □
6. What is the most aggravating thing about your pain? _____

7. How many times have you been in a hospital for back, leg, or neck problems? __
8. Have you had Myelograms? _____ yes _____ no # _____ EMG's? _____ yes _____ no # _____
9. Have you had previous back surgeries? _____ yes _____ no # _____ type? _____
                                    when? _____
10. Have you had other types of surgeries? _____ yes _____ no # _____ type? _____
                                    when? _____
11. Have any treatments ever made the pain better? _____ yes _____ no what treatments? _____
    _____
12. Have any treatments ever made the pain worse? _____ yes _____ no what treatments? _____

Fig. 2. A sample patient history questionnaire

(how much a person suffers including pain description), and pain-related interference with daily *living activities* (indicating pain activation and symptoms), as well as *pain location* exist. However, providing an exhaustive list and description of all available tools is beyond the scope of this work, therefore, only the tools that are relevant and have proven their validity, as identified in the literature, will be presented.

A) *Pain Intensity Assessment Tools*

Traditionally, three tools have been used to measure pain intensity, namely *Visual Analogue Scales (VAS)/ Graphic Rating Scale (GRS)*, *Verbal Rating Scales (VRS)*, and *Numerical Rating Scales (NRS)*.

a.   *Visual Analogues Scales (VAS)/ Graphic Rating Scales (GRS).* According to [25], the VAS (fig. 3) is one of the most common pain measurement tools, which has also been used in psychology as well. It typically consists of a 10-cm straight horizontal line with endpoints that define the limits such as "no pain" or "pain as bad as it could be".

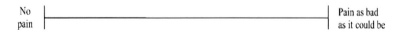

No pain ———————————————————————————————— Pain as bad as it could be

Fig. 3. A sample Visual Analog Scale

Moreover, if descriptive terms like 'mild', 'moderate', 'severe' or a numerical scale are added to the VAS, one speaks of a Graphic Rating Scale (GRS) [17]. Pain intensity thus, is determined by measuring the distance from the lower end of the scale to the mark made by the patient.

b. *Verbal Rating Scales (VRS)*. Similarly to VAS/GRS, Verbal Rating Scales also consist of two endpoints, and of a set of four-to-six adjectives that are used to describe different levels of pain (fig. 4), as explained by [17].

How much physical pain have you had during the past 4 weeks? (Please tick one box.)
- None
- Very mild
- Mild
- Moderate
- Severe
- Very severe

Fig. 4. A Verbal Rating Scale

A different form of VRS is the Behavioral Rating Scale where pain level is described by sentences indicating behavioral activities. Unlike VAS/GRS, Verbal Rating Scale is usually in the form of a questionnaire, rather than a straight horizontal line.

c. *Numerical Rating Scales (NRS)*. The last of the tools that are going to be described in this work is the NRS, where people are asked to rate their pain intensity from a scale of 0-10 or 0-100 [25]. Zero usually represents "no pain" whereas the upper limit represents "the worst pain possible". Fig. 5 shows an example of a NRS.

"If a zero (0) means 'no pain' and a ten (10) means 'pain as bad as it could be', on this scale of 0-10, what is your level of pain? Put an "X" through that number."[28]

0	1	2	3	4	5	6	7	8	9	10

Fig. 5. A Numerical Rating Scale

Although the pain assessment tools just described are all considered to be valid, there seems to be a lot of debate in literature as whether which are reliable for the purpose intended. Several studies have been conducted in order to prove their reliability similar to the one described in [30] review of pain measurement tools. In this study performed on patients with chronic pain, six different forms of the pain tools described (traditional VAS,101-point NRS, 11-point box scale, 6-point behavioral rating scale, 4-point VRS, and 5-point VRS) were compared based on the following criteria: ease of administration of scoring, rates of correct responding, sensitivity (as defined by the number of available response categories), and responsiveness to change, as well as in terms of the predictive relationship between each scale and a linear combination of pain intensity indices.

The tools produced similar results concerning their predictive validity and the proportion of patients not responding as instructed (e.g. leaving response blank, marking between two categories, marking two answers, etc.). Indeed, according to [25], several similar problems exist with the use of the aforementioned tools. Despite their apparent simplicity, approximately 7-11% of adults and up to 25% of the aged fails to complete it. Specifically, VAS methods are sometimes criticized that are being difficult to understand, with 7−16% higher failure rates being reported for VASs than for the VRSs and NRSs. The problem is found in individuals with physical or cognitive impairment and in the elderly. The VAS is also less reliable in illiterate patients [30].

When considering the remaining criteria (responsiveness to change, ease of administration, sensitivity) the 101-point NRS proved to be the most practical tool. In practice, patients prefer the NRS to the VAS since only 2% fail to complete it [25], and the feasibility of its use, as well as that it is easily possible to administer it e.g. verbally, have been proven [17]. However, in patients with a chronic disease such as osteoarthritis, "VAS and VRS responses were shown to be highly correlated ($r \approx 0.7$–0.8) and the tools produced similar effect sizes after treatment; thus, the VRS was easier to administer and interpret, and at the end the VRS emerged as the overall scale of choice in both younger and older cohorts" [30].

To this end, evidence from literature indicates that VRS, as well as NRS are the most reliable tools that patients also feel more comfortable using, however, they are not as appropriate to detect changes over time as are VAS and GRS [17]. Since pain is a disorder that in order to understand it you need to look at its development over time, VAS and/or GRS are the pain measurement tools that are going to be adopted in this work for the purpose intended.

B) *Pain Affect Assessment tools*

Accordingly, [17] also present in their review the available tools used to assess pain affect. Based on their study, the aforementioned tools (VRS, NRS, etc.) could also be used to assess affect, however, due to the fact that measuring pain affect is multidimensional in nature, that is intensity and affect are both considered in the assessment, the results show that these tools have also the same disadvantages as when measuring pain intensity alone. For that reason, more sophisticated tools have been developed for the purpose intended, specifically the *Pain-O-Meter*, and the *McGill Pain Questionnaire*.

- *Pain-O-Meter.* As described in their review, this tool "consists of a mechanical VAS and two lists of terms describing the pain affect. Each of these terms has an associated intensity value ranging from one to five. The respondents must decide, which of the 11 possible words best describe their pain. Then the associated intensity values are summed together to build the Pain-O-Meter-affective scale.

- *McGill Pain Questionnaire (MPQ)*. Similarly, they describe MPQ as a tool that consists of three main measures: pain-rating index, the number of words chosen to describe pain and the present pain intensity based on a 1-5 intensity scale. Specifically, the MPQ is administered by reading a word list to patients, and asking them to choose only those words that describe their pain at present. Pain scores are then calculated by summing the rank scores for each category [25].

In addition, several other aspects should also be taken into serious consideration when assessing a patient in pain, such as his/her pain history in order to identify how pain has developed in time and which has already been described, and *pain location*, something that can be measured by using a specific tool called *pain drawings*, and which we are going to describe in more detail in the following discussion. By doing so, the opportunity for a better understanding of pain and the factors influencing it will be granted, resulting in more effective assessment, and subsequently better treatment options.

C) Pain location

In addition to collecting pain intensity and affect related medical information, the patient is also asked to mark on a diagram, usually a two-dimensional representation of a human body, where the pain is *located*, and the *type* of pain that he or she is suffering from. This type of diagram is known in the literature as a "pain drawing" and it is shown in fig. 6.

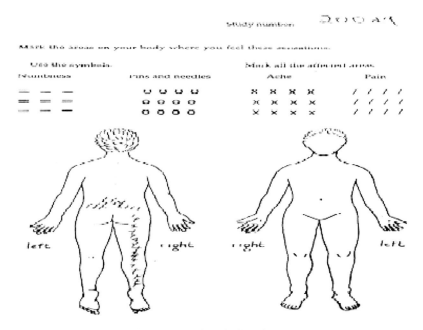

Fig. 6. A sample Pain Drawing

Specifically, pain drawing is a technique that has been used since the 1940s in the assessment of patients [34], and is considered to be a simple self-assessment method, originally proposed in back pain assessment by [43] as a visual aid tool to enable the recording of the spatial location and type of pain that a patient is suffering from.

One of the main advantages of this method is that it improves the communication between a clinician and the patient. Indeed, spoken description of pain by a patient to the clinician might not be sufficient due to educational, language, and experience differences that might occur amongst them [33]. By using pain drawings though, this two-way communication is improved by providing a common framework based on which the patient describes the pain by marking it on the pain diagram, and the clinician interprets it by examining it, enabling them in that way to overcome the afore-mentioned differences. This topographical representation of pain therefore, is very useful in summarizing patients' description of the location and type of pain, in an interpretable way for the clinician, and makes it possible to determine whether pain is of organic or non-organic nature [49].

In addition to improving communication, many more benefits of pain drawings have been described in the literature. [34] cites in her work results of studies that demonstrate consistency of patients in completing drawings, even with elderly subjects, whereas [19] highlight their importance in corresponding to imaging tests, as well as in being able to help clinicians to categorize patients into diagnostic groups (e.g. osteoporosis, tumor) based on their pain drawings. Moreover, in overall, pain drawings are considered to be economic and simple to complete, and can also be used to monitor change in a patient's pain situation as cited by [47].

As a result, based on their ability to help identify patient diagnostic groups, pain drawings have been used in various ways, including diagnosis of lumbar disc disease, evaluation of changes in pain, as well as prediction of treatment outcome [34]. To this end, because of the several uses of drawings, the need for different methods of interpreting them has also been identified. However, no standard method for *filling them out* and *scoring* them currently exists. According to some protocols, patients might be asked to mark or shade those body areas where they feel pain [17]. Slight variations of this technique also exist where the patient instead of marking or shading the pain within the outline of a blank human diagram, he or she might be asked to respond to a pre-shaded drawing, a technique that has as an advantage the controlling of the definition of the body area pre-shaded, something that should be easy for the patient to recognize and should be where most of the symptoms tend to occur [24]. Nevertheless, traditionally, according to [45], in earliest uses of pain drawings the patient would fill them out by marking the location of the pain on a blank diagram using a symbol without mentioning any sensation (pain, burning, etc.) description, as it was the clinician's responsibility to identify it through the pain discussion. More recently though, the patient is asked to also indicate their pain sensation on the drawing, with the most common way of doing it being the use of a specific symbol indicating various sensation types, as shown in fig. 6.

Similarly, there is no gold standard regarding pain sensation types that could be used to describe pain on the drawing. [47] cite in their study that there is a range of *sensation types* which have been used in literature, including [7] use of *pins and needles, burning, stabbing,* and *deep ache* in their pain drawings, and [51] use of *dull, burning, numb, stabbing or cutting, tingling or pins and needles,* and *cramping* in their drawings. Accordingly, [34] uses *aching, numbness, pins and needles, burning,*

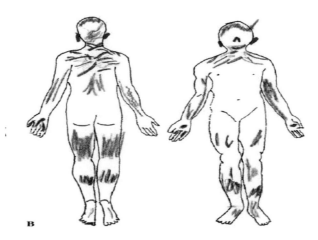

Fig. 7. A sample Pain Drawing illustrating the use of color as a representation of pain

and *stabbing,* whereas [32] further explored the use of color as a representation for the different sensation types being experienced (fig. 7). The results from this study showed that the ability of color pain drawings to express the pain experienced remained the same as with previous monochrome approaches.

On the other hand though, the usefulness of sensation in diagnosing back pain has been questioned by many studies, which conclude that pain sensation seems less reliable, most likely because it is subjective; however it was also suggested that it could assist in differentiating certain conditions [45].

Pain drawing scoring techniques

In order for the several pain drawings to be interpreted and further associated with causes of back pain and treatment suggestions, they first need to be assessed by the clinician. A very common method of assessing a drawing according to [44], is "at a glance", where the clinician usually looks to see if the pain marks or shades follow dermatome patterns. They further describe dermatomes as "a 'segmental field' of the skin that is innervated by a spinal nerve", and which could be used to determine the level of injuries that might have occurred in the spinal cord, something that makes them an accurate tool in localizing the source of certain pain types (fig. 8).

In addition to assessing a drawing at "a glance", several more manual scoring techniques have been devised that would allow for further interpretation of the pain descriptions, and which are specifically useful for studies or clinicians who would like to quantify drawings for further analysis. Generally, these techniques as described in literature broadly fall into one of four categories, namely *Penalty Point System, Visual Inspection Methods, Body Region Methods,* and *Grid Methods.* It has to be noted here that the first two methods require subjective interpretation, whilst the last two record the presence or absence of pain within defined regions [34].

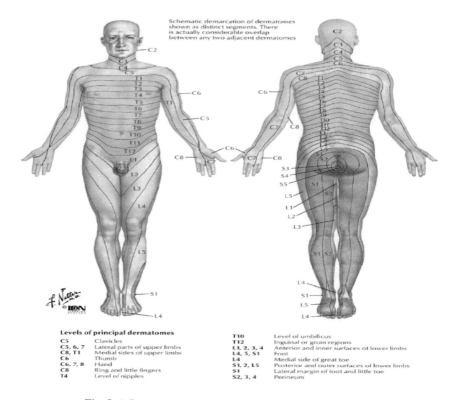

Fig. 8. A Dermatomes map used by clinicians to classify pain

• *Penalty Point Methods.* Using this method, pain drawings are scored using the penalty point system described by [43], where points are assigned for any not natural marking of pain on the diagram, which could be marking indicating pain outside the body, using extra words or symbols to describe pain or its severity, as well as pain in specific unusual body areas. The drawings then are classified as "normal" if 2 or fewer points are assigned, or as "abnormal" if the points are more than 2 [34]. Moreover, as cited in [48], by using such a penalty-point scoring method, it was found that pain drawings could also predict 93% of the patients that needed further psychological evaluation just by looking at their completed pain drawing, therefore in that case pain drawings could also be used as an economical psychological tool, besides their normal pain location recording use.

• *Visual Inspection Methods.* As cited in [48], pain drawings are usually evaluated with these methods by experienced evaluators, who are able by looking at the drawing to say what is the situation with the patient, and if further psychological testing is needed. To this end, [51] initially used these methods in their study to identify patients suffering from lumbar disc herniation. The results of their study showed that pain drawings could be classified as either *indicative* or *non-indicative* of symptomatic disc disease, depending on whether the pain was mainly in a radicular pattern from the back into one or both lower extremities (indicative), or whether it was restricted to low back only, by also been indicated by unusual marks outside the body region to describe pain (non-indicative).

- *Body Regions Method.* In this case, pain drawings are scored using a transparency of the human body divided into regions, which is laid over a drawing (fig.9) and the presence or absence of pain within a region is recorded, as described by [31].

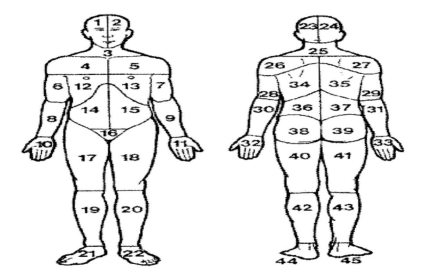

Fig. 9. The Body Regions method

However, a possible bias with this scoring system, as described by [34], is that this method includes 45 body regions, many of which probably could not be used in relation to back pain disease, therefore only regions associated with the back and other lower extremities should be used, such as regions 17 to 22 and regions 36 to 45. To this end, in another study carried out by [35], having in mind the bias possibility they limited down the division of the body into five general regions, namely low buck and buttocks, posterior thigh, posterior leg, anterior thigh, and anterior leg.

- *Grid Method.* Similarly to body regions methods, as cited in [34], first [13] described this technique by making a transparency of a grid (fig. 10) which is laid over a pain drawing. The drawing was then scored by counting the number of squares the patient indicated pain, however, in this case too, only the low back and lower extremities were included in order to again avoid bias with this scoring technique.

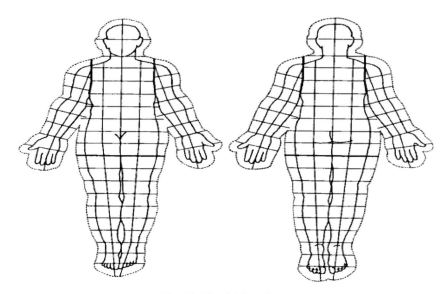

Fig. 10. The Grid method

Having said that, several studies exist in literature regarding the usefulness of the grid method in identifying various back pain patterns. [49] cite in their work results of [6] study that demonstrate the ability of grid method to differentiate of localized, mechanical and radicular or referred patterns of pain. On the other hand though, [46] found that when used grid assessment before operation in patients with spinal stenosis, the results showed a negative correlation between the outcomes of operation with the area of the body covered with symbols.

Moreover, in reality most of the pain drawing methods described can be and are used in conjunction with *sensation types,* which as has been described before, they allow for both the location of pain, as well as the type of pain to be recorded on the drawing. This is usually achieved by assigning a symbol or a color to each sensation type (e.g. yellow for pins and needles), and then mapping it on the pain drawing.

Finally, so far most of the pain drawings scoring methods were performed manually by a clinician based on his or her experience. However, various studies have taken a different approach and adopted the use of automated computer scoring by, mainly, artificial intelligence methods. To this end, [44] used artificial neural networks to assess pain drawings, whereas [18] used a computerized decision model to score them in order to identify real or imagined pain. In overall, as cited by [44] after comparing the results of the automated computer techniques to the results of experienced clinicians, generally they found that these techniques were able to classify pain drawings almost as well as physician experts.

However, based on the pain drawings discussion so far, the consensus of the literature seems to indicate that they are considered to be a valuable and useful tool in identifying pain location and sensation type, as well as identifying psychological disturbances, in both cases always when combined with the appropriate additional tools (pain assessment tools and psychological screening questionnaires). Nevertheless, the various studies that have been performed on the reliability of pain drawings have also identified that they have one major disadvantage that is worth mentioning.

Pain Drawings-Conclusions

To this end, the biggest disadvantage of pain drawings, concerns their ability when it comes to visualizing a patient's pain descriptions, which is considered to be their main purpose. Over the years there have moreover been a number of research studies to continue and extend research in respect to pain drawings. All of the studies [16], [27], [32], [37] had slight variations but were conceptually the same, using the same 2-dimensional approach. Notwithstanding their advantages, 2-D pain drawings have their limitations, as they do not capture the 3-D nature of the human body. Thus, patients are unable to visually express the pain that they are experiencing, as statements of the form "*I have a pain on the inside of my thigh*" are not easily captured in a 2-D pain drawing, constituting a limited dimension representation of the medical information, potentially resulting in a time-consuming process with possible irrelevant medical data collected that can lead to a report that obscures important information.

In back pain terms, in an experimental study performed by [12], 3D virtual images were constructed from performing computerized medical scans, in their attempt to reconstruct spinal cord injuries, with the results indicating that in this case 3D images were extremely beneficial as the models could be observed from many different viewpoints. Moreover, while recent inventions of medical imaging techniques such as computerized tomography and magnetic resonance imaging have revolutionized radiology, the development of 3-D imaging has not yet been ported across the world of pain drawings. To this end, the same feature benefit just described could be anticipated from devising a 3-D adaptation of pain drawings.

Subjective Phase-Conclusions. Finally, based on the discussion so far we can conclude that the pain tools mentioned are the standard techniques for assessing back pain, and have been proven through studies to be of a great value and use in the process. However, the consensus of the literature indicates that these pain tools are usually stored in a paper format something that makes the recording, assessment, and evaluation of the data that is stored upon it, such as areas of pain, an impractical and sometimes an arduous subject to error task. [18] argue in their study that despite the ease of administration and use of such paper-based assessment techniques, practically, they have several drawbacks. First of all, use of such tools can lead to "noncompliance, missing data, and fabrication of information if the respondents have not completed the requested information at the designated times". Moreover, the process of transferring the information from paper forms to the computer for analysis and evaluation is also a potential source of error.

Last, the paper-based solution of existing methods makes it impractical to record pain variations over time, in spite of the time-dependent nature of pain in chronic sufferers [47].

To compound the issue, the need for digitized computer applications emerged that would be able to describe the painful areas more accurately, compared with the paper-based tools, and would allow easier storing and recreating capabilities that could show changes over time using different shades, marks, and colors to identify different pain types [19]. Similarly to paper-based tools, computer-based tools have both many strengths and weaknesses. However, compared to paper-based techniques, they were found to be extremely useful in capturing time-stamped data [20], specifically necessary for recording pain variations over time. In addition, numerous advantages have been described in literature, such as their portability, ease of data sharing, instant access [20], as well as direct transfer of information, and their ability of a dynamic graphical display to visualize data [41].

Based on the above, it could be suggested that computer-based tools could easily be used for recording patient medical information. Indeed, several studies in literature indicate that electronic tools could be very practical in recording back pain information. As cited in [18], [14] digitally linked pain drawings as part of the assessment process with very positive results.

Thus, in overall, previous sections have highlighted that back pain information is mainly gathered through the use of interactive interviews by highly skilled medical personnel, supported by various *paper-based* questionnaires and tools. Yet, the 2-D representation of pain drawings constitute a limited dimension representation of the medical information, potentially resulting in a time-consuming process with possible irrelevant medical data collected that can lead to a report that obscures important information. Therefore, it seems natural to implement digitized, computer-based 3-D pain drawings, since such an approach provides an attractive opportunity for enhancing interaction between the practitioner and the patient in amore perceivable way to the natural environment.

2.3   Objective Phase

In addition to subjective testing, in order to accomplish a complete evaluation of a patient suffering from back pain, objective testing should also be used where *physical examinations* are performed to confirm or refine the preliminary diagnosis derived from the previous phase. This testing phase usually proceeds in an iterative way and may require additional subjective tests, especially when the preliminary diagnosis was not supported by the examination results [27].

Although the physical examination is not as important as the subjective phase process, as cited by [29], many authors in the literature demonstrated that impairments of trunk strength, flexibility, and endurance have been observed in many patients suffering from back pain, which result in neurological and physiological spine changes. To this end, several physical examination tests that address the aforementioned aspects should be considered, however, because presenting a thorough description of these tests is outside the scope of this work, in the following discussion only an overview of the available physical examination tests will be given.

Having said that, according to [39] and [42], a thorough musculoskeletal and neurologic examination should be the starting point of the physical examination. Specifically, it should initiate with the observation of the patient's physiologic functionalities in order to determine any abnormalities in several physiological and neurological aspects including *"algometry, gait, muscles strength, muscle tension, posture, or ROM, specifically in the trunk, thighs, and legs"*. For those aspects to be measured, several tests could be used, and which are cited in [4] and [29], as follows:

1. *Physiological tests*

> *-Cervical ROM (Range Of Motion).* With this test the clinician measures the patient's active, extension, ventral/lateral flexion and rotation of the torso.

> *-Shoulder tests.* Similarly, the shoulder muscles' strength and tension are measured by the clinician asking the patient to exert force bilaterally while having hands on the patient's arms, in one of specific eight directions at the time: lower arm up/down, external/internal rotation, upper-arm abduction, flexion, extension, and adduction.

> *-Tenderness.* Using this test the clinician measures tenderness by exerting mild to moderate pressure on 20 different areas, including spine, joints, torso, arms, and shoulders.

> *-Hypotrophy.* Additionally, hypotrophy is assessed in 8 areas including chin, neck, neck-shoulder, shoulder, upper-arms, lower-arms, hands, and chest.

As part of the physical examination, the clinician should also perform a thorough neurologic examination to assess muscle reflexes, sensation, strength, and stretch, enabling him or her in that way to determine whether a dermatomal or myotomal pattern is present. Assessing a patient based on neurological tests as well, is useful in managing pain by helping identify factors other than anatomic that could affect the condition [39]. Thus, [4] similarly to physiological tests highlighted above, they cite in their work the following neurological examination:

2. *Neurological tests*

> - *Sensibility to pain.* Pain sensation is measured from this test, in 10 indicator areas for dermatomes by pressure exerted on these areas using two pin-wheels.

> - *Strength.* Muscle strength is tested in 7 movements by asking a patient to resist force from the clinician's hand in the following movements (representing myotomes): head flexion/lateral flexion, shoulder elevation, arm abduction, elbow flexion/extension, and little finger hook.

> - *Reflexes.* Similarly, reflexes are tested in the following 5 muscle groups: suprapinatus, biceps, brachioradialis, triceps, and the Babinski reflex.

> - *Nerve stretch.* Testing of the nerve stretching is also performed for the median, radial, and ulnar nerves.

> *-Neck compression/traction.* The neck is accordingly tested for compression and traction by again the clinician having the hands on top of the patient's head and exerting increased pressure.

> *-Straight leg-raising test.* Finally, using this test the clinician evaluates the lower back and thigh muscle activation.

By completing the two initial phases of the examination (subjective and objective testing), the clinician should then be able to either confirm or refine his or her preliminary diagnosis. If the preliminary diagnosis is refined, then subjective testing should again be used in order to reach to new more accurate results. If the preliminary diagnosis is confirmed, then the clinician advances to the next phase, which is the *assessment*.

2.4 Assessment Phase

Having reached to a preliminary diagnosis, this phase involves the evaluation of the findings derived from the subjective and objective phases, especially concerning pain epidemiology, and severity of pain [27]. At this point, the clinician can also determine whether further imaging testing is needed to assist in the evaluation, or rule out clinical suspicions that he/she might have, since as it has already been mentioned, due to limitations of pain drawings and pain measurement tools, the results that would derive from the subjective and objective phases might as well be vague.

Imaging Techniques. There are various imaging techniques that could assist in the diagnosis and assessment process, but they normally vary in purpose that they could be used. So, [11] in his review outlines the following most common imaging tests:

X-rays. This diagnostic test is considered to be fast, economical and convenient; however its use in the diagnosis and assessment of back pain does not yield any important findings. Nevertheless, for specific cases it is a valuable tool to use [38].

Computerized Tomography (CT) Scanning. CT scan is one of the most valuable tools for assessment of back pain. It is also said to be really efficient in providing valuable information regarding the bony architecture [39], and combined with plain X-rays, it could be sufficient to provide enough data for back pain diagnosis and proposed treatment [38].

Magnetic Resonance Imaging (MRI). MRI scanning has almost become the gold standard in the assessment of patients suffering from back pain. Its advantage over CT scanning is its ability to provide clear high-definition images of the soft tissues that the bony architecture consists of, and the low radiation emission. However, drawbacks of this technique also exist, including its cost and complexity of use [38], [11]. In overall, it is argued that CT and MRI scans are generally only helpful in evaluation of patients for whom surgical procedure has been considered [55].

Discography. Discography is considered to be an invasive technique with notable risks in the assessment of back pain, as it normally involves the injection of contrast material in the disc area, something that usually cause low back pain [11]. Consecutively, there has been a lot of controversy in literature about its use in the assessment process, with most of the current literature supporting the use of discography in specific situations, as cited in [38]. Similarly to MRI, discography should be considered to patients undergoing a surgical procedure.

Ultrasound imaging. According to [11], ultrasound imaging is a flexible technique used to assess the pathogenic disc. In studies that have been conducted, it was found to be able to detect changes in the pathogenic area; however it was not considered reliable due to its low specificity. It could, nevertheless, be used as a cost-effective method prior to CT/MRI scan or discography.

Nuclear scans. Finally, the least commonly used technique is the nuclear scanning, which includes single-photon emission CT to produce three dimensional spatial images, valuable for the exclusion of tumor, fracture, and infection. Although it can be helpful in select cases, in overall it was found not adequate to assess back pain [11].

Besides the imaging techniques just described, others also exist, but since the intention of this work is not to provide a thorough description of them, only the most commonly used have been mentioned. In addition, although they are a valuable tool in the assessment of back pain, currently available imaging techniques also have several limitations, so they usually provide only partial conclusions in the process. This is the main reason that imaging tests are recommended only as a supplementary method that should be used in conjunction with other assessment techniques [11]. Moreover, [52] in their study argue that it is a fact that imaging testing is frequently used in the assessment of back pain despite recommendations and guidelines on limitation of its usage. Excessive usage naturally causes increased healthcare costs, in addition to the theoretical health risk that implies due to the high emission of radiation.

Finally, based on the overall findings from the assessment process, the clinician then categorizes patients in one of three groups, according to the Agency for Health Care Policy and Research guidelines (AHCPR): 1) *patients with a potentially serious underlying problem,* 2) *patients with possible neurological involvement,* and 3) *patients with nonspecific back pain* [55]. Such categorization of patients into the aforementioned groups is considered to be of high importance for the assessment process, as eventually, when the potential group has been identified, and if necessary, imaging tests have been performed, plausible therapeutic protocols that could be used for treatment planning are determined and finally selected/designed in the following last phase, always in accordance to the assessment phase findings [27].

2.5 Planning Phase

The final phase of the patient management process involves the design or selection of an appropriate therapeutic protocol, which the clinician administers to the patient by continually monitoring and assessing the response to the treatment plan and then revises the diagnosis and/or treatment plan accordingly, if necessary, until the process terminates with satisfactory patient recovery [27].The treatment plan is designed or selected based on the information built up during the previous phases.

However, it should be noted that there is no sure treatment of back pain disorders. Therefore, the main aim of the treatment plan should be the right pain management by trying to a) *relieve pain,* b) *to return normal muscle function,* and c) *to eliminate factors that could advance pain into a chronic disorder* [42]. This could be achieved using a multidimensional approach to pain management, meaning that sometimes the use of treatment options from various complementary disciplines might be required. To this end, when developing a treatment plan, a clinician normally considers any appropriate treatment option available, which could be characterized as of either a *conventional* or *alternative* nature.

Conventional Treatment. Conventional management of back pain is considered the standard of care [39]. The basic elements of conventional treatment, according to [5], are the following:

Nonsteroidal Anti-inflammatory Drugs (NSAID). Such anti-inflammatory drugs are usually used in order to reduce the inflammatory reaction as well as the pain level of the patient [22]. One systematic review of 51 randomized controlled trials comparing NSAIDs with placebo showed that NSAIDs significantly improve pain control, so they are recommended for the treatment of back pain, as cited in [21].

Muscle relaxants. It is maybe the most common drug therapy and involves the use of muscle relaxants mainly for pain relief purposes. Similarly to NSAIDs, evidence from studies and trials showed that they are helpful in the treatment of back pain, especially when combined with NSAIDs. However, there might be side effects depending on each person using them, something that might limit the usefulness of these drugs, so they should be used with caution, as cited in [21].

Local injections. There is a wide variety of injections that could be used for both diagnostic and therapeutic purposes, and are considered an alternative to the oral methods of NSAIDs and muscle relaxants [22]. One of the most common injections used is the Trigger Point (TP) injection, which is considered to be one of the most effective methods by most clinicians, as described by [42], since it is directly inserted until it reaches the pain trigger point resulting in immediate pain relief.

Controlled physical activity. This treatment plan refers to a short period of bed rest, progressive mobilization, and exercise as the patient's pain improves [5]. However, using bed rest as treatment is found to be controversial [39], thus, suggestions from literature indicate that a patient should not stay in bed for longer than two days [21], [5], [39]. As far as patient exercise is concerned, although it is usually suggested as a treatment option, a meta-analysis of 10 trials of structured exercise therapy compared with no exercise showed that there was no improvement in pain using back exercises, so they are not considered helpful.

Physical modalities. The main physical modalities used are cryotherapy or thermotherapy, meaning applying ice or heat on the pain point. Probably the most commonly used is the application of ice, however, there is minimal evidence regarding the use of ice as a treatment option, whereas the application of heat was found to be helpful in reducing pain and increasing function, as cited in [21].

Alternative Treatment. In addition, patients many times turn to alternative options that could be used either in parallel to conventional therapy, or alone in order to cope with pain that was not previously relieved using conventional treatment. These options are usually one, or more of the following:

Acupuncture/acupressure. This method is considered to be one of the oldest forms of local injection therapy, and it is usually used by physicians or chiropracticioners. Treatment-wise, there is limited evidence regarding the use of acupuncture in back pain, however in overall, higher-quality trials provide evidence that it is not beneficial, as cited in [21].

Transcutaneous Electrical Nerve Stimulation (TENS). Accordingly, TENS is a quite popular physical modality method amongst patients and physicians alike, however, as with previous modalities evidence of its effectiveness is sparse [22]. It is worth mentioning at this point that Acupuncture/acupressure and TENS are both part of the injection therapy and physical modalities methods respectively, however, they are not considered conventional therapy methods. The reason behind that is a set of recommendations for back pain therapy that the AHCPR arrived at, and which it specifically emphasizes that the use of Acupuncture/acupressure and TENS are not included [5].

Massage. Massage therapy is considered safe and it is quite popular amongst patients, since it can release tension in the muscles resulting in some pain relief. Two systematic reviews though, found insufficient evidence to make a reliable recommendation regarding massage for back pain treatment [21].

Surgery. Although surgery cases are considered to be very common and are many times used for back pain treatment, in reality are not recommended by clinicians and should only be used when it is absolutely necessary.

Patient education. Finally, patient education focusing on "activity, aggravating factors, the natural history of the disease, its relatively benign etiology, and expected time course for improvement" is also considered to be of great importance in speeding patient recovery and educating for chronic pain prevention.

Moreover, since this is not a thorough review of the back pain treatment methods that exist, it is highly possible that more treatment options are available and are used for back pain treatment, however, for the purpose of this work only those that are considered to be the most common for therapy have been presented.

2.6 Need for a Mobile Solution

Bearing in mind the discussion so far, because of the complexity and sensitivity of back pain problems, every sufferer needs individual treatment options. However, unavoidable situations such as queues at hospitals or practitioners' individual places of treatment, which are prioritized based on the level of emergency or sickness, cause type 2 patients (abdominal pain, chronic back pain, etc.), who are not considered as urgent cases, to have to wait excessively long, in order for their health-related information to be collected and/or distributed. Moreover, assuming that individual treatment and prescription has been given, it is natural that the patients want to be informed regularly of their health situations, and the doctors on their part to be able to monitor their patients' medical situation, therefore, to have both easy and relatively fast access to such health information.

Sadly enough, conditions such as the hospital queues mentioned before, among others of course (since this is only a very simple example to demonstrate the situation), do not allow an effective and efficient use of health information that would provide both parts with the necessary means for disorder, specifically, back pain disorder in our case, diagnosis, and treatment. The rapid acquisition and distribution of such information is definitely a priority, but most of the times, the professionals responsible for such activities often operate under tight time constraints. Therefore, health-related information collection and allocation in an effective and systematic way must be balanced with the fact that they need to attend to all patients as promptly as possible [54].

Because of the enormous impact of the aforementioned conditions, there have been efforts [16], [26], [47] to guide the patient's diagnosis, treatment, and monitoring outside clinics in a way that health-related issues can be efficiently manipulated and used in a timely manner, since time and space constitute barriers between health care providers and their patients, and indeed, among health care providers themselves. One of these directions has been to empower the patient to become a stakeholder in the management of pain. Moreover, bearing in mind the need for an anywhere, anytime connection for medical information access, a more flexible and mobile telemedicine system could be developed that would be able to overcome the current health-related information limitations discussed so far. This is precisely what we address in this work, and describe our experiences with the design of a PDA-based solution for mobile data collection of 3-D pain data.

2.7 Summary

To date, there is no standard procedure for collecting and assessing back pain related medical information. Currently, the healthcare industry is investing a lot of money and resources in identifying ways for the prevention and monitoring of chronic diseases, one of which is back pain. However, by reviewing the current literature, we have seen that the existing back pain assessment methods cannot be considered adequate in providing the best quality treatment for back pain patients. Current statistics regarding the numbers of back pain sufferers, as well as the expenses in terms of money and resources, demonstrate that such methods do not provide an effective solution to this worldwide chronic phenomenon, as they do not overcome the limitations identified regarding their ability to effectively visualize pain and store it for further analysis, in the case of pain drawings. To this end, the implementation and experiences of a wireless-enabled monitoring system for back-pain patients will be presented in this work that will improve the relative paucity of the existing tools and techniques in ways that the total quality of treatment will be considered more effective than the to date practices.

3   Prototype Design and Implementation

In this chapter, the work will be focused on the design aspects of the application, which will be presented by proposing and demonstrating a system structure and architecture. This proposed model will then be the fundamental basis for the applications' implementation. Thus, this work will be now taken a step further by initially identifying the users and their requirements that will help us complement the knowledge acquired during the thorough review of the various tools and methods available in the back pain field performed in the previous section. Our work will continue then by coming up with the proposed system structure and architecture, and a high level description of its functionality.

3.1 User Requirements

The design of the prototype was conducted in collaboration with a team of clinicians from the Rheumatology Department of the Northwick Park Hospital, London, who would potentially use the system, and the purpose was twofold: first interviews with these stakeholders were held to identify aspects of the application such as usability, flexibility, and privacy, and second to come up with deficiencies of the existing back pain assessment approach, and identify areas of opportunity for the 3-D tool to possibly exploit.

Similarly, the same interviews were also carried out on people suffering from back pain conditions, all volunteers from the Rheumatology Clinic of Northwick Park Hospital, London, and from the U.K. National Forum of Wheelchair User Groups. Again, the aim of this study was to identify aspects regarding the usability, flexibility, and privacy of the proposed prototype, this time, however, from a patient's point of view. In brief, the identified requirements were to:

1. provide a 3D model of the human body;
2. provide fully navigational controls enabling the ability to Zoom, Rotate, Drag for depth perception;
3. allow individually selectable regions of the body to demonstrate the location of pain;
4. use color to represent different types of pain;
5. allow the details to be saved for later analysis by physician and for record keeping on a patient's file
6. provide the patient with the ability to input back pain data ubiquitously and upload it to a central server
7. provide a handheld solution for data collection, since many back pain patients for example, due to associated disabilities, are confined to wheelchair or beds, and would not have easy access to desktop systems
8. include personal medical information collection capabilities in the form of a questionnaire allowing also for pain intensity and factors to be shown
9. create an easy to use and navigate graphical environment

3.2 Prototype Proposed Architecture

With the user requirements derived, the following approach was identified as the most suitable solution. Our proposed prototype will combine a 3D representation of a pain drawing with the possibility for the user to directly navigate and select the type and location of pain in the 3D representation. In addition, it will provide the capability to the user to also support the drawing with specific back pain related medical data collection (personal profile, pain factors, pain intensity, etc) in a questionnaire format. The collected information will then be saved to a backend database for further analysis and preview.

For all these, our system will provide a user-friendly GUI that will support this behavior by allowing the user to touch and select the information and object of interest using a finger or a pointing device such as the PDA stylus, which is a wireless device chosen to fulfill our goal of overcoming time, space, and further constraints. Finally, all the information recorded will be accessible by a clinician regardless his/her location, as they will be securely uploaded and be available from a server.

3.3 Prototype Building Components

From the above proposed architecture we can safely derive an initial system structure that consists of 3 main building components: The *User (patient), the Hospital*

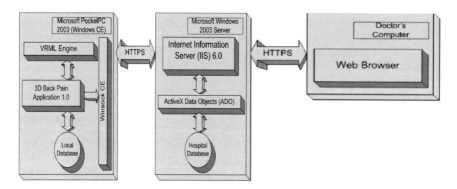

Fig. 11. Prototype system architecture and building components

Web/Database Server, and the *Clinician* components. Fig. 11, as taken from [47] and expanded to meet our needs, shows the system building components mentioned.

User Component. This is considered to be the most important component of the prototype proposed, and it could be reasonably characterized as the heart and backbone of our prototype, as this is where the main PDA 3D application responsible for the recording and transmitting of back pain information resides.

Consequently, the developed 3-D back pain application was designed and implemented by combining the efficiency of Microsoft embedded Visual Basic, a language specifically geared to help developers build applications for the next generation of communication-and-information access devices running Windows for Mobile Devices, and the functionality of the Cortona SDK, a development component that enables Virtual Reality Modeling Language (VRML) browsing.

To this end, this module will allow the user to interact with our proposed application by enabling any patient to collect medical information through a specifically designed for the purpose intended questionnaire, regarding his/her medical profile, pain type, location of pain on the body, and pain intensity. Specifically, pain intensity is inputted for a particular region of the body via a visual analog scale (implemented in our prototype via a scroll bar), as we can see in fig. 12.

Similarly, using the VRML component, our application displays a 3-D human mannequin (fig. 13) whose surface was segmented into clinically appropriate regions after consultations with the medical staff involved in this work. Based on these consultations, we have also color coded four different types of pain (*numbness, pain, pins and needles,* and *ache*) to be used for pain pinpointing, as previous studies [37], [40] indicated that it was an efficient way of communicating pain.

The user has zoom-in and zoom-out buttons for manipulating the mannequin, whereas rotations are implemented through user stylus input. In order to input the type of pain that s/he is currently experiencing, the user employs the stylus to first select the pain type, after which s/he manipulates the mannequin to the desired level of detail, and with the help of the touch-sensitive screen, indicates the particular region of the body that is affected (fig. 14 and fig. 15).

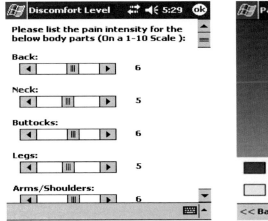

Fig. 12. Pain intensity measured by the use of Visual Analog Scales

Fig. 13. Our proposed 3D Pain Drawing

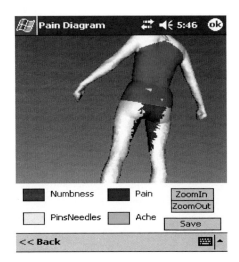

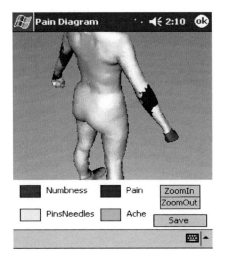

Fig. 14. Pain regions selected on the 3D Pain Drawing (1)

Fig. 15. Pain regions selected on the 3D Pain Drawing (2)

This is then recorded to a *local Microsoft Pocket Access database* file. It is notable to mention that even though data input is mainly done on the 3-D mannequin, the data that are saved are not pictorial, but numerical (location of pain—each body region had a unique identifier, type of pain, intensity of pain, and time of day). As such, database sizes could be kept relatively small and can be uploaded using standard dialup connection speeds (under 45 s using a 56-kb/s modem to transfer a typical day's worth of collected data).

Data can finally be *uploaded* (fig. 16) either through the standard synchronization tools via the PDA cradle, or when the user is within wireless Internet coverage. In

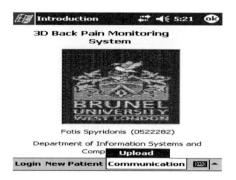

Fig. 16. Medical data collected can then be uploaded to the Hospital Server

both cases, the application uses Winsock CE 3.0 (Windows CE Sockets) to send its database content to a central hospital database server (fig. 12).

In overall, the 3D Back Pain Application was implemented on an HP iPAQ 5450 PDA with 16-bit touch-sensitive transflective thin film translator (TFT) liquid crystal display (LCD) that supports 65,536 colors. The display pixel pitch of the device is 0.24 mm and its viewable image size is 2.26 inch wide and 3.02 inch tall. It runs Microsoft Windows for Pocket PC 2003 (Windows CE) operating system on an Intel 400 Mhz XSCALE processor and contains 64MB standard memory as well as 48MB internal flash ROM. The reason a Microsoft Windows based PDA was chosen is because it is a more popular platform than its main competitors Palm OS and Symbian.

Hospital Database Server Component. With the back pain recording finished, the data will then be sent after the patient's demand to the hospital's database server (fig. 12) which acts as the intermediate between the clinician and the patient. So, the data will remain on this server until further requested by either party.

Due to the sensitivity of the data sent from the patient's handheld device, all the information is sent through WiFi Protected Access–Pre-Shared Key (WPA-PSK) encrypted radio broadcast at wireless level. At software level, the information privacy is maintained by the use of 128-b Secure HyperText Transfer Protocol (HTTPS). In addition to all of the above, to prevent identity theft, rotating-password approach is utilized, which requests five random characters of predefined 16-letter password, and creates a unique keyword combination for every transfer.

To this end, the Web server was implemented on an Intel Pentium IV running at 3.4 GHz, with 1-GB RAM and a 250-GB hard disk. The operating system was Windows 2003 Server and Internet Information Server (IIS) 6.0 with an Open Database Connectivity (ODBC) service. Finally, throughout our trials, a Netgear DG834PN 108-Mb/s RangeMax ADSL Modem Wireless Router was used.

Clinician Component. The final component of our proposed system architecture is the clinician's application. With the data uploaded to the hospital server, the clinician can now access the database uploaded and retrieve and analyze the medical data stored for back pain assessment and diagnosis. Although the clinician component is not the main focus of this work, it could be mentioned that two applications to retrieve the data from the hospital server have been developed. The first one is a standalone application that could run on any Windows operating system, offering the clinician the ease to retrieve the medical information uploaded by the patient regarding pain location, intensity, etc. and further analyze it. Similarly, the second application has been developed as a web application with the exact capabilities as the standalone version, and which the clinician could access from any location that Internet access is offered.

3.4 Summary

Concluding this very important part of this work, so far we have discussed the proposed architecture of the system to be developed, as well as we have seen the implemented solution in the form of screenshots that demonstrate the functionalities identified in the user requirements collected by the clinicians and the patients alike. In the following section, we will proceed to the prototype's evaluation, where all these functionalities will be evaluated against a number of patients and clinicians.

4 Prototype Evaluation

In this section the prototypes will be evaluated against their potential users i.e. patients and clinicians alike, in order to help us achieve our goal of examining the system's functionality, and obtaining information on its usefulness, in order to better understand the potential and problems in its use. The purpose of this initial evaluation of the prototype was twofold: first, to gain feedback from the clinicians involved in developing the requirements, and second, to gain an understanding of how usable the interface was by potential patients.

4.1 Clinical Evaluation

Four clinicians were asked to review the prototype. One was a back-pain specialist from a London hospital; another was a palliative care specialist from a different London hospital, with the prototype also being evaluated by two physiotherapists. This review was to ascertain whether this approach to pain visualization could be used in practice, by professionals with considerable experience in the use of existing 2-D pain drawings. In general, all clinicians surveyed approved of the visual appearance of the system, and suggested that the prototype would be usable in a clinical environment. They provided a number of interesting observations on limitations and improvements that could be made.

The back pain specialist noted that the 3-D interface covered almost all aspects of existing pain drawings. He was impressed by the level of detail and navigation control. However, he did note that users with disabilities might find it difficult to interact with the PDA. While he was "excited" by the possibility of patients collecting their own data, especially at set times of the day (and thus, being able to remotely monitor the progression and type of pain, vis-a-vis the prescribed medication/treatment), he did highlight that 1) users should be given appropriate training and 2) appropriate personnel and facilities should be made available to interpret this wealth of data, otherwise it would ultimately be a futile exercise.

These concerns were also echoed by the palliative-care clinician, who was, however, impressed by the opportunity that the application gave patients to become stakeholders in managing their pain. Moreover, he was also of the opinion that even though the tool did not provide a diagnosis as such, it could have important and benefic psychological effects on patients eager to record their pain diaries.

Both physiotherapists interviewed had no concerns with the usability of the prototype, but did suggest that 1) the feet should point downward rather than be in a standing position to allow for ease of marking and analysis and 2) we could, in future versions of the prototype, consider having a more fine-grained division of the mannequin body surface. The physiotherapists were impressed by the potential ability of the prototype for anytime, anywhere data collection, and hinted that even if the prototype would have had usability issues, in practice, most patients would overlook this, as the convenience factor associated with it would outweigh such considerations—for one, there would be less hospital visits!

4.2 Patient Evaluation

Forty-five patients (26 males, 19 females, mean age 46.1 years) have evaluated the prototype between September 2006 and January 2007. Out of these, 13 were patients at the Rheumatology Clinic of Northwick Park Hospital and volunteered to take part in the study. The remaining 32 participants were members of the U.K. National Forum of Wheelchair User Groups.

The only qualifying condition was that participants had to have broadband access at home and allow us to install the wireless router over the five-day evaluation period (although wireless connectivity is not necessary for pain data upload, it was considered essential in order to evaluate this aspect of our prototype). Patients were given a three-page user manual and asked to record pain data at three set times a day, subsequently uploading the information at the end of each day to the hospital server. At the end of the evaluation period, patients were asked to complete a questionnaire (Table 2) in which their opinions over a range of statements were recorded on a 5 point Likert scale, where 5 corresponded to the most positive response and 1 to the most negative. Users were also asked to note any other comments they might have had in respect of the developed application.

Table 2. Patient evaluation questionnaire with responses

Question	Mean Response	Standard Deviation
Q1. How effective did you find the controls to navigate the model?	4.24	0.83
Q2. How would you describe the overall layout of the interface?	4.31	1.00
Q3. Were the tool tips helpful?	4.29	0.89
Q4. Was the use of the color notation clear?	4.29	0.94
Q5. It is important to be able to record my pain on a PDA.	4.38	0.86
Q6. It is useful to be able to log pain data across time.	4.40	0.78
Q7. It was difficult to input pain data on a PDA	2.07	0.75
Q8. Process of transferring data from PDA to the main database could be easier	1.98	0.72

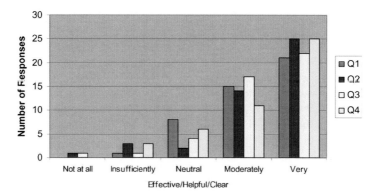

Fig. 17. Breakdown of survey responses: questions 1-4 from questionnaire

In general, the results were positive. Users found the color notation clear, and found it easy to navigate and control the 3-D model used in the PDA application (fig. 17). These results with respect to the developed interface are especially encouraging, since the majority of the users were wheelchair patients, many of whom wore glasses, and whose condition was compounded by other disabilities (such as motor ones).

Strongly positive results were obtained with respect to the ability of the prototype to record pain data anywhere, anytime, and especially, with the fact that it allows the patient to show clinicians how their pain varies across the day, in this respect, the trend confirming earlier results of [47]. Furthermore, patients generally disagreed with statements regarding the difficult of data input and upload (fig. 18).

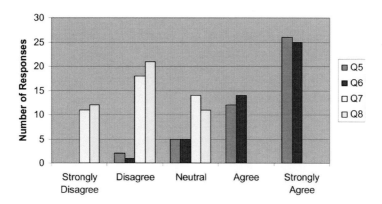

Fig. 18. Breakdown of survey responses: questions 5-8 from questionnaire

Some of the comments made by patients when evaluating the application include:

"The application allows me to correlate more closely the pain I am experiencing with the activities that I had been doing . . ."

The patient then remarked that, as a result of self-monitoring of how activities impacted his/her pain levels, he/she could manage the pain much better by reducing those activities that led to intense pain.

Another patient remarked: *"The software made me realize that I was taking my medication at the wrong time of the day . . ."*

This observed discrepancy between medication intake and experienced peaks of pain, as well as a better understanding of the link between activities undertaken during the day and pain intensities and patterns in the end resulted in the patient reducing his medication (strong analgesic) by 25%, with no deterioration in the pain levels encountered. Indeed, the reduction of medication intake as a result of self monitoring of pain was not a singular observation, as this was reported by five other members of our study group.

Yet another patient highlighted: *"Being able to rotate, zoom-in and out makes me feel that I have a much better control of my pain . . ."*

This observation seems to show that even though pain levels of the individual in question had not necessarily decreased as a result of the developed application, at least it offered him a perceived leverage of control over his suffering. Indeed, as remarked earlier, surveyed users were most enthusiastic about the ability to log data and its variation in time.

In rounding off our analysis of participants' comments, we mention that we were particularly pleased with the statement to the effect that:

". . . 3-D on a PDA allows me to accurately pinpoint any location I choose. Now, I would never go back to 2-D (pain drawings) again!"

Lastly, we remark that, from the additional written and oral comments that we have received, the general trend was that patients were enthusiastic about the application, with the only suggestion for further improvements being a finer division of the body mannequin, so that pain locations could be better pinpointed and the possibility of having more than one type of pain for each selected body region. These suggestions are currently being addressed in the new version of the 3D pain drawing that we have been developing in order to meet the patient and clinician recommendations for improvement.

4.3 Summary

In this section we have seen the importance of a system's evaluation in identifying any usability and effectiveness issues or problems. Specifically, we have gone through an evaluation of our prototype application, from which we have concluded that both the patients' and the clinician's attitudes towards the application where very positive and they both highlighted its great potential in the field.

In the next and final section, we will present our conclusions regarding the work done, and also propose further work that could be done in order to extend, or even improve, our system's current functionalities.

5 Conclusion

This work has presented a novel, PDA-based application for ubiquitous upload of pain data gathered using a 3-D pain drawing. Our evaluation with a cohort of 45 users has revealed encouraging results, with patients appreciating the advantages that self-monitoring of pain offers in managing this complex phenomenon, while clinicians especially liked the ability of the developed application to remotely monitor pain.

Moreover, both patients and clinicians indicated positive views toward the developed interface, platform, and functionality.

We realize that the cost (of equipment and software) is a potential issue toward large-scale adoption of our work. However, we are heartened by two aspects in this respect: the prices of PDAs are decreasing, while their computational capacity is increasing, as is their connectivity. Moreover, any potential initial investment in equipment and software could be offset by the reduction in health care costs (better pacing of medication intake, as our study has highlighted; potentially fewer hospital visits) as well as by increased patient satisfaction due to the opportunity to become a stakeholder in the management of pain (again, as shown by our study, although we realize that it is difficult to put a price on patient satisfaction).

5.1 Contributions

The work undertaken so far has proved us that this project can have very important contributions that need to be taken into consideration, both in the academia and industry areas.

Academic Contributions. The main focus of this work was 3D visualization, demonstrated by the use of a 3D mannequin for back pain diagnosis and treatment purposes. Currently, researchers in the field are increasingly exploiting this relatively new and promising technology, something that shows the huge potential that exists for it in disease treatment. To this end, 3D mannequins such as the one developed in this work could be further exploited in the field and used for several purposes such as surgery simulation and training. So, the 3D model could be manipulated and extended in a way that it will represent a virtual patient allowing both visualization and navigation inside the body's structure i.e. muscle and internal organs simulation, in accordance to real medical images. Furthermore, besides the healthcare field, very important research could also be carried out by other research fields as well, that could exploit our proposed technologies.

Industry Contributions. The motivation behind this work lies in the fact that, while back pain is a worldwide problem with considerable implications on countries' healthcare budgets and national economies, there is a relative paucity of tools for the effective collection and digitization of back-pain data, as discussed in this work. The disabling pain experienced by back-pain sufferers means that in many cases, such data collection cannot take place unless medical personnel is present at the patient's domicile, a situation which, in most cases, is both unrealistic and impractical. Considering the above discussion, we foresee that the work produced by this study will hopefully be able to overcome the aforementioned limitations, by improving healthcare services for people suffering from such long term conditions, something that will definitely have a beneficial impact on care, waiting lists, demand, workforce, hospital admissions, costs, and prescribing [8].

Therefore, at the end this work, it is expected to come out with a fully developed and evaluated tool that may be commercialized and/or utilized in further research projects on related domains. For example, the digitization and conversion of the 2D pain drawings described could be further used for people with multiple sclerosis to record the pain suffered from this disease.

5.2 Limitations and Future Work

The work reported in this chapter has raised interesting future directions, chief of which is the use of color to code multiple pain types for a particular body region. While our proof-of concept prototype has not taken into consideration issues such as application-level security and scalability; clearly, these are avenues for future work, as are more fine-grained subdivisions of the 3-D mannequin. The application could also be ported to other clinical areas (such as patients recovering from surgery or being treated for cancer). Our research is, of course, prototypical. It has not been tested in a large-scale setting, nor has its impact on health care processes been assessed. All these efforts constitute an essential part of our future endeavors.

References

1. Adams, A.A.: The Biomechanics of back pain. Churchill Livingstone, Edinburgh (2002)
2. American Chiropractic Association (2008),
   http://www.amerchiro.org/level2_css.cfm?t1id=13&t2id=68
   (Accessed: April 4, 2009)
3. Backcare (2008),
   http://www.backcare.org.uk/335/Facts%20and%20figures.html
   (Accessed: April 3, 2009)
4. Bertilson, B., Grunnesjö, M., Johansson, S., Strender, L.: Pain Drawing in the Assessment of Neurogenic Pain and Dysfunction in the Neck/Shoulder Region: Inter-Examiner Reliability and Concordance with Clinical Examination. Pain Medicine 8(2), 134–146 (2007)
5. Borenstein, D.G.: A Clinician's Approach to Acute Low Back Pain, Spine, pp. 16–22 (1997)
6. Capra, P., Mayer, Y.G.: Adding Psychological Scales to your Back Pain As-sessment. J. Musculoskel. Med. 2, 41–52 (1985)
7. Chan, C.W.: "The pain drawing and Waddell's nonorganic physical signs in chronic low-back pain,". Spine 18(3), 1717–1722 (1993)
8. Colin-Thome, D., Belfield, G.: Improving Chronic Disease Management, Department of Health, pp. 1–6
9. Department of Health, Departmental Report 2008, pp. 1–251 (2008)
10. Dixon, J., Lewis, R., Rosen, R., Finlayson, B., Gray, D.: Managing Chronic Disease: What Can We Learn From the US Experience. King's Fund, 1–54 (2004)
11. Finch, F.: Technology Insight: imaging of low back pain. Nature Clinical Practice Rheumatology 2(10), 554–561 (2006)
12. Frank, A.O., De Souza, L.H.: Conservative management of low back pain. Int. J. Clin. Pract. 55(1), 21–23 (2001)
13. Gatchel, R.J., Mayer, T.G., Capra, P., Diamond, P., Barnett, J.: Quantifica-tion of Lumbar Function: Part 6: The Use of Psychological Measures in Guiding Physical Functional Restoration. Spine 11, 36–42 (1986)
14. Ghinea, G., Gill, D., Frank, A.O., De Souza, L.H.: Using geographical in-formation systems for management of back pain data. Journal of Manage-ment in Medicine 16, 219–237 (2002)
15. Ghinea, G., Magoulas, G.D., Frank, A.O.: Intelligent multimedia communi-cation for enhanced medical e-collaboration in back pain treatment. Transac-tions of the Institute of Measurement and Control 26, 223–244 (2004)

16. Gomez, E.J., Caceres, C., Lopez, D., Del Pozo, F.: A web-based self moni-toring system for people living with HIV/AIDS. Comput. Methods Programs Biomed. 69(1), 75–86 (2002)
17. Haefeli, M., Elfering, A.: Pain assessment. European Spine Journal, 17–24 (2006)
18. Jamison, R.N., Fanciullo, G.J., Baird, J.C.: Computerized Dynamic Assess-ment of Pain: Comparison of Chronic Pain Patients and Healthy Controls. American Academy of Pain Medicine 5(2), 168–177 (2004)
19. Jamison, R.N., Fanciullo, G.J., Baird, J.C.: Usefulness of Pain Drawings in Identifying Real or Imagined Pain: Accuracy of Pain Professionals, Non-professionals, and a Decision Model. The Journal of Pain 5(9), 476–482 (2004)
20. Jamison, R.N., Raymond, S.A., Slawsby, E.A., McHugo, G.J., Baird, J.C.: Pain Assess-ment in Patients with Low Back Pain: Comparison of Weekly Recall and Momentary Elec-tronic Data. The Journal of Pain 7(3), 192–199 (2006)
21. Kinkade, S.: Evaluation and Treatment of Acute Low Back Pain. American Family Physi-cian 75(8), 1181–1188 (2007)
22. Kirkaldy-Willis, W.H., Bernard, Jr., T.N.: Managing Low Back Pain, 4th edn. Churchill Livingstone, USA (1999)
23. Koelink, F.C.A.: Chronic Back Pain: Assessing the Patient at Risk. Can. Fam. Physi-cian 36, 1173–1177 (1990)
24. Lacey, R.J., Lewis, M., Sim, J.: Presentation of pain drawings in question-naire surveys: influence on prevalence of neck and upper limb pain in the community. Elsevier 105, 293–301 (2003)
25. Lee, S.J.: Pain measurement: Understanding existing tools and their applica-tion in the emergency department. Emergency Medicine, 279–287 (2001)
26. Lin, C.H., Young, S.T., Kuo, T.S.: A remote data access architecture for home-monitoring health-care applications. Med. Eng. Phys. 29(2), 199–204 (2006)
27. Lin, L., Hu, P.J., Sheng, O.R.: A decision support system for lower back pain diagnosis: Uncertainty management and clinical evaluations. Science Direct, 1152–1169 (2006)
28. Lurie, J.D.: What diagnostic tests are useful for low back pain? Best Practice & Research Clinical Rheumatology 19(4), 557–575 (2005)
29. Malliou, P., Gioftsidou, A., Beneka, A., Godolias, G.: Measurements and evaluations in low back pain patients. Scandinavian Journal of Medicine and Science in Sports, 219–230 (2006)
30. Mannion, A.F., Balague, F., Pellise, F., Cedraschi, C.: Pain measurement in patients with low back pain. Nature Clinical Practice Rheumatology 3(11), 610–618 (2007)
31. Margolis, R.B., Tait, R.C., Krause, S.J.: A Rating System for Use with Pa-tient Pain Draw-ings. Pain 24, 57–65 (1986)
32. Masferrer, R., Prendergast, V., Hagell, P.: Colored pain drawings: prelimi-nary observa-tions in neurosurgical practice. European Journal of Pain 7(3), 213–217 (2002)
33. Mooney, V., Cairns, D., Robertson, J.: A system for evaluating and treating chronic back disability. West J. Med. 124, 370–376 (1976)
34. Ohnmeiss, D.D.: Repeatability of Pain Drawings in a Low Back Pain Popu-lation. Spine 25(8), 980–988 (2000)
35. Ohnmeiss, D.D., Vanharanta, H., Duyer, R.D.: The association between pain drawings and computed tomographic/ discographic pain responses. Spine 20, 729–733 (1995)
36. O'Sullivan, P.: Diagnosis and classification of chronic low back pain disor-ders: Maladap-tive movement and motor control impairments as underlying mechanism. Science Direct, 242–255 (2005)

37. Parker, H., Wood, P.L., Main, C.J.: The Use of the Pain Drawing as a Screening Measure to Predict Psychological Distress in Chronic Low Back pain. Spine 20(2), 236–243 (1995)
38. Patel, V.: Diagnostic Modalities for Low Back Pain, vol. 2, pp. 145–153. Elsevier, Amsterdam (2004)
39. Prather, H., Foye, P.M., Cianca, J.C.: Industrial Medicine and Acute Muscu-loskeletal Rehabilitation: Diagnosing and Managing the Injured Worker with Low Back Pain. Arch Physical Medicine Rehabilitation 83(1), 3–6 (2002)
40. Prkachin, K.M., Schultz, I., Berkowitz, J., Hughes, E., Hunt, D.: Assessing pain behavior of low-back pain patients in real time: Concurrent validity and examiner sensitivity. Behav. Res. Therapy 40(5), 595–607 (2002)
41. Provenzano, D.A., Fanciullo, G.J., Jamison, R.N., McHugo, G.J., Baird, J.C.: Computer Assessment and Diagnostic Classification of Chronic Pain Patients. Pain Medicine 8(S3), 167–175 (2007)
42. Raj, P.P., Paradise, L.A.: Myofascial Pain Syndrome and Its Treatment in Low Back Pain, pp. 167–174. Elsevier Science, Amsterdam (2004)
43. Ransford, A.O., Cairns, D., Mooney, V.: The Pain Drawing as an Aid to Psy-chologic Evaluation of Patients with Low-Back pain. Spine 1(2), 127–134 (1976)
44. Sanders, N.W., Mann, N.H.: Automated scoring of patient pain drawings us-ing artificial neural networks: efforts toward a low back pain triage application. Computers in Biology and Medicine, 287–298 (2000)
45. Sanders, W.N., Mann, N.H., Spengler, M.D.: Pain Drawing Scoring Is Not Improved by Inclusion of Patient-Reported Pain Sensation. Spine 31(23), 2735–2741 (2006)
46. Sanderson, P.L., Wood, P.L.R.: Surgery for lumbar spinal stenosis in old people. J. Bone Joint Surg. 75, 393–397 (1993)
47. Serif, T., Ghinea, G.: Recording of Time-Varying Back-Pain Data: A Wire-less Solution. IEEE Transactions on Information Technology in Biomedicine 9(3), 447–458 (2005)
48. Serif, T., Ghinea, G., Frank, A.O.: A Ubiquitous Approach for Visualizing Back Pain Data, pp. 1018–1027. Springer, Heidelberg (2005)
49. Takata, K., Hirotani, H.: Pain drawing in the evaluation of low back pain. International Orthopaedics, 361–366 (1995)
50. Uden, A., Astrom, M., Bergenudd, H.: Pain Drawings in Chronic Back pain. Spine 13(4), 389–392 (1988)
51. Uden, A., Landin, L.A.: Pain drawing and myelography in sciatic pain. Clin. Orthop. 216, 124–130 (1987)
52. Van den Bosch, M.A.A.J., Hollingworth, W., Kinmonth, A.L., Dixon, A.K.: Evidence against the use of lumbar spine radiography for low back pain. Clinical Radiology 59, 69–76 (2004)
53. Vaughn, M.L., Cavill, S.J., Taylor, S.J., Foy, M.A., Fogg, A.J.B.: Using Di-rect Explanations to Validate a Multi-layer Perceptron Network that Classifies Low Back Pain Patients, pp. 692–699. IEEE, Los Alamitos (1999)
54. Warren, J.R., Warren, D.E., Freedman, R.W.: A Knowledge-based Patient Data Acquisition System for Primary Care Medicine. Communications of the ACM, 547–553 (1993)
55. Wong, Y.E., Deyo, A.R.: Acute low back pain. Elsevier Science 8(5), 171–174 (2001)

Appendix

Following, a list of several key Journals and Conferences in the area is provided, which may be a valuable source of information for the studied field to be further explored

Journals in the area of Computational Intelligence in Medicine

1. IEEE Transactions on Information Technology in Biomedicine [Available at: `http://ieeexplore.ieee.org/xpl/RecentIssue.jsp?punumber=4233`]
2. Telemedicine and E-health [Available at: `http://www.liebertpub.com/products/product.aspx?pid=54`]
3. Journal of the American Medical Informatics Association [Available at: `http://www.jamia.org/`]
4. Communications of the ACM [Available at: `http://cacm.acm.org/`]
5. Computer Methods and Programs in Biomedicine [Available at: `http://www.elsevier.com/wps/find/journaldescription.cws_home/505960/description#description`]
6. Computers in Biology and Medicine [Available at: `http://www.elsevier.com/wps/find/journaldescription.cws_home/351/description#description`]
7. The Journal of Pain [Available at: `http://www.jpain.org/home`]

Key conferences in the area of Computational Intelligence in Medicine

1. IEEE Engineering in Medicine and Biology Society (EMBS) [Available at: `http://embs.gsbme.unsw.edu.au/`]
2. American Medical Informatics Association [Available at: `http://www.amia.org/`]

Author Index